Medicine, the Market and the Mass Media

It is sixty years since the end of the Second World War, but historians have only just begun to explore thoroughly the postwar history of health and its interwar antecedents. Most research and literature has focused on health services and the arrival of the NHS; where public health is concerned many historical surveys ignore the recent past and base their investigations on the nineteenth-century public health legacy.

This collection opens up the postwar history of public health to sustained research-based, historical scrutiny. *Medicine, the Market and the Mass Media* examines the development of a new view of 'the health of the public' and the influences that shaped it in the postwar years. The book looks at the dual legacy of social medicine through health services and health promotion, and analyses the role of the mass media along with the connections between public health and industry. These essays take a broad perspective examining developments in Western Europe, and the relationships between Europe and the USA.

Virginia Berridge is Professor of History and head of the Centre for History in Public Health at the London School of Hygiene and Tropical Medicine, University of London. She has published books and articles on health and society in the twentieth century.

Kelly Loughlin is a lecturer in History at the London School of Hygiene and Tropical Medicine and the main focus of her research is the history of health and medical communications in the UK.

Routledge Studies in the Social History of Medicine

Edited by Joseph Melling, University of Exeter, and Anne Borsay, University of Wales at Swansea.

The Society for the Social History of Medicine was founded in 1969, and exists to promote research into all aspects of the field, without regard to limitations of either time or place. In addition to this book series, the Society also organises a regular programme of conferences, and publishes an internationally recognised journal, *Social History of Medicine*. The Society offers a range of benefits, including reduced-price admission to conferences and discounts on SSHM books, to its members. Individuals wishing to learn more about the Society are invited to contact the series editors through the publisher.

The Society took the decision to launch 'Studies in the Social History of Medicine', in association with Routledge, in 1989, in order to provide an outlet for some of the latest research in the field. Since that time, the series has expanded significantly under a number of series editors, and now includes both edited collections and monographs. Individuals wishing to submit proposals are invited to contact the series editors in the first instance.

Medicine, the Market and the Mass Media

Producing health in the twentieth century

Edited by Virginia Berridge and Kelly Loughlin

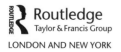

Routledge
Taylor & Francis Group

LONDON AND NEW YORK

First published 2005
by Routledge
2 Park Square, Milton Park, Abingdon, Oxon OX14 4RN

Simultaneously published in the USA and Canada
by Routledge
270 Madison Ave, New York, NY 10016

Routledge is an imprint of the Taylor & Francis Group

Typeset in Times NR MT by Taylor & Francis Books
Printed and bound in Great Britain by
The Cromwell Press, Trowbridge, Wiltshire

British Library Cataloguing in Publication Data
A catalogue record for this book is available from the British Library

Library of Congress Cataloging in Publication Data
Medicine, the market and the mass media : producing health in the
twentieth century / edited by Virginia Berridge and Kelly Loughlin.--
1st ed.
 p. cm. -- (Routledge studies in the social history of medicine)
 ISBN 0-415-30432-6 (hardback)
 1. Public health--Europe--History--20th century. 2. Social medicine--
Europe--History--20th century. 3. Health education--Europe--
History--20th century. 4. Mass media in health education--Europe--
History--20th century. I. Berridge, Virginia. II. Loughlin, Kelly, 1968-
III. Series.
 RA483.M43 2005
 362.1'094'0904--dc22
                          2004025147

T&F informa

Taylor & Francis Group is the Academic Division of T&F Informa plc.

Contents

Illustrations

Tables

Figures

Contributors

Stuart Anderson is a senior lecturer at the London School of Hygiene and Tropical Medicine. He is editor of *Making Medicines: a Brief History of Pharmacy* (Pharmaceutical Press, 2005), Chair of the Society for the Social History of Medicine, and President of the British Society for the History of Pharmacy.

Luc Berlivet is Chargé de Recherche with the Centre National de le Recherche Scientifique (CNRS), based at the Centre de Recherche Médecine, Sciences, Santé et Société (CERMES, Paris). His research focuses on the 'reproblematisation' of health issues into risks during the twentieth century, with a special interest in the history of epidemiology.

Virginia Berridge is Professor of History at the London School of Hygiene and Tropical Medicine, University of London. She is head of the Centre for History in Public Health and headed the Wellcome Trust-funded 'Science speaks to policy' programme of research of which this book is an outgrowth. Her publications are on recent public health: drug, alcohol and smoking policy; the history of HIV/AIDS; and the relationship between research and policy.

Tony Cutler is Professor of Public Sector Management, Royal Holloway College, University of London. His books include *Keynes, Beveridge and Beyond* (with K. and J. Williams) (Routledge, 1986, reprinted 2003) and *Managing the Welfare State* (with B. Waine) (Berg, 1997). His research interests include the financial history of the NHS and the history of the application of 'management' techniques in public sector services.

Lesley Diack is a Joint Research Fellow at the School of Pharmacy at the Robert Gordon University and the School of Medicine at the University of Aberdeen researching and developing shared learning. She has published a number of articles on the Aberdeen typhoid outbreak, women's health issues and oral history.

Jean-Paul Gaudillière is a senior researcher at the Institut National de la Santé et de la Recherche Médicale, France. He has been working on the history of biomedical research after the Second World War in France and the USA. He is currently writing a history of biological drugs focusing on the changing relationship between biomedical researchers and industry, *L'Invention de la biomédecine: la France, l'Amérique et la production des savoirs du vivant après 1945* (La Découverte, 2002) (English translation forthcoming, Yale University Press).

Mark Jackson is Professor of the History of Medicine and Director of the Centre for Medical History at the University of Exeter. After qualifying in medicine in 1985, he pursued research on the social history of infanticide and the history of 'feeble-mindedness'. More recently, he has been researching and writing on the history of allergic diseases, such as asthma, hayfever and eczema, in the modern world. His publications include *New-Born Child Murder: Women, Illegitimacy and the Courts in Eighteenth-Century England* (Manchester University Press, 1996), *The Borderland of Imbecility: Medicine, Society and the Fabrication of the Feeble Mind in Late Victorian and Edwardian Britain* (Manchester University Press, 2000), and *Allergy: the History of a Modern Malady* (in press, 2005), as well as numerous edited volumes and articles.

Martin Lengwiler is at the Social Science Research Centre in Berlin. He has published on the history of medicine and the history of the Welfare State, including: 'Psychiatry beyond the asylum: the origins of German military psychiatry before the First World War' (*History of Psychiatry*, 2003); 'Technologies of trust: actuarial theory, insurance sciences, and the establishment of the welfare state' (*Information and Organization*, 2003).

Ilana Löwy is a senior researcher at the Institut National de la Santé et de la Recherche Médicale, France. She is interested in the history of the 'Pasteurian sciences' – bacteriology and immunology, links between the laboratory and clinical medicine, colonial medicine, and gender studies. She is working now on the history of breast cancer risk, and is the author of *Between Bench and Bedside: Science, Healing and Interleukin-2 in a Cancer Ward* (Harvard University Press, 1996); French translation, *Cancer des chercheurs, cancer des cliniciens: trajectoire d'une innovation thérapeutique* (Archives d'Histoire Contemporaine, 2002).

Lion Murard is a senior researcher at the Centre de Recherche Médecine, Sciences, Santé et Société (CNRS-INSERM-EHESS) in Paris. He co-authored with Patrick Zylberman *L'Hygiene dans la Republique: la sante publique en France ou l'utopie contrariee 1870–1918* (Fayard, 1996). He is currently working on the history of public health in Europe in the period between the wars, and has recently published on the Rockefeller Foundation, and French social medicine in the 1930s.

David Smith lectures in the History of Medicine at Aberdeen University. He edited *Nutrition in Britain* (Routledge, 1997) and co-edited *Food, Science, Policy and Regulation in the Twentieth Century* (Routledge, 2000), with

Jim Phillips. A book on the Aberdeen typhoid outbreak will be published by Boydell & Brewer in 2005.

Penny Starns was awarded her doctorate at the University of Bristol in 1997. Since that time she has worked as a researcher and writer for BBC history programmes and as a Research Fellow. Penny has a particular interest in oral history and was responsible for the BBC Radio 4 series *Frontline Females* and the award-winning *Evacuation: the True Story*. Her written works include *Nurses at War* (Sutton, 2000), *Medicine and Warfare* (*Modern History Review*, 2002) and the *Evacuation of Children during World War Two* (DSM, 2004).

Carsten Timmermann is a Wellcome Research Associate at Manchester University's Centre for the History of Science, Technology and Medicine. He has worked on medicine in Germany in the interwar period and on the history of cardiovascular disease in Britain and Germany. Currently he is researching the history of lung cancer in Britain.

Viviane Quirke is a Wellcome Trust Postdoctoral Research Fellow at the Centre for Health, Medicine and Society, Oxford Brookes University. Her doctoral research at Oxford University was on the changing relations between scientists and pharmaceutical companies in Britain and France *c*. 1935–65. Her current research interests include the development of drug treatments for chronic diseases in Britain and France after the Second World War.

Foreword

This book covers a crucial period in the development of modern public health policy and practice, covering half a century or so during which there were dramatic advances in knowledge with accompanying improvements in public health.

The conference on which this book is based is unusual in having attracted both historians with a particular interest in public health and researchers from a range of disciplines relevant to improving understanding of the determinants of health and effective public health policies and practices.

The book has a strong contemporary resonance, not least because of its in-depth examination of two areas often neglected by researchers, the roles of industry and the mass media. It draws on a range of experiences from industrialised countries. Importantly, it demonstrates to researchers and practitioners without a background in history that many contemporary debates such as those driven by differing perspectives on the role of the state in promoting health and preventing disease are not new but have deep historical roots. For historians too there is much rich material here, for example on the ascendancy of individual behavioural determinants of health in the postwar period and the contrasting emphasis on social and environmental determinants of health, exemplified by the WHO Healthy Cities programme. The emergence of international agencies and major philanthropic organisations in the interwar years heralded the rise of WHO postwar and the subsequent entry of a range of international donors into an increasingly complex global health arena. The development of clean-air legislation in the 1950s presaged the reintegration of environmental concerns with public health in the latter part of the last century, echoing the earlier concerns of public health pioneers with the environmental causes of disease in the nineteenth century.

Public–private partnerships have frequently been promoted in recent years as vehicles for the advancement of health internationally. As this book clearly demonstrates, there were many important interactions between public and private sectors stretching back decades that influenced, for example, health education, quality assurance, the organisation of healthcare and international health. Although relations between industry and public health have not always been hostile there have inevitably been some tensions between public health professionals and the interests of the private sector, which are well described in the book. Public health advocacy groups have over the years become increasingly skilled at using the media to influence public opinion and thus public policy, sometimes operating independently of the academic public health community.

The transfer and transformation of ideas, organisational innovations and technologies internationally is a pervasive theme of the book. In France the mass media became a tool for health education of the population, particularly on the dangers of smoking, and in Britain both smoking and road safety were the foci of media campaigns using influences from US advertising theory. The differences in the evolution of pharmaceutical regulation between the USA and UK are illuminating, driven for example by concerns about accidental and deliberate poisoning in the UK and the adulteration of imported drugs in the USA.

I am delighted that the London School of Hygiene and Tropical Medicine has been able to play a central role in this carefully researched and thought-provoking book, which will be of interest not only to historians but also to those concerned with public health research, policy and practice.

Professor Sir Andy Haines
Director
London School of Hygiene and Tropical Medicine,
University of London

Acknowledgements

This book originated in a conference organised by historians working in a school of public health – the London School of Hygiene and Tropical Medicine. The conference, 'Science, policy and practice: historical dimensions', held in 2001, took its theme from 'Science speaks to policy', a programme of historical research based at the London School.

The idea of dialogue, implicit in 'science speaking to policy', provides a useful description of the cross-disciplinary context of the conference and the research programme. Numerous possibilities for exchange across the disciplines and between past and present are generated in a context where historians work alongside epidemiologists, policy analysts and a range of public health specialists. The conference attracted a mixed audience of historians and public health researchers, with non-historian colleagues providing input as nominated discussants. We are grateful to all of the speakers and to the discussants, Ben Armstrong, Dave Leon, Judy Green, Margaret Thorogood, Tony Fletcher, Jon Turney, Kelly Loughlin and Jenny Stanton.

We are also grateful to the Wellcome Trust, who funded both the programme of historical research and the conference based upon it, and to the Society for the Social History of Medicine, which also provided conference support. Our thanks are due to colleagues at the London School who have provided the basis for the broadening of our ideas about public health and its history. Our particular thanks go to Ingrid James, who has provided organisational and secretarial support for the programme, conference and book.

The original research presented in Stuart Anderson's chapter was supported by a project grant in the history of medicine awarded by the Wellcome Trust. Luc Berlivet started the research for his chapter during postdoctoral work at the London School, which was also supported by a Wellcome Fellowship. The chapter by Virginia Berridge and Penny Starns is in part based on research on the Wills Archive, work carried out under the auspices of a Wellcome pilot project. Lesley Diack and David Smith's chapter stems from work undertaken in connection with a Wellcome-funded project into the history of the Aberdeen typhoid outbreak, and the authors would like to thank their colleagues Professor Elizabeth Russell and Professor Hugh Pennington, along with archivists and interviewees connected with the project. The research for Mark Jackson's chapter was also supported by the Wellcome Trust, and he would like to thank Andrew Thorpe for providing key references and insights into the politics of the 1950s.

The Swiss National Science Foundation provided funding for the research presented in Martin Lengwiler's chapter. Carsten Timmermann expresses his gratitude to Professors Ernst Georg Krause, Hans-Dieter Faulhaber, Heinz Bielka and Jens Uwe Niehoff, as well as Dr Rainer Hohlfeld, for sharing vital information on the academic life in Berlin Buch and on cardiovascular research in the GDR. Jonathan Harwood, John Pickstone and Michael Worboys provided comments on early versions of this chapter, and the research was also supported by a Wellcome Postdoctoral Fellowship. The research presented in Viviane Quirke's chapter was supported by a Wellcome project grant awarded to Judy Slinn for a study on 'Innovation in the UK pharmaceutical industry, 1948–78'. She would also like to thank Carsten Timmermann for pointing out some of the sources on the history of the beta-blockers.

All contributors would like to thank the editors for comments and suggestions during the development of this volume.

The editors would like to thank Her Majesty's Stationery Office for permission to include Table 8.1, reproduced from C. Webster, *The Health Services since the War, Volume II: Government and Health Care, the National Health Service 1958–79* (1996), the Office of Health Economics for permission to include Table 8.2 and Fig. 8.1, reproduced from N. Wells, *Medicines: 50 years of Progress 1930–1980* (1980), and Thomson Publishing for permission to include Table 8.3, reproduced from S.C. Anderson, 'The historical context of pharmacy', in K. Taylor and G. Harding (eds), *Pharmacy Practice* (2001).

Abbreviations

ABPI	Association of the British Pharmaceutical Industry
APHA	American Public Health Association
ASCO	American Society of Clinical Oncology
ASH	Action on Smoking and Health
BGs	Boards of Governors
BMA	British Medical Association
BSE	Bovine Spongiform Encephalopathy
CAP	Committee on Administrative Practice
CDC	Centers for Disease Control
CFES	Comité Français d'Éducation pour la Santé
CHSC	Central Health Services Council
CJD	Creutzfeldt Jakob Disease
CLCC	Centre de Lutte Contre le Cancer
CLIA	Clinical Laboratory Improvement Amendments
CNRS	Centre National de la Recherche Scientifique
CRC	Cancer Research Campaign
CVD	Cardiovascular disease
EBM	Evidence-Based Medicine
ELSI	Ethical, Legal and Social Implications
FAO	Food and Agriculture Organization
FDA	Food and Drug Administration
FSA	Food Standards Agency
GDR	German Democratic Republic
GMSC	General Medical Services Committee
HMCs	Hospital Management Committees
HMO	Health Maintenance Organization
HMSO	Her Majesty's Stationery Office
HSR	Health Services Research
HTC	heat-treated cellulose
HU	Humboldt University
ICI	Imperial Chemical Industries
IDL	Imperial Developments Limited
IGL	Imperial Group Limited
IGR	Institut Gustave Roussy

INSERM	Institut National de la Santé et de la Recherche Médicale
ISCSH	Independent Scientific Committee on Smoking and Health
ITG	Imperial Tobacco Group
ITGL	Imperial Tobacco Group Limited
KF	King's Fund
KWI	Kaiser Wilhelm Institutes
LN	League of Nations
LNHO	League of Nations Health Organization
LSHTM	London School of Hygiene and Tropical Medicine
MAFF	Ministry of Agriculture, Food and Fisheries
MH	Ministry of Health
MONICA	Monitor trends in Cardiovascular Disease
MP	Member of Parliament
MRC	Medical Research Council
NBCC	National Breast Cancer Coalition
NHS	National Health Service
NIH	National Institutes of Health
NPHT	Nuffield Provincial Hospitals Trust
NPM	New Public Management
NRT	Nicotine Replacement Therapy
NSC	National Safety Council
NSM	New Smoking Material
OECD	Organization for Economic Co-operation and Development
ORTF	Office de la Radio et de la Télévision Française
PMSA	Provincial Medical and Surgical Association
RCP	Royal College of Physicians
RCT	Randomised Controlled Trial
RF	Rockefeller Foundation
RHBs	Regional Hospital Boards
RM	Resource Management
RoSPA	Royal Society for the Prevention of Accidents
SACGT	Secretary's Advisory Committee on Genetic Testing
SCOTH	Scientific Committee on Tobacco and Health
SED	Socialist Unity Party
SEITA	Service d'Exploitation Industriel des Tabacs et Allumettes
SERM	Selective Oestrogen Receptor Modulators
SOFRES	Société Française d'Études pour Sondages
TAC	Tobacco Manufacturers Advisory Committee
TDAC	Tobacco Distributors Advisory Committee
TID	Tobacco Intelligence Department
TRC	Therapeutic Research Corporation
UCSF	University of California, San Francisco
UNICEF	United Nations Children's Fund
USPHS	United States Public Health Service
WDTA	Wholesale Drug Trade Association
WHO	World Health Organization

Introduction

Virginia Berridge and Kelly Loughlin

This book is about the nature of change over time in post-1945 public health and the influences that have impacted on it, in terms above all of its knowledge base and dominant ideologies. Within this overall framework we examine the role of two important but neglected topics – of industry and the mass media. Our focus is on public health within different national contexts, and the role of those specific national contexts in the exchange between public health sciences and policy-making. We also analyse the importance of models from outside the health sector, from industry, disseminated at the national and the international level, and at the role of the international sphere in the process of 'policy transfer', of moving knowledge and policy models from one national location into another. This is a process that has been studied by political scientists, but rarely historically.[1]

Our overall aim is to deepen understanding of the nature of postwar public health and the forces that have shaped it. To date, this topic has received surprisingly little sustained historical attention, despite the growth in writing on more distant public health history.[2] We should explain that by public health we mean the efforts of societies and individuals to prevent disease, prolong life and promote health, a definition we have adapted from that used in the 1988 Acheson Report, a British policy document produced at a time when HIV/AIDS seemed to offer new possibilities for public health; these are words reiterated by the more recent Wanless Report on public health (2004).[3] Writing on the contemporary history of health has expanded in recent years, although not to the same extent as that on the contemporary history of science, where developments in microbiology and genetics provide a focus for popular and scholarly interest.[4] When health is the focus there is a tendency to concentrate primarily on health services and their history, rather than the wider issue of the health of society and its determinants, and the way this relationship has been conceptualised over time. This perhaps mirrors the way in which health services in practice have always attracted the lion's share of policy attention.

Published commentary on current public health policy is far from history free. But it uses history in distinct and limited ways. One tendency is to assume history is distant events – that the history is 'background' which stops some while before the present day.[5] In Petersen and Lupton's valuable book on the 'new public health', for example, the role of history is that of a bystander, the supplier of important background, but not central to their analysis of recent ideological changes.[6] Other commentary does use the history of recent events but takes it to be just the ever-changing parade of policy documents and initiatives emanating from central government.[7] Such surveys tell us what happened but they do not begin to address the important historical question of why it did – what interests, issues, activities were important.[8] In the UK, another history-using style is the role given to recent history in polemics against the emergence of the 'nanny state'. The perceived huge role of the state in health promotion is presented as historically specific to the postwar period, a dangerous intrusion of central government into the lives of individuals, supported by an increasingly dominant media.[9] In this book we are concerned to develop an understanding of the impact and history of the media within public health that moves on from the 'media injection' model of media effect.

Of course, historians have also written about postwar public health. Lewis's excellent analysis argues that public health doctors tended to justify their activities in relation to whatever health tasks they had assumed at the time, and takes that story into the 1970s, with some further commentary on changes in the 1980s.[10] Porter talks about public health as health services or concepts of the 'healthy body', while Webster and others have mapped out the contours of a recent history of public health and health promotion.[11] Yet it is still possible for public health specialists to ignore this historiography.[12] Textbooks from within the field provide a survey of history that is incomprehensible in the face of historical research.[13] This may be because there is not much in-depth research and the same material tends to be used and reused. But it is also of concern because practitioners in the field are educated with this material and thus emerge with an incomplete, indeed distorted, appreciation of the historical roots of their current activity.

In this book we aim to start expanding the understanding of public health change through the insights of original historical research. This is research that takes us into areas rarely covered in the standard surveys – industry, the media, for example. Chapters in the book also look outside the UK and at the international level, demonstrating an awareness of the cross-national and international roots of public health developments. In particular we seek to develop an overall synthesis that links aspects of the postwar history, such as evidence-based medicine (EBM) and health services research (HSR), with developments in public health and health promotion that are often seen as entirely separate and never discussed together.

The postwar stages of change

Public health change can be characterised in three ways, or at three levels: formal institutional change; professional change; and changes in the knowledge base. This book looks in particular at the latter area, and how it has meshed with defined changes in policy.[14] The overall framework within which such changes can be placed shows some definite stages for public health in the postwar period. A dual legacy can be traced from prewar social medicine, leading into EBM/HSR on the one hand, public health/health promotion on the other, with linkages between the two. These lineages have corresponded to some extent to the technician–manager/activist dichotomy that has been identified by analysts of postwar public health.[15] For both strands, EBM and health promotion, significant developments on the international scene fed into British developments and cross-national transfer of ideas and practice was important.

Social medicine, derived in the UK from the work of Titmuss and Ryle, failed to consolidate its influence at the broader level.[16] Its postwar legacy lay in epidemiology. The focus on chronic rather than epidemic disease in the 1950s saw the rise of chronic disease epidemiology as the primary technical tool of public health. The resultant rise of the 'risk factor' in epidemiology was central to new styles of public health that focused on risk rather than direct causation.[17] This change in focus and approach was epitomised by the emergence of smoking as the central issue for postwar public health from the 1950s.[18] In the UK the new-style public health came to fruition in the 1960s and 1970s, with an awareness of the possibilities of the mass media in public health initiatives.[19]

We can identify three stages of this reconfiguration of postwar public health, all of which are represented in the chapters in this volume. A 'new public health' was emergent in these years. Initially, the 'new public health' that emerged postwar concentrated on the role of behavioural determinants of health at the individual level. In Britain, this strand was represented in policy documents like *Prevention and Health, Everybody's Business* (1976); these were criticised for adopting the 'victim blaming' approach.[20] In the 1980s came a second version of the new public health. The international influence of social medicine, derived in part from the historian Henry Sigerist's role in social medicine in the 1940s and translated into North America and the newly established WHO, re-emerged in policy documents such as the Ottawa Charter of 1986.[21] The international health promotion movement began to stress the environmental and structural determinants of health and the need for 'healthy public policy', rather than simply encouraging individual behaviour change. In the 1990s we can identify a third stage of public health that we have termed elsewhere 'pharmaceutical public health', because it draws on drug and vaccine responses to public health issues, on relationships with the pharmaceutical industry and also on 'new' genetic insights into health.[22]

This is a brief history of our public health/health promotion strand. What of the technician role of public health? 'Formal public health' saw the relocation of public health professionals in health services in the UK.[23] Health services research (HSR) with its focus on the randomised controlled trial was the legacy of social medicine in those new configurations.[24] The subsequent rise of the EBM/health movement represented another international influence, with strong North American, in particular Canadian, input.[25] These movements were the twin legacies of prewar public health and social medicine. Commentators argued that they represented the twin polarities of the 'activist' and 'technician manager' roles towards which public health professionals inclined.[26] Of course these tendencies cannot be entirely separated. Bartley, for example, has drawn attention to how public health practitioners adopted 'activist' issues, such as health inequalities, because professionally they were excluded from power in health service decision-making, but resumed the technician role once their position became more central within services in the late 1980s.[27] Often, language derived from one strand of public health masked activities that derived from the other; public health professionals used the language of activism while dealing with technical health service management realities.[28] The public health literature treats these developments as entirely separate; the new public health and EBM are barely linked. We argue here that they are both key legacies of social medicine and are distinct and related tendencies in postwar public health.

Let us represent this diagrammatically (see Table 0.1).

The chapters in this book tell us more about these periods and underline key themes within them.

First let us look at:

The interwar influences on postwar public health

International influences were strong in postwar public health and on the rise of health services research from the 1960s. But chapters in the book show how the international milieux of the interwar years also fostered precursors of 'new' developments postwar. International health in the interwar years

Table 0.1   Lineages in postwar public health

Public health/health promotion stages	EBM stages
1940s social medicine	1940s social medicine
1950s rise of risk factor and chronic disease epidemiology	1950s rise of risk factor and chronic disease epidemiology
1960s health education and media, social survey, market research	1960s rise of RCT
1970s new public health 1, Lalonde, WHO Health for All	1970s Cochrane, relocation of public health in health services in UK
1980s new public health 2, Ottawa Charter	1980s EBM, AIDS and directed research
1990s new public health 3	1990s NHS R&D

has been widely discussed by historians.[29] The period has been characterised in terms of two key developments, the emergence of permanent international organisations, epitomised by the League of Nations and its Health Organization (LNHO), and the rise to prominence of a new style of international corporate philanthropy – in the Rockefeller Foundation (RF), the Milbank Memorial Fund, the Sage Foundation and similar organisations. The LNHO was the agency responsible for public health and social medicine, although its primary concern in the 1920s was the scientific universalism of standard setting, in terms of biologicals and mortality/ morbitity data. By 1937 approximately 72 per cent of the world's population was covered by LNHO statistics.[30] The depth and degree of interlinkage between the LNHO and the RF has been a central theme in discussions of international health between the wars. The relationship has been described as a 'public–private partnership' that shaped a global biomedical/public health infrastructure.[31] Although the USA was not a member state of the League of Nations, it was significant that the LNHO drew between a half and a third of its budget from a US foundation, the RF.[32] This Foundation also pursued initiatives through its own International Health Commission, as well as providing support for clinics, training schemes, schools of public health and laboratory services throughout the world.[33] Through its focus on training and institution building the RF was fundamental in creating an international network of public health experts. This approach could be seen as the scientisation of social policy, on the one hand, and the primacy of professionalised, increasingly technocratic solutions to public health problems, on the other. The LNHO itself became increasingly narrow in the quest for standardised instruments and measures. The involvement of US foundations in international health during this period of US political isolationism can be seen either as benign philanthropy or as US imperialism by private means.

Lion Murard's chapter shows how many of the aspects we think of as 'new' in postwar public health in the 1950s and 1960s were foreshadowed by developments in US health and their transfer through international organisations into the European health field. Rural health was the key issue across European nations before the Second World War. It was in this connection that instruments for measuring community health performance originated in the USA as the American Appraisal Form for Community Health work and were reframed internationally as the League of Nations' collection of life environment and health indices. The US model, significantly, derived from those designed under the auspices of insurance companies; here was a business impetus, whereas the Geneva index wanted to bring together the range of factors affecting a population's standards of well-being and ways of life. Murard's example of cross-Atlantic international co-operation in the prewar years is also a 'concrete history of abstraction', which demonstrates how the tools of measurement within public health were themselves expressions of specific and changing political projects. These tools recall the roots of EBM and health services research within public health, and of the postwar call for epidemiology to provide 'community diagnosis'.[34] These indices and their transformation provide us with an example of prewar 'policy transfer'.[35]

Martin Lengwiler's chapter also shows how, at a national level, in Switzerland, before the war, elements of the postwar configuration of public health were already prominent. The field of occupational health, often forgotten, or marginalised postwar, was the pacemaker here. Methodological innovations in accident prevention acted as a 'laboratory' for innovative media-based prevention strategies. Lengwiler contrasts the European technical models of work-based accident prevention with the psychological models emanating from the USA. He argues that these began to impact in some European countries like Switzerland through the US 'Safety First' campaign and that discussion of psychological models first permeated health education strategies in this way. Lengwiler, too, is discussing a process of 'policy transfer' whereby US models are being transferred and refined in the European context; the origin of the psychological model within the commercial/business sector was, as with Murard's health indices, an important component. Psychology was an important 'public health science' whose role was beginning to expand in the interwar years.[36]

The importance of the media in postwar public health

Lengwiler's paper also introduces us to the role of the media in public health. The styles of current public health history and commentary that we surveyed at the start have paid little attention to this important component. Yet medicine, and health overall, have become involved postwar in what media analysts have termed a 'circuit of mass communication'.[37] Medico-scientific and health news is now part of a process of production and dissemination that can have enormous and reciprocal policy impacts. The role of the media in the early crisis of HIV/AIDS and the impact on politicians is one example.[38] BSE, foot and mouth, and other crises have followed. This media health field is largely a creation of the postwar years. Health correspondents did not exist before the 1950s and media punditry by doctors could fall foul of measures of professional status such as restrictions on advertising.[39] The role of the mass media in public health has been a central concern in the postwar decades. This concern has been double-sided. The mass media has been enlisted as a public health tool through the development of mass advertising campaigns, and it has been the focus of opposition and control due to the use of mass advertising by commercial interests such as tobacco and alcohol.[40] Moreover, public health pressure groups such as the UK's Action on Smoking and Health saw the media as the key platform for mobilising claims and counterclaims, and media 'spin' became more important for them than mass membership or local campaigns.[41]

Chapters in the book analyse the different national origins of such approaches and the dilemmas that they raised. Lengwiler's chapter compares campaigns in accident prevention in Switzerland before and after the Second World War; the latter demonstrated a greater emphasis on the role of the individual in matters of personal/public health. For occupational health this focus represented the privatisation of safety and a stress on the individual responsibility of workers. Media-based methods profited from the growing influence of scientific research, in particular the propaganda studies of applied psychology during and after the Second World War. It was in the postwar years, he argues, that such techniques expanded into the wider field of public health, which looked to make use of mass advertising and new communication media.

Lesley Diack and David Smith's chapter shows how the media entered in to the management of a food crisis in the 1960s in Scotland. The Aberdeen typhoid outbreak in 1964 was notable for its high media profile. The local Medical Officer of Health, Dr Ian McQueen, deliberately raised the media temperature of the outbreak in order to reach the citizens of Aberdeen and to convey the importance of the measures he was advocating. Later criticised for an over-sensationalist approach that exaggerated the problem and created panic, McQueen's handling of the crisis was also symbolic of the choices that faced public health in Britain in the 1960s. He was using 'modern' technologies of mass communication within the context of the local remit of the Medical Officer of Health, based in local government structures. So, modern media techniques had a new place within old local government structures. Just a few years later a different model of media-based public health emerged, of centralised mass media campaigns and of public health doctors relocated within health services and clinical medicine. McQueen's initiative could be seen as a 'path not taken'. The fact that this initiative emanated from public health in Scotland is also significant, as Scotland had an organisation and style of public health different from that of England and Wales.[42]

Luc Berlivet's chapter shifts our attention to France and to the next decade, to the emergence of mass-media advertising as a key strategy within health education in the wake of policy activity on smoking and health. Berlivet shows how the policy significance of smoking paved the way for an emphasis on the centrality of mass communication and for the modernisation of the French health education organisation. The reformulation of health education strategy subsequently took social science on board both in the guise of academic publication and in applied form through market research. Here was a model for the 'modern' public health of the 1970s, based on international transfer of experience in health education and on French road safety advertising in the early 1970s. Berlivet's analysis of the adoption of mass-media strategies in France shows similarities with the British experience. In Britain, smoking was also the springboard for the new approach although developments took place earlier, in the late 1960s and early 1970s, and the models came from US advertising theory, from 'hidden persuasion' rather than from safety or occupational health campaigns, although road safety and drink driving campaigns did use the new models as well.[43]

Industrial models, public health and health services

In Switzerland, industrial models had been important in the emergence of a psychological approach to accident prevention through the location in occupational health. Health indices in the USA in the interwar years also derived from insurance industry models, as did early studies of smoking-related risk.[44] Our second major theme in this book is the more general interconnections between industry, public health and health services post-1945. Commercial and industrial sectors, as we have already seen, were important in providing the frameworks for concepts of measurement and evaluation in interwar public health, and also through industrial psychology, which spread from dealing with the health of employed workers into population health more generally.

But connections with industry have a wider application for public health. Contemporary public health is hostile to some industries – tobacco, the food and alcohol industries. Being anti-industry is emblematic of a correct public health stance. Yet the papers in this volume show some different relationships have operated in the past and that current hostile relationships have not always been the case. Our studies link also with historical discussion on the role of 'the invisible industrialist' in histories of science and technology.[45] Such work has concentrated on connections between industrial R& D on the connections between research, academics and industry. The generalisability of scientific knowledge and the replication of local results were dependent on industrially produced items such as laboratory animals or laboratory kits for analysis.[46] The interconnection of industrial interests with the new directions in postwar public health and health services have, however, been little studied.

Tony Cutler's chapter shows how the managerialist project in health, which later became central to new public management in health services and a concern of health services research, had its origins in the 1950s, not the 1980s. It stemmed from the attempt to introduce models of standard costing in industrial applications of management accounting to health services, hospitals in particular. The 'standard patient' was needed in order adequately to cost out treatment. Here again we have the application of industrial and commercial models in health, also a feature of other papers in this volume (Murard, Lengwiler, Berlivet).

Viviane Quirke's chapter stresses the role of pharmaceutical innovation in the postwar change towards lifestyle public health. She explores in particular ICI's late but successful move into pharmaceuticals that led them to explore new approaches and niches for drug development in the context of the postwar shift from infectious to chronic disease. Quirke shows how this arose from a drop in sales of antimalarials and a climate of optimism about the victory over infectious disease. ICI's cardiovascular programme and the development of beta-blockers illustrated the close ties between companies and government that had developed in the scientific-military-industrial complex during the war and sustained within the biomedical complex afterwards. Quirke argues that industry scientists were active players in the move from infectious to chronic disease, rather than simply observing and responding to governmental policies. A situation of mutual interdependence was created between these companies and the state, which continues to underpin public health and other policies in the twenty-first century.

Scientists within ICI had considerable freedom within the company's management structure in the 1940s and 1950s. They had the ability to make their mark on research, and development and also on research policy overall. *Virginia Berridge and Penny Starns's* chapter also demonstrates the role of industry scientists for a slightly later date – the 1960s and 1970s – and for a different industry, tobacco. The tobacco industry is currently the central 'evil empire' for contemporary public health. Its earlier involvement in harm reduction strategies in British public health in the 1970s has been largely 'hidden from history'. In the 1970s industry, government and public health forged alliances round the issue of 'safer smoking' and the development of tobacco substitutes. Such collaboration grew, as with the pharmaceutical industry, out of the patterns of wartime collaboration and government/industry interdependence. The policy agenda of reduction of risk from smoking, rather than its elimination, was one that was also shared with public health interests. A government expert committee, the Independent Scientific Committee on Smoking and Health, adjudicated in the 1970s on possible guidelines for the development and marketing of safer cigarettes or tobacco substitutes. There are parallels here with the later promotion of nicotine replacement therapy (NRT) as a harm reduction technology, in alliance with the pharmaceutical industry rather than with tobacco.

Had the initiatives of the 1970s borne fruit, then tobacco could have been regulated like other medicines. *Stuart Anderson's* chapter shows how the pattern of drug regulation differed between Britain and in the USA. In the former, drug regulation had its origin in concerns about poisoning, both accidental and deliberate. In the USA, it was the adulteration of imported drugs that was the central initial concern. In the decades following the establishment of the NHS, the relationship between the Ministry of Health, the pharmaceutical industry and the medical profession was dominated by the costs of drugs and little attention was paid to the regulation that might be needed for increasingly potent medicines reaching the market. As a result the thalidomide tragedy produced different responses in Britain from the USA. The latter tightened the existing federal system; while in Britain, there was overhaul of the entire framework. The relationships between government and industry cemented at the time of the Second World War entered a new phase.

Changing models and different national styles

Models of public health have changed over the 50-year postwar period and continue to do so. The change to lifestyle public health was central, although there have been some more recent reformulations. These are taken account of in the final section of the book.

Lifestyle public health replaced an earlier environmental concern. *Mark Jackson's* chapter shows how the 'great fog' of 1952 in London led to the 1956 Clean Air Act, which fitted a traditional public health interest in the environmental causes of disease. He sees the 1956 Act as a nascent form of modern environmentalism, which anticipated the environmental turn in public health towards the end of the twentieth century. But Jackson recognises that environmental concern from the 1960s to the 1980s and beyond was a separate movement expressed through single-issue pressure groups rather than mainstream public health. It was not until the late 1980s that environmentalism and public health began to reintegrate, often with reference to the nineteenth century rather than the more recent history of public health in the 1950s.

Carsten Timmermann's chapter shows the rise of another component of the 'new public health' of the 1970s – the concern about cardiovascular disease (CVD). How CVD was framed scientifically was dependent greatly on political and structural circumstances. Timmermann contrasts the work in the German Democratic Republic (GDR) of two research institutes on CVD launched in the 1950s, one led by Albert Wollenberger, a returned *émigré* from the West, whose work was aimed at that audience, the other by Rudolf Baumann, a proponent of the Pavlovian approach to medical science. Epidemiology, which provided the cornerstone for the refocusing of medical concern towards chronic disease in the West, played no part in their work. Moreover, the epidemiological approach present in the country owed more to social medicine traditions, which emphasised life conditions, rather than reductionist 'risk factors'. The 'forced marriage' of the two institutions in the 1970s saw the greater predominance of US-style epidemiology under the influence of political factors: the changed landscape of domestic politics, and the desire for international co-operation under the umbrella of the World Health Organization (WHO).

Timmermann's paper reminds us of political factors that underpin changes in public health science and the role both of national context and cross-national transfer of ideas.

The market played little part in the changes that occurred in East Germany, although the idea of the patient as consumer was important in the changes of the 1970s. But the final chapter, by *Jean-Paul Gaudillière and Ilana Lowy*, draws several of the themes of this volume together. The development of testing for breast cancer predisposition arose from the patenting of the sequence of BRCA genes and illuminates the role of innovation and regulation within different healthcare systems and medical cultures, in this case France and the USA. The authors show how, in the USA, the 'start up' model of genetic testing that prevails is based on the activities and commercial strategies of the new biotechnology companies. Arguments are based on views of individual autonomy, consumer choice and the supposed link between markets and technological efficiency, supported by highly organised consumer groups. In France, cancer genetic services are part of cancer centres, at the interface between public and private. They perform tests for mutations and do not concern themselves with predisposition. The distinctions and strength of national medical cultures comes to the fore here, with French clinicians paying little attention to profit motive or proprietary issues.

Gaudillière and Lowy's comparison shows how contemporary reorganisation of the research system has created new ways of defining public health that compete with older professional regimes of biomedical regulation. Genetic testing offers the possibility of a 'new public health' of the late twentieth and early twenty-first century in which 'embodied risk' has begun to create a reorganisation of the knowledge base of public health. Concern about regulation and access to genetic goods and services, along with access to personal genetic information, has led to the routine incorporation of Ethical, Legal and Social Implications (ELSI) in discussions of public health genetics.

Conclusion

The chapters in this volume underline how postwar public health has a much more nuanced history and complex set of lineages than standard surveys suggest. In Western countries we associate the history of health from the 1970s onwards with economy and management, with the concepts of evidence and evaluation. Chapters here show that the interwar years were a seed bed for those aspects of public health often considered as more recent, post-1970 developments. Take for example the role of health indices, of evaluation and effectiveness demonstrated in the interwar emphasis on health statistics. The role of 'public/private' partnerships in health, seen as a development of the last few years, also has its interwar antecedents. This was demonstrated in the relationships that operated at many levels between health personnel, academia and industry, and the crossover between industrial and health models. The role of the insurance industry has been particularly important here as a crossover location.[47] Occupational health was an area that linked pre- and postwar public health, and provided the original location for many of the new postwar developments, both in Switzerland and the UK. Yet this is a neglected area historically, and one that, in the UK, developed separately from public health postwar.[48]

Policy transfer and the cross-national movement of models and ideas has been important, not only in the way this is addressed in the standard histories, with their ritual mention of Lalonde and the Ottawa Charter. Our studies show how these were only the most visible 'landmarks' standing out from a general *mélange* of cross-cutting influences. US models of industrial psychology affected accident prevention campaigns in Switzerland; health indices travelled from the USA to Europe and back again. The falling market for antimalarials in low-income countries impacted on pharmaceutical company R&D policies and the generation of drugs and markets in high-income countries. East German styles of public health and uses of epidemiology were affected by US models through the agency of the WHO. The role of the WHO, and its forerunner the LNHO, as a key crossover location for the exchange of ideas, programmes and policies is central to public health.[49]

The *media* was a component of this cross-national transfer of styles and ideas. Our chapters show how the role of the media was more significant and more complex than the standard 'media brainwashing' style of discussion. Swiss campaigns used US models and the road safety campaigns seem to have been important precursors of later mass media-based health education campaigns. How far the drink driving issue in the interwar years was also a dynamic here remains to be investigated. British public health initially used the new style of media at the local level, but new centralised technocratic styles of health education campaigns became the norm both in Britain and in France. The media was a central defining part of the 'modernising' project of public health in the UK postwar, first epitomised in the smoking issue, and later expanding into health activism more generally. Visual politics played out in the media became central to many activist causes. Activism redefined itself through its media image from the 1970s.

These campaigns also draw our attention to *new styles of research* and uses for the social sciences within health in the postwar years. The social sciences became important technical tools for health campaigns, impacting through commercial routes and models, as in the market research used in evaluation and in campaign preparation. The social survey assumed importance within public health, and paralleled the rise in importance of the randomised controlled trial within EBM.

Market models and the marketisation of social science in this way is just one aspect of the entwined relationships between *industry, commerce and postwar public health*. Given the assumed hostility of public health activism post-1970s to relationships with industry, it is important to note the role of these public/private relationships historically. Public health reorientation to chronic disease was underpinned by pharmaceutical innovation; marketing models were introduced into health education, providing the basis for the later tools of evaluation and social marketing; and drug regulation was an area of interaction in the 1960s and 1970s between public and private sectors. Tobacco regulation was planned to follow this model too. In health services, industrial models (the costing of the 'standard patient') arrived much earlier on the scene, in the 1950s, than standard historical surveys assume.

And, of course, such models of public health were not static. The chronic disease, individual behaviour focus of the 1970s was giving place in the 1980s to a greater environmental emphasis within public health, although the roots of that re-entry remain to be investigated. Environmentalism developed separately from public health for much of the postwar period as a series of single-issue campaigns and it is only latterly that formal public health has begun consciously to revert to an earlier environmentalist legacy. In doing so, it has used the legacy of the nineteenth century rather than that of the 1950s.[50] And public health has assumed different forms, even different modes of science in different national and political contexts, as for example in the clear differences between East German epidemiology and that practiced in the West. The role of the WHO here was as the agent of Westernisation in standard-setting.

The papers in this volume thus open up a huge number of new windows on twentieth-century and in particular post-1945 public health. Public health is much more than the chronological lists of policy documents with which public health practitioners are routinely presented. Its history is a complex and often surprising intersection of influences at the national and international levels; contemporary public health needs to take account of a history of which it is only just beginning to be aware.[51]

Notes

1 D.T. Rodgers, *Atlantic Crossings: Social Politics in a Progressive Age*, Cambridge, MA: Belknap Press of Harvard University Press, 1998; David P. Dolowitz and David Marsh, 'Learning from abroad: the role of policy transfer in contemporary policy making', *Governance* 13(1), 2000: 5–24; G. Walt, L. Lush and J. Ogden, 'International organisations in transfer of infectious diseases policy: iterative loops of adoption', *Governance* 17(2), 2004: 189–210.

2 C. Hamlin, *Public Health and Social Justice in the Age of Chadwick. Britain, 1800–1854*, Cambridge: Cambridge University Press, 1998; D. Porter (ed.), *The History of Public Health and the Modern State*, Amsterdam: Rodopi, 1994.

3 *Public Health in England: the Report of the Committee of Inquiry into the Future of the Public Health Function* (Acheson Report), London: HMSO, 1988; D. Wanless, *Securing Good Health for the Whole Population. Final Report*, Norwich: HMSO, 2004.

4 On the contemporary history of health, see for example C. Webster, *The Health Services since the War. Volume I. Problems of Health Care. The National Health Service before 1957*, London: HMSO, 1988; C. Webster, *The Health Services since the War. Volume II. Government and Health Care. The British National Health Service, 1958–1979*, London: The Stationery Office, 1996. See also L.V. Marks, *Sexual Chemistry. A History of the Contraceptive Pill*, New Haven and London: Yale University Press, 2001; R. Davidson, *Dangerous Liaisons. A Social History of Venereal Disease in Twentieth Century Scotland*, Amsterdam: Rodopi, 2000. See V. Berridge, *Health and Society in Britain since 1939*, Cambridge: Cambridge University Press for the Economic History Society, 1999. For studies on the contemporary history of science, see for example I. Lowy, *Between Bench and Bedside: Science, Healing and Interleukin-2 in a Cancer Ward*, London: Harvard University Press, 1996; S. de Chadarevian, *Designs for life: Molecular Biology after World War Two*, Cambridge: Cambridge University Press, 2002; P.J. Westwick, *The National Labs: Science in an American System, 1947–1974*, Cambridge, MA: Harvard University Press, 2003.

5 For example Rob Baggott's excellent survey of recent public health policy has two chapters (2 and 3) that cover history. The book then has a number of topic-specific chapters which assume that the history has been covered in the initial contextual chapters. R. Baggott, *Public Health. Policy and Politics*, Basingstoke: Palgrave, 2000.

6 A.R. Peterson and D. Lupton, *The New Public Health. Health and Self in the Age of Risk*, London: Sage, 1996, pp. 28–30.

7 D.J. Hunter, *Public Health Policy*, Cambridge: Polity Press, 2003; D.J. Hunter, 'Public health policy', in J. Orme, J. Powell, P. Taylor, T. Harrison and G. Buckingham (eds), *Public Health for the 21st Century*, Maidenhead: Open University Press, 2003, pp. 15–30.

8 The survey of recent history in the Wanless Report (2004) is one example of the use of historical events in this way. Wanless's survey seems to be taken in part from Hunter's analysis.

9 J. Le Fanu, *The Rise and Fall of Modern Medicine*, London: Little Brown, 1999; M. Fitzpatrick, 'Take two aspirins and thank your caring PM', *Times Higher,* 19–26 December 2003: 28–9. See also his *The Tyranny of Health: Doctors and the Regulation of Lifestyle*, London: Routledge, 2001.

10 J. Lewis, *What Price Community Medicine? The Philosophy, Practice and Politics of Health since 1919*, Brighton: Wheatsheaf Books, 1986; J. Lewis, 'Public health doctors and AIDS as a public health issue', in V. Berridge and P. Strong (eds), *AIDS and Contemporary History*, Cambridge: Cambridge University Press, 1996, paperback edition, 2002, pp. 37–54.

11 D. Porter, *Health, Civilization and the State: a History of Public Health from Ancient to Modern Times*, London: Routledge, 1999; C. Webster and J. French, 'The cycle of conflict: the history of public health and health promotion movements', in L. Adams, M. Amos and J. Munro (eds), *Promoting Health. Politics and Practice*, London: Sage, 2002, pp. 5–12; D. Blane, E. Brunner and R. Wilkinson, 'The evolution of public health policy – an anglocentric view of the last fifty years', in D. Blane, E. Brunner and R. Wilkinson (eds), *Health and Social Organization: Towards a Health Policy for the Twenty First Century*, London: Routledge, 1996, pp. 1–17.

12 See for example J. Crown, 'The practice of public health medicine: past, present and future', in S. Griffiths and D. Hunter (eds), *Perspectives in Public Health*, Abingdon: Radcliffe Medical Press, 1999, pp. 214–22.

13 For example Naidoo and Wills, a well-known textbook in health promotion, which has as its historical stages: 1800–1900 public health movement; 1900–40 health education; 1940s to 1970s rise of prevention; 1980s rise of individual; 1990s rise of market; 1997 onwards rise of social responsibility and the new public health. None of this is referenced to the work of historians. See J. Naidoo and J. Wills, *Health Promotion. Foundations for Practice*, London: Bailliere Tindall, 1994, p. 138.

14 See acknowledgements at the start of this volume.

15 For example M. Bartley, *Authorities and Partisans: the Debate on Unemployment and Health*, Edinburgh: Edinburgh University Press, 1992.

16 D. Porter, 'Changing disciplines: John Ryle and the making of social medicine in Britain in the 1940s', *History of Science* 30, 1992: 137–64; D. Reisman, *Richard Titmuss: Welfare and Society*, London: Heinemann, 1977; D. Porter (ed.), *Social Medicine and Medical Sociology in the Twentieth Century*, Amsterdam: Rodopi, 1997.

17 W.G. Rothstein, *Public Health and the Risk Factor: a History of an Uneven Medical Revolution*, Rochester, NY: University of Rochester Press, 2003. See also L. Berlivet, '"Association or causation?" The debate on the scientific status of risk factor epidemiology, 1947–1965', in V. Berridge (ed.), *Making Health Policy. Networks in Research and Policy after 1945*, Amsterdam: Rodopi, 2005.

18 V. Berridge, 'Post war smoking policy in the UK and the redefinition of public health', *Twentieth Century British History* 14(1), 2003: 61–82.

19 V. Berridge and K. Loughlin, 'Smoking and the new health education in Britain, 1950s to 1970s', *American Journal of Public Health* 95, 2005: 956–964.

20 *Prevention and Health, Everybody's Business: a Reassessment of Public and Personal Health*, London: HMSO, 1976.

21 M.I. Roemer, 'Henry Ernest Sigerist: internationalist of social medicine', *Journal of the History of Medicine and Allied Sciences* 13, 1958: 229–43; E. Fee and E.T. Morman, 'Doing history, making revolution: the aspirations of Henry E. Sigerist and George Rosen', in R. Porter and D. Porter (eds), *Doctors, Politics and Society: Historical Essays*, Amsterdam: Clio Medica, 1993, pp. 275–311.

22 V. Berridge 'Historical evaluation of health promotion', in M. Thorogood and Y. Coombes (eds), *Evaluating Health Promotion: Practice and Methods*, Oxford: Oxford University Press, 1999, pp. 11–24.

23 Lewis, *What Price Community Medicine?* pp. 110–24.

24 Jeanne Daly, *Evidence Based Medicine and the Search for a Science of Clinical Care*, Berkeley: University of California Press, 2005.

25 P.K. Rangachari, 'Evidence-based medicine: old French wine with a new Canadian label?' *Journal of the Royal Society of Medicine* 90, 1997: 280–4

26 For example W.W. Holland, 'A dubious future for public health?' *Journal of the Royal Society of Medicine* 95, 2002: 182–8. See also W.W. Holland and S. Stewart, *Public Health, the Vision and the Challenge*, London: Nuffield Provincial Hospitals Trust, 1998.

27 Bartley, *Authorities and Partisans*.

28 Public health professionals in the late 1990s and early 2000s adopted inequalities as an issue again through government policy in the UK, but seemed to spend much time in practice dealing with other more technical matters such as waiting lists.

29 Comprehensive collections on international health between the wars can be found in P. Weindling (ed.), *International Health Organisations and Movements, 1918–1939*, Cambridge: Cambridge University Press, 1995, and in I. Lowy and P. Zylberman (eds), 'The Rockefeller Foundation and biomedical sciences' (special issue) *Studies in the History and Philosophy of Biological and Biomedical Sciences* 31, 2000. There are also numerous specific area studies. See for example M. Cueto, *Missionaries of Science: the Rockefeller Foundation and Latin America*, Bloomington: Indiana University Press, 1994.

30 P. Mazumdar, 'In the silence of the laboratory: the League of Nations standardizes syphilis tests', *Social History of Medicine* 16(3), 2003: 437–59.

31 M. Dubin, 'The League of Nations Health Organisation', in Weindling (ed.), *International Health Organisations and Movements*, pp. 56–80.

32 P. Weindling, 'Social medicine at the League of Nations Health Organisation and the International Labour Office compared', ibid., pp. 134–53, see p. 137.

33 J. Farley, *To Cast out Disease: a History of the International Health Division of the Rockefeller Foundation, 1913–51*, Oxford: Oxford University Press, 2004.

34 See J.N. Morris's views postwar, quoted in Lewis, *What Price Community Medicine?* p. 103. On Jerry Morris and his contribution to postwar public health, see V. Berridge, 'Jerry Morris', overview for special issue of *International Journal of Epidemiology* 30, 2001: 1141–5; K. Loughlin, 'Epidemiology, social medicine and public health. A celebration of the 90th birthday of Professor J.N. Morris', *International Journal of Epidemiology* 30, 2001: 1198–9. V. Berridge and S. Taylor (eds), *Epidemiology, Social Medicine and Public Health*, London: Centre for History in Public Health, 2005.

35 For studies of this process in relation to current issues, see the papers emanating from the ESRC's Future Governance Programme, Lessons from Comparative Public Policy. See the website of the London School of Economics, www.lse.ac.uk/collections/government/research/resgroups/futgovprog.htm.

36 N. Rose, *The Psychological Complex: Social Regulation and the Psychology of the Individual*, London: Routledge and Kegan Paul, 1985; M. Thomson, 'Mental

hygiene as an international movement', in Weindling (ed.), *International Health Organisations and Movements*, pp. 283–304.

37 D. Miller, J. Kitzinger, K. Williams and P. Beharrell, *The Circuit of Mass Communication: Media Strategies, Representation and Audience Reception in the AIDS Crisis* (Glasgow Media Group), London: Sage, 1998.

38 V. Berridge, 'AIDS, the media and health policy', in P. Aggleton, P. Davies and G. Hart (eds), *AIDS, Rights, Risk and Reason*, London: Falmer, 1992, pp. 13–27.

39 K. Loughlin, 'Networks of mass communication: reporting science, health and medicine from the 1950s to the 1970s', in Berridge (ed.), *Making Health Policy*, 2005; K. Loughlin, 'Spectacle and secrecy: press coverage of conjoined twins in 1950s Britain', *Medical History* 49(2), 2005: 197–212.

40 Berridge and Loughlin, 'Smoking and the new health education'.

41 V. Berridge, 'New social movement or government funded voluntary sector? ASH (Action on Smoking and Health) science and anti tobacco activism in the 1970s', in M. Pelling and S. Mandelbrote (eds), *The Practice of Reform in Health, Medicine and Science, 1500*–2000, London: Ashgate (forthcoming).

42 D. Dow (ed.), *The Influence of Scottish Medicine: an Historical Assessment of Its International Impact*, Carnforth, Lancs: Parthenon, 1988.

43 Berridge and Loughlin, 'Smoking and the new health education'.

44 A. Brandt, 'The cigarette, risk and American culture', *Daedalus* 119, fall 1990: 155–76.

45 J-P. Gaudillière and I. Lowy (eds), *The Invisible Industrialist. Manufacturers and the Production of Scientific Knowledge*, London: Macmillan, 1998; T. Schlich, *Surgery, Science and Industry: a Revolution in Fracture Care, 1950s–1990s*, Basingstoke: Palgrave, Macmillan, 2002; P. Vagelos and L. Galambos, *Medicine, Science, and Merck*, Cambridge: Cambridge University Press, 2004.

46 T. Wilkie, *British Science and Politics since 1945*, Oxford: Basil Blackwell, 1991; S. Horrocks and D. Edgerton, 'British industrial research and development before 1945', *Economic History Review* 47, 1994: 213–38.

47 M. Dupree, 'Other than healing: medical practitioners and the business of life assurance during the nineteenth and early twentieth centuries', *Social History of Medicine* 10(1), 1997: 79–103.

48 T. Carter, 'Fifty years of medicine in the workplace', *Journal of the Society of Occupational Medicine*, 1985: 4–22.

49 K. Lee, *Historical Dictionary of the World Health Organization* (Historical dictionaries of international organizations series, no. 15), London: Scarecrow Press, 1998; J.N. Ruxin, 'Hunger, science, and politics: FAO, WHO, and UNICEF nutrition policies, 1945–1978', unpublished Ph.D. thesis, University College London, 1996.

50 The transcript of a witness seminar on the London fog of 1952 is available on the website of the London School of Hygiene and Tropical Medicine, www.lshtm.ac.uk/history/bigsmoke.html. See also V. Berridge and S. Taylor (eds), *The Big Smoke: Fifty years after the 1952 London Smog*, London: Centre for History in Public Health, 2005.

51 Transcript of witness seminar held at the Wellcome Trust, London, 12 October 2004, 'Public Health in the 1980s and 1990s: decline and rise?' To be published with V. Berridge, D.A. Christie and E.M. Tansey (eds) in Wellcome Witness Seminar Series.

Part I

Interwar influences on postwar public health

1 Atlantic crossings in the measurement of health

From US appraisal forms to the League of Nations' health indices

Lion Murard

Article translated from French by Noal Mellott (CNRS, Paris, France).

International transfer of expertise during the interwar period has been the subject of sustained academic scrutiny.[1] A US phenomenon, corporate philanthropies gained attention in this area through their worldwide involvement in developing public health infrastructure and standards, and in forming an elite of medical 'statesmen'.[2] The Rockefeller Foundation's International Health Board, arguably the world's most important disease-control agency until the creation of WHO, was primarily interested in 'backing brains'.[3] Imbued with the utopian vision that an applied science could unite a divided world, the 'Rockefeller medicine men' declared that 'to make a country safe for democracy, we must first make it healthy'.[4] In their opinion, nothing was more urgent than to help in the creation of an elite of change-inducing officials in each nation, and even more, the creation of an '*esprit de corps*' among these 'translocal' professionals.

From its inception on the eve of the First World War, the Rockefeller pattern of mounting a mass attack on hookworm infection,[5] or the Gambian mosquito, broadened into far-flung schemes involving demonstration projects and education, on an ever-widening international front.[6] It was war, however, that gave relevance to this wholesale diffusion of proper methods of administration. 'Philanthropic globalism' emerged from the conflict as a special branch of that unofficial, technical diplomacy which was being carried out in war-stricken Europe by such theoretically apolitical agencies as Herbert Hoover's American Relief Administration, or Henry Davison's League of Red Cross Societies.[7]

The Rockefeller enterprise fit so well with that of the newly formed League of Nations Health Organization (LNHO), that the Foundation ended up financing 35–40 per cent of its budget.[8] A truly 'special relationship'[9] was formed, leading to a delegation of authority so sweeping in character, that one could sometimes imagine the Geneva organisation as no more than a simple 'appendix' of the Rockefeller Foundation.[10] The official USA sulked behind its oceans like Achilles in his tent, but the competing entrepreneurism of these philanthropic agencies mitigated the effects of isolationism. Sanitation by proxy was provided by 'the truly amazing extension' of the League of Nations' (LN) health work in such diverse areas as the exchange of public health personnel, the improvement of national health systems, or intelligence on epidemics.[11] By 1937, for instance, 72 per cent of the world's population was covered by the LNHO's medical statistics.

Rather than seeing the interwar period as characterised by an isolationist USA, which turned its back on socialised forms of European healthcare, a Foundation-based approach reveals constant interactions. At times the US work was pioneering, and at times it was seeking to transpose and adapt initiatives worked out elsewhere. Here, I focus on local, reciprocal schemes of innovation in public health measurement, which were conducted simultaneously on both sides of the Atlantic.

This chapter examines cross-currents in the ideas and influences that led, in the 1920s, to the drafting of a tool for local health administrations, the American 'Appraisal Form for Community Health Work',[12] and, in the 1930s, to its being reframed transnationally as the LN's collection of 'Life, Environment and Health Indices'.[13] Both artefacts were empirical, policy-oriented, but significantly different: the former was limited to gauging the effectiveness of public health departments whereas the latter extended 'their subject matter to include such topics as medical services, housing and nutrition, all of which were excluded in the American schemes'.[14] While the geocentric US form was primarily a measuring rod for community health work, 'a methodical self-analysis by the health department of its own organization',[15] its European counterpart was intended to provide an aeroplane view of 'a given community's living standard and health balance-sheet'[16] that could be used for 'international or even intranational comparisons'.[17]

Borrowing from procedures used in manufacturing and industry, measurement in the USA was to be primarily based on the standards designed under the auspices of life insurance companies, corporate philanthropies, field health officers and the Chamber of Commerce. Meanwhile, a quite different numerical instrument was taking shape in Geneva:

> In place of the inert figures standing in the columns of statistical directories, and in the stead of the impressionistic notes and thick details contained in the surveys, the League's index claimed to account for variations in certain quantities and thus, at least to a degree, in collective Life, so shifting and hard to grasp.[18]

This claim, perhaps inordinate, definitely stemmed from a failing historical memory. Nonetheless, 'planned and carried out as a joint undertaking by the LNHO and the [US] Milbank Memorial Fund',[19] it deserves attention as 'an ideal type of international cooperation'.[20]

This chapter intends to shed light on these 'Atlantic crossings',[21] the making and unmaking of an Atlantic era in health measurement. The US forms drew inspiration from the earlier British General Registrar Office's 'healthy standards', in that they aimed at boosting intercommunity competition. As they were being transposed internationally, however, they were at risk of tilting

unsteadily towards social medicine. My goal is to explore the striking variations in the motives for producing and using such instruments.

Assessing local public health performance in the USA: the APHA's Committee on Administrative Practice (1920–56)

Invigorated by the spirit of Wall Street, the Progressive Era's all-encompassing
endeavour to set standards for housing, working conditions and welfare
exposed the inability of city governments to provide minimal services. How
stark the landscape sketched by the economist Irving Fisher of a continent so
soiled that: 'the Ohio River represents a thousand miles of typhoid fever, and
the Hudson River a *cloaca maxima* from Albany to the sea' – a land where
'out of 80,000,000 of our people, 8,000,000 must perish from tuberculosis!'[22]

Local authorities who did so little to implement epoch-making medical
discoveries were 'inexcusably blind to their own, best economic interests', since
bacteriology provided them 'with such full knowledge that the determination of
the average death rate is in their hands'.[23] In their role as social corporations
for boosting community services, local governments had to be 'forced into good
habits' and, above all, to replace their old grab-bag budgets with ones planned
along scientific guidelines. In 1908, the New York Bureau of Municipal
Research, the flagship of the 'City Manager Movement', sponsored the first
budget exhibition in the USA. It would even go so far as to conduct surveys in
city management on budget-making, accounting, auditing, revenues and public
works, as well as on the police, fire and other municipal departments.[24]

Still in search of their own distinctiveness, sanitarians borrowed from
Taylorists the new ethos of '100 per cent efficiency', '100 per cent
Americanism'. In his monumental 1915 survey of state boards of health,
Charles Chapin (1856–1941), Superintendent of Health in Providence,
Rhode Island, broke new ground: 'There is probably not a single large
municipal health department in the country which is operated along strictly
logical lines....Much is done that counts little for health and much is left
undone which would save many lives.'[25]

This sowed 'a good deal of consternation'[26] in the ranks of the American
Public Health Association (APHA). Poor in both numbers and funds, the
APHA was losing any hope of improving the effectiveness of local health
departments. Despite a few dazzling advances against backwardness,
'barbarous America'[27] still provided a stark contrast between dreams of
cosmopolitan success and an awareness of its parochialism.

Implementing organisational practices in local public health services
would have lain beyond the strength of the sanitary movement were it not
for life insurance companies. The latter had long been showing interest in
teaching the masses how to live longer. The word 'waste' insulted its quantitative ethics. As of 1909, the Metropolitan Life Insurance Company
launched welfare services for its 10 million industrial policy-holders. It
entrusted this programme to a well-known social worker at the Russell Sage

Foundation, a former manager of New York City's United Hebrew Charities, Lee Frankel (1867–1931).[28] He was assisted by Louis Dublin (1882–1969), a New Yorker born in Lithuania and raised in the Lower East Side's 'Babel of noise and filth', who ran the Metropolitan's Statistical Bureau. Did the insurer and insured not share a common interest? If the latter realised that 'better care of his health will result eventually in savings to his pocket-book',[29] he would directly benefit in terms of less illness and premature death, and 'the insurer would profit from lower mortality'.[30] Metropolitan Life's programme sparked a phenomenal increase in its free visiting-nurse services, and its welfare budget flew up into the millions of dollars. Concerned about health work all over the country, Frankel and Dublin did not hesitate to throw their lot in with the APHA. Frankel, in the position of treasurer, put the association back on its feet. Membership had risen from 500 in 1890 to 700 in 1912, but shot up to 3,400 in 1919 when he was elected president. In May 1920, Dublin recommended setting up a special committee for advancing health procedures by measuring their effectiveness throughout the country.[31]

As an outgrowth of the City Manager Movement, the Committee on Municipal Health Department Practices set up by the APHA in September 1920 followed up Chapin's proposal to formulate public health activity and achievements 'in terms of simplified numerical scores or grades which would be combined into a single total score'.[32] This idea, as suggested, would never have thrived had Metropolitan Life, spurred on by its welfare division, not financed the committee's entire annual budget. Changing the committee's name to the Committee on Administrative Practice (CAP) in 1925 signalled that its scope was expanding to state and rural programmes, once the Milbank Memorial Fund joined Metropolitan Life in supporting its work. This pioneering committee brought together a wide range of talents. It was chaired by Charles-Edward Amory Winslow (1877–1957), professor and chairman of Yale University's Department of Public Health, the first public health leader in the USA to recognise the importance of 'medical economics'.[33] The secretary was Dublin, a biostatistician attracted by the British Biometric School,[34] who would be the committee's kingpin.

In unison with William Farr orchestrating competitions between 'healthy' and unhealthy districts, Chapin had appended to his survey a score of major activities (vital statistics, laboratory, communicable disease control, etc.) totalling 1,000 points for a complete, ideal programme. To rank cities by the merits of their health programmes, he formalised science-based performance standards for localities to use to measure how far they were lagging behind. Using this approach to tell efficient and wasteful procedures apart, the CAP conducted a systematic study of how health was organised in the eighty-three largest cities in the USA. Dated July 1923, this 'first comprehensive comparative review of health practice in the world' was published as *Bulletin 136* by the Federal Public Health Service.[35] It also included the essentials for a 'normative, standard community program'.[36]

Table 1.1 The US appraisal of administrative health practice: maximum total points for each of the local public health department's major activities

Sections	City health work (1926)	City health work (1929)	Rural health work (1932)	City health work (1934)	Local health work (1938)
Vital statistics	60	50	50	60	40
Laboratory	70	60	–	45	–
Popular instruction	20	40	–	–	–
Communicable disease control	175	160	170	155	160
Venereal disease	50	50	55	65	90
Tuberculosis	100	90	100	90	90
Cancer	–	20	–	–	–
Heart disease	–	20	–	–	–
Maternity hygiene	–	80	90	90	90
Infant hygiene	200	80	90	90	170
Preschool hygiene		80	90	90	
School health	150	120	140	110	140
Sanitation	80	80	90	80	90
Food and milk control	75	70	75	75	80
Sanitary inspection	20	–	–	–	–
Balanced programme	–	–	50	50	50
Total	1,000	1,000	1,000	1,000	1,000

Notes:
NB: 'It is noteworthy that the coefficients of the Appraisal Form refer to the importance of eacl service instead of its purpose. For instance, since supervising drinking water is easy in most cities this service has a low coefficient even though the importance of drinking water is of the firs magnitude', Anon., L'appréciation des services d'hygiène au moyen de *l'Appraisal Form* APHA, 1929', *Bulletin mensuel de l'Office International d'Hygiène Publique* 23(6), 1931: 1116.

Source: C.-E.A. Winslow, 'The appraisal of administrative health practice', *Journal of the Roya Sanitary Institute* 47(2), 1926: 142; Anon., L'appréciation des services d'hygiène au moyen d· *l'Appraisal Form*, APHA, 1929', *Bulletin mensuel de l'Office International d'Hygiène Publique* 23(6) 1931: 1114; R.-H. Hazemann, 'Application de la méthode des indices en vue de l'établissement, d· l'exécution et du financement des programmes sanitaires', *Bulletin de la Statistique Générale de l· France* 28(4), 1939: 675.

Borrowed from 'businessmen's precise methods',[37] in particular from the forms that fire insurance companies had been using since 1916 to assess risks in a locality,[38] the balanced scoreboard worked out by the CAP during the 1920s and 1930s was to serve for grading city and rural health programmes according to accepted standards of practice.[39] Designed to provide a reasonably accurate picture of the services performed, a series of self-assessment instruments were made public in two versions, the 'Appraisal Form for City Health Work' (1925, revised in 1926, 1929 and 1934)[40] and the 'Appraisal Form for Rural Health Work' (1927, amended in 1932). In the summer of 1938, the two were combined into the 'Appraisal Form for Local Health Work', a systematised report on work done and work outstanding, with items arranged for easy comparison. At a glance, the reader could see how a locality rated for each of eleven major health activities (raised to fourteen in 1929, see Table 1.1).

Let us take the example of sanitation, a section rating for up to 80 of the 1,000 maximum points. Robert-Henri Hazemann (1897–1976), a Rockefeller fellow trained at Johns Hopkins in biostatistics and the founder of France's first health centre, described it:

> The first item has to do with sanitary inspection: 10 points is granted for 3,000 annual visits per 100,000 inhabitants. The second item refers to water, with 35 points at most, 30 if the water supply meets up to the laboratory standards set in Washington. Swimming pools carry 5 points at most, including 1 point if all bathers shower and wash with soap before entering the pool. Educating people about sanitation carries 5 points, of which 2 are granted if more than 150 brochures per 100,000 inhabitants are distributed annually, 1 if at least 3% of the population attends health lectures, and 2 if newspapers carry at least two articles a year.[41]

As we see, the intention was to measure not a community's health status but, instead, the 'immediate results attained',[42] such as statistics properly obtained and analysed, vaccinations performed, infants followed up in clinics, or physical defects among school children discovered and remedied. In the section on home visits by school nurses, the standards were: 400 visits a year per 1,000 primary school children, which was worth 10 points, whereas 200 visits was worth only 4 and there were no points for fewer than 100 visits.[43] Out of all this would be drawn a numerical rating score based on aggregated points awarded across these key administrative areas. Table 1.2 lists the criteria of progress in tuberculosis control, which could amount to 100 points.

Local planners could use this measuring rod to rationalise services (in the 1930s, the New York City Health Commissioner had more than 2,500 employees), argue for more means, and victoriously push back budgetary restrictions, which, otherwise, would be blindly made. Hazemann, who, while working in a suburb near Paris, had tried to design 'poverty indices' and would soon head the technical cabinet of the Popular Front's Ministry of Health, clearly saw these advantages. In 1936, he emphasised how much the US scoring procedure 'standardises' responses so as to help 'hygienists find their way', 'politicians take their bearings' and 'public opinion form on technical ground'.[44] Comparable ratings often attracted interest from the media, resulting in good and bad publicity for local agencies: 'National

Table 1.2 The US appraisal of administrative health practice: tuberculosis control (total points 100)

Item	Standard	Value
Reporting (10 points)	2 new cases (all forms) reported last year per death	10
Field nursing service (25 points)	Number of visits: 5,000 visits by nurses per 100 deaths last year	20
	Follow-up of post-sanatoria cases: 20% of total tuberculosis field nursing visits	5
Clinical service (25 points)	Number of clinic visits: 3,000 visits per 100 deaths	15
	Ratio of 3 visits per patient registered	10
Hospitalisation (25 points)	25,000 patient days per 100 deaths	15
	25% of total admissions are incipient cases	10
Open-air classrooms, preventoria or day camps (15 points)	10 children per 1,000 grade school population (public and private)	15

Source: C.-E.A. Winslow, 'The appraisal of administrative health practice', *Journal of the Royal Sanitary Institute* 47(2), 1926: 145–6.

magazines commented exclusively upon the results. More importantly, the cities concerned took steps to make needed improvements.'[45] The CAP cited a mayor who, upon learning that his city ranked low in diphtheria prevention and that full credit could be secured at a cost of $175 for antitoxin, made the sum available at once from special funds.[46] These ratings thus became an instrument for decision-making.

More generally, the appraisal method provided a yardstick that was adopted in 1924 by social services and charities,[47] and worked out in the 'Appraisal Form for Industrial Health Service' that, by 1932–3, was spreading to businesses, such as the American Telephone and Telegraph Company. From there, it was examined by the American Management Association.[48]

It is difficult not to draw a parallel with economics trying to build a model of the business cycle at this time. In the early twentieth century, several organisations specialising in consultancy sprung up in the USA, for example Babsonian Statistical Organization or Brookmire Economic Service. They were trying by trial and error to combine numerical data into an index for assessing general trends in the economy. Purely empirical, short-term forecasts abounded at Harvard University, where, in 1917, the first business cycle observatory was set up to design an economic barometer out of statistics. Though applied more flexibly in Berlin by Ernst Wagemann's Institut für Konjunkturforschung as of 1925,[49] and later in Moscow, this approach suffered ever more injurious setbacks. Harvard's predictions continually turned out wrong: its barometer was stuck on fair weather on the eve of the 1929 stock market crash!

This idea of automatically measuring economic fluctuations with a prefabricated tool was, even as economics was gradually giving it up, being transposed into the field of health administration. In both economics and health administration, such tools could assess deviations from what was deemed to be a normal level of performance. For instance, the American Child Health Association reminded health officers of the form's 'similarity of purpose and effect, which it has in common with the spectrometer of the physicist and astronomer'.[50] Earlier, in the Victorian era, the General Registrar Office had used quarterly or even weekly death statistics to quantify what we might call the negligence of major cities. Health thus became a purchasable commodity as, week after week, the 'barometer of comparative national health' run in major newspapers was spread out on the breakfast table.[51] Barometer, thermometer, spectrometer, these terms reflected the deep aspiration of the appraisal technique to 'automatically produce social truth'.[52]

In an era of measurable returns, public opinion could be won over by promising dividends: a longer life and better health. As the British epidemiologist Wade Hampden Frost (1880–1938), visiting professor at the Johns Hopkins School, noted, the health officer is to be the adviser of the man in the street, hardly to be told apart from 'a fiscal agent' to whom the public entrusts public money to be invested so that it would yield 'the best returns in health'.[53] Since this money comes from the public, he is expected to render accounts for each investment and estimate the expected returns. Nor should he be upset to gain or lose clients' confidence in proportion to the returns.

Perhaps, as in the age of Chadwick, few people actually believed the sanitarians' claims of lives and money saved; perhaps few really cared.[54] Disease prevention had no constituency, and the money-value-of-a-man concept lacked the power to convince. Nonetheless, Louis Dublin and Alfred Lotka argued: 'Health work pays....Though it is impossible to state in dollars and cents just what are the economic returns on the money invested in health work, there can be no doubt that the profit is very large.'[55]

In charge of evaluating the New York demonstrations sponsored by the Milbank to help communities repeat the Framingham demonstration on a larger scale, Winslow had no reluctance about using Dublin and Lotka's *The Money Value of a Man* figures to translate death rates into monetary terms. He went so far as to calculate the savings that the Syracuse Health Program made in 1931 on: infant diarrhoea (126 lives saved at $7,000/infant = $900,000); acute communicable diseases (seventy lives at $10,000/life = $700,000); and tuberculosis ($1,574,000, see Table 1.3).[56] The appraisal form was presented in such terms: as a 'method for increasing the return on public health expenditures', it embraced 'the point of view of the taxpayer who wants the more he can get from a tax dollar'.[57]

Performance measurement classified localities by their 'ability to purchase health protection'.[58] As early as 1929, the CAP was predicting that life, health and accident insurance companies would come to use the appraisal

Table 1.3 Accomplishments of the Syracuse Health Program: lives saved by the reduction of tuberculosis, rates at various ages period with corresponding money gain

Age period	Lives saved	Mean value of net future earnings ($)	Monetary gain ($)
Under 5	9	10,000	90,000
5–14	8	14,000	112,000
15–19	3	20,000	60,000
20–44	46	20,000	920,000
45 and over	49	8,000	392,000
Total	115	–	1,574,000

Source: C.-E.A. Winslow, *A City Set on a Hill: the Significance of the Health Demonstration at Syracuse*, New York: Doubleday, Doran & Company, 1934, p. 357.

technique to 'differentiate in their rates between cities with organized business-like health service and those ill-equipped'.[59] That very year, the first Health Conservation Contest, inaugurated in association with the US Chamber of Commerce, crowned ten years of unrelenting action by the APHA's vanguard. With the financial backing of the Prudential, Metropolitan and Equitable life insurance companies, the Chamber relied on the CAP to launch a nationwide 'health conservation contest between cities along the lines of its fire prevention contests which have been so useful in the past'.[60] In a letter to John Kingsbury (1876–1956), director of the Milbank Memorial Fund, Winslow predicted that this outstanding event would provide, 'a unique opportunity to stimulate public health work throughout the country and to translate the experience of the Milbank demonstrations into terms of general practice'.[61]

As the channel whereby health officers pooled experiences, the CAP willingly presented itself as a 'broadcasting agency for the Milbank demonstrations', a launching pad for a programme with the goal to 'not just help Cattaraugus County, Syracuse and Bellevue-Yorkville, but to use them as levers to change health practice in the United States'.[62] Yearly contests opened a way to achieve this goal. Broadcasting the forms signalled that it was high time to use them in an organised effort to improve the efficiency of the whole health system. The Chamber of Commerce worked to this end, endorsing Dublin's endlessly repeated advice that a 'good health record is a business asset for a city'.[63] Civic pride and business interests were goaded to the quick: 108 cities submitted their candidacy for the 1929 contest, 171 in 1931, and 97 in 1934. Raised to the level of a national sport, these contests, which had been renamed the National Honor Roll, were, in 1934 with the Kellogg Foundation's backing, extended to rural areas. As a consequence, the CAP's budget exploded: from $5,000 dollars in 1920 to $1 million in 1956, when the committee dissolved. In Dublin's words, 'What began as a shoestring venture in 1920, financed by the Metropolitan Company, was transformed into a large operation with unprecedented effects on public health.'[64]

It has been shrewdly observed that the USA's 'common national history' probably starts with the 1930s Depression.[65] In 1935, Winslow declared for all to hear:

> A professional group of public functionaries has determined to pool the resources of its knowledge to establish and maintain the highest possible standards of scientific attainment and of public service. They have transformed administrative health practice from a medley of local and accidental enterprises into a concerted national program.[66]

But in early 1936, Edgar Sydenstricker (1881–1936), Chief of the Public Health Service's Office of Statistical Investigations and Milbank's Scientific Director, critically remarked that the CAP yardsticks were not always 'accurately calibrated', nor 'continually put to the test of actual efficiency'.[67] Worse yet, 'the entire list of public health procedures might well be viewed in the light of a healthy skepticism'.[68] And Isidore Falk (1899–1984), his closest assistant, scoffed at the obvious shortcomings of a ready-made outline to which 'some (many?) health officers adjust the practices of their communities so that their scores are increased to be the maximum for minimum effort and expenditure'.[69]

Joe Mountin (1891–1952), chairman of the CAP's Subcommittee on Current Health Department Practices, remarked that an organisation 'may be rendering adequate service and yet not be efficient, or the converse'. This future assistant Surgeon General of the United States Public Health Service (USPHS) regretted, already in 1929, that since the appraisal form 'throws no light on personnel and budget requirements', it 'cannot state whether a low score is due to the inefficient health organization or to the niggardliness of the community'.[70] Earlier studies 'dealt with description of existing resources rather with suggested norms',[71] and even when normative studies were later conducted, they mainly sought to 'stimulate mutual emulation in fields previously chosen as holding promise of results'.[72] And the Commonwealth Fund reported that the forms were 'less valuable as a scoreboard, than as a guide for the analysis of the year's work'.[73]

What Winslow attractively described as a 'unique example of scientific self-evaluation of a public service'[74] turned out to be unsuited for a 'spill-over' from the local to the national level – for the nationwide public health programme that New Dealers were longing to launch. The proof of these shortcomings came through the 1935–6 National Health Inventory, the first nationwide survey of the health status, needs and problems of 2.5 million persons:[75] 'The American people are not so healthy as they have a right to be…the policy of placing the responsibility for public health upon communities and states has failed ignominiously.'[76]

Never has a people been so 'health conscious', and yet only about a fifth of rural-dwellers benefited from organised health care. Sydenstricker railed against the 'niggardly appropriations for public health [that are] grudgingly made'[77] – a fiasco that did not fail to ricochet onto the CAP, 'the originator and the warden of the Appraisal Forms'.[78]

As we shall see, the Atlantic crossing of the US appraisal forms to the LN's Life, Environment, and Health indices shifted the cargo about in two major ways. First of all, there was a shift in the scope and contents. Scoring health practices tended towards 'over-standardisation' – a characteristically US vice.[79] After all, the appraisal forms had not aroused much interest when presented to British health officials.[80] Besides, they were restricted to 'administrative' activities: thirty nurses per 100,000 inhabitants in a city, eight visits for each and every case of whooping cough, etc. In contrast, the health indices would intend to cover any subject reasonably presumed to have a bearing on health. Winslow enthusiastically wrote in June 1936:

> The [LN's] Health Section is now adapting our American idea of quantitative health appraisal to use in a wider field. It has replaced our rigid standards by flexible sanitary indices; and it has supplemented the appraisal of routine administrative practice by a whole group of new indices relating to housing, nutrition, physical education, economic status and literacy which measure the fundamental social bases with which we must reckon in our newer concepts of public health.[81]

Shifting attention away from the 'anatomy of existing functional arrangements for health services'[82] towards the periodic assessment of health conditions, problems and service needs entailed a critique of the data. As a consequence, the indices took, for instance, little account of the death rate, since it had become a 'highly refined statistical index at the expense of its value as an administrative guide'.[83] Instead, emphasis was laid on the quite new notion of a balance sheet, or synthetic diagnosis, which, drawn up by regularly observing a community's customs, mores and economy, could be periodically tested and revised.[84] Thus took shape – and this was the second shift – 'a problem-solving approach'[85] that would 'encourage local authorities to think in terms of local needs, not in terms of any standard pattern'.[86]

Although it was worthwhile evaluating public health efforts in monetary terms, the crucial test and ultimate measure of success, as Sydenstricker had pointed out in 1926, would have 'but one standard', namely the population's health. Not the amount of work done, so many children weighed and reweighed, so many nurses' visits, but, denoted in numerical 'indices', 'changes or contrasts in the state or condition of public health itself'.[87]

The League of Nations' sanitary index, or the cosmopolitan progressives' moment

'An outstanding landmark in the history of public health'[88] was how Winslow praised the International System of Health Indices framed between 1935 and 1939 in the context of the Great Depression, which was cruelly exposing the utter incomparability of existing information on the relations between social deprivation and health. 'We are still a long way off from international vital statistics,' sadly declared Sydenstricker, the USPHS's first statistician, after, in 1923, he was sent to organize the LN's Service of Epidemiological Intelligence and Public Health Statistics, which the Rockefeller Foundation was sponsoring.[89] This demand for a common language was being voiced ever louder in the early 1930s, when Geneva noticed a yawning gap between official statistics, which, in country after country, 'reveal a healthier state than ever', and the widespread feeling that the 'crisis must have deleterious effects'.[90] In 1932, Frank Boudreau, an American working in the LN's Health Section, called for a 'statistical method which gets to the bottom of the mystery', a method that, coming to the aid of health administrations threatened with cost-cutting, would point out 'authoritatively the folly of reducing health services at the very time they were most needed'.[91] Geneva pointed this out: 'Only objective numerical indices of public health, of social and economic conditions and of sanitary activities could, by eliminating official optimism, help establish the desired correlations.'[92]

Envisioning a complete system for appraising health conditions, the LN's Health Section followed in the steps of Edwin Chadwick, Lemuel Shattuck and, even more, John Billings, a military doctor whose detailed form for a sanitary survey of the USA in 1875 contained the germinal idea of 'a comprehensive evaluation of all the health aspects of community life': nearly 500 questions ranging from population and climate to water supply, habitations, garbage and excreta.[93] Five hundred 'indices of health in relation to environment and sanitation' was also the number put forward in the first publication on the subject, a 1936 paper from the LNHO's *Bulletin* immediately republished with a preface by Winslow in the *Milbank Quarterly*.[94] Isidore Falk, the main author of this article, informed the APHA:

> We have finally developed a procedure which goes beyond the field of the Appraisal Form in that it attempts to measure health conditions, the vitality of a people, the sanitary and environmental conditions relating to health, as well as to measure administrative practices. Our scheme does not embrace either standards or scores.[95]

'Coined' by Ludwik Rajchman (1881–1965), the LN medical director,[96] the plural underscored the difference from a single overall index of the sort imagined by demographers (in line with Hersch's 1920 linkage of inequality in the face of death to an 'index of ease')[97] or statisticians (such as Roesle in 1933 who recommended calculating an 'index of health' for the jobless and their families).[98] Geneva's concept was drawn from Alfredo Niceforo's 'numerical indices of civilization and progress',[99] which were to be transposed from describing a specific civilisation to figuring a certain 'life-capital'

Table 1.4 A summary of the subjects included in the League of Nations' system of health indices (three topics, forty-four subtopics)

A Indices of vitality and health	C Indices of administrative activity
I Population	I Community expenditures on sickness and
II Natality	public health
III Stillbirths, infant and maternal	II Sanitary personnel
mortality	III Vital statistics
IV General mortality and causes	IV Laboratory services
V Morbidity	V Acute communicable diseases
VI Invalidity	VI Venereal diseases
VII Insanity and mental defects	VII Tuberculosis
VIII Alcoholism and drug habits	VIII Other diseases
IX Accidents	IX General public health nursing
X Suicides and homicides	X Maternity hygiene
XI Examinations of physical fitness	XI Infant and preschool hygiene
	XII School hygiene
	XIII Physical education (outside of schools)
B Indices of environment	XIV General sanitation
I Climate	XV Food inspection and nutrition
II Topography and density of population	XVI Housing
III Occupation	XVII Industrial hygiene
IV Distribution of wealth	XVIII Health instruction
V Cultural level	XIX Care of the insane and feebleminded
VI Illegitimacy and prostitution	XX Hospital facilities
VII Housing	XXI Health insurance
VIII Nutrition	XXII Free medical assistance
IX Consumption of alcoholic	XXIII Invalidity care
beverages, etc.	XXIV Care of the aged

Source: K. Stouman and I.S. Falk, 'An international system of health indices. A preliminary report', *American Journal of Public Health* 27(4), 1937: 365.

and the interacting factors affecting it, namely: natural, economic and social conditions, as well as the efficiency of health services.[100]

In a flicker of light from the New Deal in the dark 1930s, Rajchman was, in the spring of 1935, making plans for such an international system. Eager to increase the USA's contribution to the League's technical activities,[101] he talked about this with Falk, a vital statistician trained by Dublin, who was now research associate at the Milbank.[102] He had carefully made his choice of whom to talk to. Falk was both 'Winslow's protégé'[103] on the ground-breaking Committee on the Costs of Medical Care, and Sydenstricker's right-hand man on Milbank's scientific staff. In this period of a rush to Washington, Falk, along with Sydenstricker, had been appointed to FDR's Committee on Economic Security in 1934, where he was working on the Social Security bill, finally passed in August 1935. This assignment brought this liberal internationalist to Europe in May 1935 to examine public health and health insurance. During this visit, Rajchman asked him to concentrate on health indices. Immersed in the socio-economic aspects of sickness and medical care, Falk finalised two preliminary memoranda while touring Scotland and England, and visiting Copenhagen, Stockholm, Vienna, Prague, Bratislava, Brussels and Nancy during the summer. 'Merely dictated by a desire of comparability with the American Appraisal Form',[104] the comprehensive survey coming out of the Rajchman–Falk discussions contained 500 indices, 'a reasoned selection from the unwieldy mass of public health statistics',[105] grouped under three main topics – vitality and health, sanitary conditions, and administrative practices – and forty-four subtopics (Table 1.4). It condensed into: a 'detailed' list for brief, intensive, periodic surveys; an 'abridged' list of about a hundred items for the routine measurement of health conditions; and even a 'short' list of sixty indices sufficient for an 'aeroplane view of the entire field'.[106] Experiments were planned for Denmark or Sweden, England or Scotland, and a few areas in France. All this depended on Sydenstricker's 'approval of the program in general'.[107]

The first field trial suggested by Rajchman in the autumn of 1935 as an 'essential preliminary before the schedule is submitted to public health administrators in European countries',[108] was, conveniently, carried out in New Haven, an average-sized town and Winslow's home patch for community health experiments.[109] Knud Stouman (1889–?), former chief of the LN Vital Statistics Department, was paid by the Milbank to conduct the survey. Falk advised him: 'You could work more productively with Professor Winslow in New Haven than with the staff of the CAP.'[110] Somewhat motivated by frustration with the CAP, this advice was, above all, evidence of the New Dealers' interest in a study that, combining European imports with homegrown ingredients, boldly addressed the issue of planning in community health on the basis of international standards. Falk openly discussed this with Rajchman in early 1936. The APHA Committee on Rural Health Work:

> now believes that the American Appraisal Forms should be changed in precisely the ways which are fundamental to our study for the Health Section....Thus, while we have been making extensive use of the American experience of the past 15 years, the APHA is now influenced by the plans which we have projected.[111]

We do not know what the much less outspoken Stouman, who had experience in Danish and British statistical offices, and had worked on mortality tables for the Prudential Insurance Company, thought.[112] On reading his 17 January 1936 lecture at Yale Medical School, we wonder whether he would not have been satisfied with a simple nomenclature of health indices, a catalogue without any explanatory value similar to Bertillon's classification of causes of death.[113] This would have been heresy to Falk, who, seeing in statistics the science of an order to be created, claimed to 'construct out of numerical data *aggregates*, indices'.[114] He wrote to Sydenstricker, 'Dr Stouman seems to have forgotten that these indices were not to be designed merely according to what information is available and can be obtained now.'[115]

Tensions would mount no higher. Sydenstricker's sudden death in March 1936, on the eve of the Milbank's Annual Conference on 'Measurement in Public Health', brought 'the American part of the job' to an end.[116]

Rural Europe, especially in the east, would be next. This is not surprising. Geneva-backed indices were borne by a 'new wave of holistic thinking on health care'.[117] As international tensions flared, vitamins turned into political facts. Emblematic of this was the June 1935 LNHO report, *Nutrition and Public Health*, signed by E. Burnet and W. Aykroyd. By pointing out that a better diet was a 'factor of growth and productivity', it took an opposite approach to the single concrete proposal advanced by the 1932 World Monetary and Economic Conference, which had called for curbing production, creating scarcity and waiting for prices to rise. For the report, the Depression that, 'for a long time, has been taken to be a crisis of overproduction, must be considered instead to be a crisis of underconsumption'.[118] These ideas were spreading in 1935, when Rajchman commissioned Falk to work on the indices. They pulled the new science of nutrition out of the laboratory into world affairs. Home economics, school cafeterias, food budgets and co-operatives: Geneva soon resonated with talk about 'protective' foodstuffs rich in vitamins, the family's purchasing power and consumer economics. This was in line with the pleas by Frank McDougall, who would later head the FAO and was 'guided and inspired by John Boyd Orr',[119] for a 'deliberate association of the agricultural and health problems'.[120]

Following up on a proposal by the Australian delegate (Stanley Bruce, inspired by his economic adviser, McDougall), the LN Assembly called for the League to 'marry health and agriculture'.[121] Again, in 1937, it called for orienting activities towards 'raising living standards, especially of the eastern European peasantry'.[122]

How could bread and butter not be the issue? Fascist welfare states were teaching democrats that granting individual liberties was not enough to secure people's loyalties.[123] Attempts to lower the temperature in the continent's seething hinterland would little by little set a European order at odds with the rising German one. What happened to the indices in this sphere of high politics?

Back from the USSR, where the Health Committee's Bureau, presided by Thorvald Madsen, a Dane, had met from 22 to 28 June 1936,[124] Rajchman was pleased to learn that the indices were still arousing 'considerable interest' in the USA, Stockholm and Copenhagen. Referring to the New Haven study, he declared: 'Winslow and I had little doubt that in well-selected urban and suburban districts of Moscow and Leningrad a similar investigation could well be undertaken'[125] – doubts that he should have had, not so much because of a (new) Stalinist wave of terror but because 'of the priority now given to the general economic and social lifting of rural areas'.[126] From Moscow in June 1936, Jacques Parisot (1882–1967), who held the chair of Social Medicine in Nancy, France, called for: 'penetrating the intimacy [of peasant life], improving the fate of country-dwellers [and] fighting against their exodus, preparing the movement back to the earth'.[127]

The staggering agenda for the far-reaching European Conference on Rural Life (instead of Rural Hygiene, as in 1931) proposed by the Health Committee's Bureau during its Moscow and Paris sessions included nothing less than:

> 1. The rural ambiance: peasant culture, peasant art and folklore, farm loans, agrarian reform, the cooperative movement, repeopling the countryside, rural development, community planning, transportation, electrification, local administration; 2. Food and produce; 3. The rural house and its outbuildings; 4. Peasant education: general, technical, hygiene, homemaking; 5. Peasants at work: new farming methods, rural industries; 6. Peasants at rest: organization of leisure activities, physical education, libraries, radio, cinema; 7. Medical and social policy: maternal and child care, birth control, nurseries and kindergartens in rural areas, malaria, alcoholism, health personnel, midwives, *feldscher*, etc.[128]

The indices were supposed to 'contribute efficiently' to the success of this conference that, had it not miscarried, would have taken place in July 1939.[129] In the quest for methods to 'determine the food state of a population' or 'identify the fundamental data about sanitary, low-cost housing',[130] the commission preparing the conference proposed unknotting the tangled geographical, economic and social factors affecting the state of health in a region. 'Since mortality and morbidity statistics are in this respect notoriously inadequate,' as Rajchman said, the LNHO was to design an instrument for assessing 'the very conditions wherein health problems turn up'.[131]

By the autumn of 1936, the New Haven page had turned, but a new chapter was opening in Hungary in early 1937 thanks to the Milbank's financial assistance, which was forthcoming once Bela Johan (1889–1983), undersecretary of the Hungarian Home Office and former director of the State Hygienic Institute, declared he wanted to 'express in brief the state of public health in a rural district, and to measure later the progress of our work'.[132] Given his longstanding interest in the 'cost of a rural hygiene service per inhabitant',[133] Johan, whom the Rockefeller Foundation considered the 'best public health administrator in Europe', reported to the Health Section that he wanted to use the indices for a 'practical application, and this would be here mainly in the case of rural health work'. This request was passed on to the Health Committee where Parisot, who had replaced Madsen as chair, immediately asked that Bruce's recent suggestions about simple methods for evaluating progress in public health be followed up.[134] Work should begin right away on the indices, a job turned over to the directors of Rockefeller-sponsored institutes and schools of hygiene, who were meeting in Geneva the same month. Falk informed Stouman, 'Winslow likes the Hungarian report. The evidence is clear that the system of health indices lends itself to the rural survey technique.'[135] In fact, except for Brussels, where Stouman was carrying out a final survey in the summer of 1937,[136] field studies would no longer be conducted in cities.

The indices clearly took on a Austro-Hungarian hue. The geopolitical evidence of this is the list of nations that, in November 1937, wanted to experiment with them: the group of countries born out of the collapse of the Habsburg Empire – Hungary, Poland, Romania, Czechoslovakia and Yugoslavia – as well as Turkey, Belgium, France and the Netherlands.[137] The USA was missing, Surgeon-General Hugh Cumming having withdrawn, although saying he was interested because attempts to set up indices in the USA had yielded but 'mediocre results'.[138] As for Great Britain, Major Greenwood was quite sceptical,[139] and William Jameson even more reserved on a question to be handled, in his opinion, not by the London School of Hygiene but by the Ministry of Health.[140] Similar reserves were voiced by Denmark, Sweden and Latvia, which figured among the twelve nations (out of the twenty-eight European nations that wanted to take part in the future Rural Life Conference) willing to prepare for the conference a study on their rural populations' state of health. The indices were left to French-speaking countries and the defunct 'Green International' in the east.

It is not surprising that, also in November 1937, a subcommittee on health indices (chaired by the Belgian René Sand) was set up at the Geneva meeting of directors of institutes and schools of hygiene. Hazemann, the secretary, wanted to continue developing this composite standard 'from the angle of rural hygiene' so as to complete it with data from human geography, rural economics, social work, urbanism and sanitation.[141] Over Stouman's objection ('The Nancy schedule is an aide-memoire for surveys and can never be looked on as a proposal for a system of health indices'),[142] miscellaneous items from the form used in Lorraine were added on: peasant housing, lighting, ventilation, dunghills, flies, mosquitoes and rodents, food safety, control of fresh produce, diseases affecting both people and animals, work hours, the organisation of leisure, surveillance and control of sports, etc.[143] In a return to the spirit of the medical topographies[144] but without any narrative text, the inventory was 'objective', apparently, 'because numerical'.[145]

The aim was to observe '*in situ* how peasants lived'.[146] At a time when half of Europe was rural, how to overlook the affinities drawing social medicine toward 'open-air geography'?[147] Field surveys, excursions and travels like Montesquieu's were ways of learning 'as indispensable to the health officer as clinical observation is to future doctors'.[148] Hygienists had to be thoroughly familiar with the community's mores, customs and economy, as in the 'health inventories' of several rural communes in Seine-et-Marne Department, France, drawn up around 1930 by Hazemann. This former Rockefeller fellow, now an expert in Geneva's Health Section, filled more than fifty tables with numbers, ranging from the 'quantity of meat consumed per week and per person' to the 'distance of wells from unsanitary outhouses', not to forget the 'legal status of property' or 'ventilation at night'.[149] Doctor-sociologist, doctor-geographer, all were one. And let us not forget the tirelessly conducted 'health surveys' in the USA (more than 4,000 during the interwar period),[150] the 'case study campaigns' carried out in Romania by students under the Social Service Act or in Central and Southern Europe via the schools of hygiene, which a Rockefeller field officer said were 'much weaker in epidemiology' than their counterparts in the USA but 'much stronger in public health practice and administration'.[151] Nor should we overlook the qualitative monographs of about 600 pages that Parisot demanded of his students in Nancy on topics such as life and health in a given locality in Lorraine during the past thousand years, or the farming economy, water, milk, manure, and other snapshots of peasant life.[152]

While meeting in Geneva to define the geographical unit for applying the indices, the aforementioned directors of schools and institutes of hygiene did not hesitate at all: it would be the 'natural region', a key concept borrowed from the French school of geography. This choice indirectly criticised Karl Haushofer's *Wehrgeopolitik*, which, thinking only in terms of borders seen as ethnic or political isobars, calculated the demographic pressure per square kilometre on each side. Geneva's attempts to formalise medical and social phenomena countered this racialisation of public health. 'Geomedicine', a word coined in 1931, would take the Slavic region from the Baltic to the Black Sea to be a distinct epidemiological unit.[153] In contrast, the curves, or 'isohygies', drawn in 1939 by Gustavo Pittaluga, the president of the 1931 European Conference on Rural Hygiene, were intended to depict on a map the conditions of, and especially the possibilities for, hygiene among the planet's peoples.[154] Climate, population density, local customs in food and housing – in other words, 'ways of life' – were the opposite of the 'indices of social biology' used by the German, or Romanian, school of sociology.[155]

Given the tension between political arithmetic and descriptive topography, this 'epistemological facies' did not at all differ very much from Soviet statistics, which also jerked back and forth between case studies of peasant budgets and farm surveys carried out in 'typical areas'.[156] As a graph of a community's life and an inventory of its strong and weak points, the indices were merely the 'numerical expression of monographic surveys',[157] with which they shared the same empiricism. Maximilien Sorre, the only one of Vidal de la Blache's students who showed interest in the items listed by Stouman and Falk, saw them as the 'major chapter headings for any study of rural geography'.[158] As a 'practical guide for rural health and general administration', they took in other respects an axiomatic turn that brought them close to being frameworks of interpretation, or of prediction, with probabilistic implications about what would be 'presumably effective' measures.[159] Their designers, Falk and Stouman, pointed this out at the very start: the indices were to have an operational, experimental value, to be strategic variables for 'basing plans on'.[160] This scientific instrument thus took on a fully normative sense as a means of knowledge and administration. The hard part was to achieve an overall understanding of a community's customs and life-ways so as to formulate a rational programme for action – a 'medico-social' regional plan, of which the best example was the one operated in seven southern states under the Tennessee Valley Authority's director of Health, E.L. Bishop, who would be Winslow's successor as chairman of the CAP (1936–41).[161]

Geopolitics and the limits of international co-operation

While informing Rajchman of the modifications being made in the APHA's rural appraisal form so as to 'embody a short list of health indices', Falk did not bridle his enthusiasm:

> Thus we will have run the circle. The concept of health indices was originally developed by an adaptation of the technique of the appraisal forms. Now the technique of the health indices is moving into the appraisal forms to modify them in turn.[162]

Did this circularity involve a transplant of methodology? One might think so, as the APHA had allowed imports from across the Atlantic to be grafted onto homegrown ingredients. In 1938, it corrected the Americanocentrism of its appraisal forms by selecting indices to provide a 'bird's eye view' of the type of community, its facilities, etc.[163] Another opportunity was the first edition of its *Health Practice Indices* in 1942–3, an intriguing booklet that used seventy-one charts to present the health practices of 243 communities in the USA and Canada: these data, such as local health expense per capita, 'analyzed on the basis of median and quartile distributions of various types of activity, are of great value to the local health administrator in planning his own program'.[164] Another opportunity appeared in 1944, when the Association's progressive wing briefly embraced the hope of a National Reporting Area with emphasis 'on problems and accomplishments rather than volume of work'.[165] In a striking reversal from the earlier Honor Rolls, which had mainly emphasised health department efforts, lessons learned abroad seemed temporarily to bring attention to resulting health protection as a whole – temporarily indeed, since the USA and Europe were reverting to being the alien civilisations they were before the First World War.

This ambivalence stands out when reading the praise that W.F. Walker, chairman of the Appraisal Form Committee, heaped on the list to be included in the new 1938 form: fifty-seven indices selected for 'brief, readily made summaries of the health conditions and needs'.[166] Nonetheless, as director of the Commonwealth Fund's Division of Health Studies, he was refusing to fund further studies of what was still nothing other than an experimental tool for periodic surveys and comparisons.[167] Impressed with

the number of indices and 'the fact that in so few instances is there any definite evidence of effect upon the health status of the community', Walker
announced that 'the CAP did not feel that it was a subject which should
engage its first attention'.[168] With Sydenstricker gone, and with him the
cosmopolitan progressives' moment, illusions were dissipating like fog. 'The
CAP does not think very highly of the indices,'[169] Boudreau noted when
he became director of the Milbank. A month earlier, Falk himself had
consoled 'poor Stouman' that 'nothing can be done through the CAP'.[170]

How do we explain this widening rift? Not by Geneva's agrarian shift.
More determined than ever to 'begin, support and speed up' rural development, the directors of European schools and institutes of hygiene were
prodded on by ministers, experts (including McDougall) and peasant party
leaders who were sitting on the commission preparing the Rural Life
Conference. Under Parisot's guidance, they proceeded in the spring of 1938
to overhaul the indices 'for rural uses'. This produced a 'minimal list' with
explanatory notes by Hazemann.[171] This decision contrasted with the efforts
by US sanitarians who were busily combining the city and rural appraisal
forms.[172] But these technical points of divergence did not influence
prevailing opinions on either shore of the Atlantic: the 'rural problem [was
still] of course the great unsolved problem of public health'.[173] Proof of this
was the appointment in 1938 of the APHA's executive secretary, Reginald
Atwater (previously commissioner of Health in Cattaraugus County, NY),
as chairman of an LNHO special committee on health indices. This
committee, despite the absence of Parisot and Höjer, met on the shores of
Lake Geneva in mid-October 1938 with Kacprzak (Warsaw), Tomcsik
(Budapest) and Paterson (replacing Major Greenwood) present, a meeting
held a few days after Munich.

Nor did this rift have to do with the purpose of using the indices for a
general (and not just medical) reorganisation of rural administration.[174]
Assessing ratios of actual to standard performance was the very reason why
the CAP existed. What attracted it to the New Haven experiment was
precisely the 'possibility of developing some simple survey schedules which
can be used everywhere in the country'.[175] 'Statesmanlike' developments in
Hungary in the spring of 1938 rearoused interest across the Atlantic.
Convinced that the methods whereby the country's 160 health centres
reported results were 'inadequate', J. Tomcsik, the director of the Hungarian
State Hygienic Institute, selected forty-eight indices for chief health officers
to use in their monthly reports. Borrowing from the list of sixty-eight indices
drawn up by Stouman in Mezökövesd district (Table 1.5), he sent these officers an abridged list for standardising their 1937 annual reports, whence a
national report was to be drawn.[176]

Given all this, the Atwater committee, in October, did more than just
draw up a modified series of indices for rural areas. In a significant advance,
it proposed a 'Skeleton of a standard report on the state of health of the
population and factors influencing it'.[177] Conceived as a 'means of stimulating

Table 1.5 Hungary, 1937: an abridged list based on a field survey, twenty environmental indices out of a total of sixty-eight health indices

1 Temperature (1928–36)	
Maximum monthly average	22.6°C
Minimum monthly average	2.1°C
2 Annual rainfall (1901–30)	52 cm
3 Population density per km² (1936)	94.5
4 Percentage of the population dwelling in the district's chief town (1936)	29.8
5 Percentage of the population dwelling outside villages (1930)	4.5
6 Percentage of inhabitants living on agriculture (1930)	81.3
7 Percentage of inhabitants in commerce (1930)	2.2
8 Percentage of the farming population belonging to the category of small peasants (1930)	28
9 Percentage of the farming population belonging to the category of farm hands who do not own land (1930)	46.4
10 Percentage of the farming population doing seasonal work outside the district (1936)	37.3
11 Percentage of farmers owning less than 5.6 hectares	78.8
12 Percentage of the land belonging to big landowners (1930)	0.5
13 Number of telephones per 1,000 inhabitants	2.7
14 Number of automobiles per 1,000 inhabitants	0.4
15 Percentage of illiteracy at the age of 6 and over (1930)	11.9
16 Primary school attendance (1936)	93
17 Probability that a single woman between 15 and 44 years old will have a child, divided by the probability that a married woman in the same age group will have one (1936)	0.14
18 Percentage of unbaked brick houses (1930)	66.6
19 Percentage of houses built in rock (1936)	5.4
20 Number of inhabitants per ordinary peasant household (main room, kitchen and storeroom) (1936)	5

Source: K. Stouman, 'Les indices de santé, essai d'application dans un district rural de
Hongrie, Mezökövesd', Bulletin trimestriel de l'Organisation d'Hygiène de la
SDN 6, 1937: 880–1.

hygienists on such important questions as demographic movements, infant
mortality, cases of typhoid, etc.',[178] this outline with selected numerical
indices integrated in its various chapters would hardly have represented
anything other than a US-style standardisation. But more was to be
expected from an instrument intended to provide a 'panoramic view from
one end of Europe to the other of the everyday life of those who work the
land'.[179] It could be expected to 1) facilitate 'expeditious comparisons'[180] of
localities with each other and, over time, of the same locality with itself; 2)
identify 'types' of an ideal health organisation given the geographical,
climatic, cultural and even political environment; 3) contribute to the 'automatic self-standardization' of practices,[181] which the 'demonstration
method' had failed to do on a wide scale; and 4) include observation and
decision-making in a single methodology. This advanced beyond mirroring
the best practices in Danish folk high schools, the Italian *dopolavoro*,

Yugoslavian health co-operatives or Chinese village health workers. Questions were now arising about how to reproduce these prototypes.

What is one to think of the contempt expressed by the director of the Warsaw Institute following a cautious effort to apply the indices in Plock District with its 135,000 habitants: 'New Haven cannot serve as an example for our country'?[182] This backs up Arthur Newsholme's assertion that economic practicability formed the baseline for planning in community health.[183] This statement is in line with Joseph Mountin's suggestion, as head of the USPHS Office of Studies of Public Methods, to retain as criteria of progress not so much the 'standards of performance commonly spoken of as representing good practice' as the 'effectiveness and economy of different procedures for accomplishing desirable purposes'.[184] Presuming, for example, that a mother's care for her baby can benefit from guidance from a public health nurse, questions could be asked about the types of contact, and their optimum number, between nurse and mother that are actually effective. The question could also be asked whether the same purposes could not be accomplished at a lower cost by using improved techniques in mass education instead of nurse visits. This intention to clarify the links between input and output, between activities and accomplishments, motivated Geneva's efforts to use indices to study how much local services cost per inhabitant.[185]

Besides, diffusing the best practices and having them adopted depended on a 'local technical consciousness'.[186] The Rockefeller Foundation in the new US south, Andrija Stampar in Croatia, the Mass Education Movement in Ting-Hsien and elsewhere, all, regardless of national borders, resorted to crafty tactics. To convince mothers on the Hungarian plain to bring their children to clinics, Johan procured forty wagon loads of sugar, an expensive foodstuff, and let the word spread that the children who came would receive two pounds of sugar per month.[187] Another tactic was to distribute vegetable seed with the hope that peasants would modify diets.[188] Understandably, Johan was busily comparing the indices from Stouman's 1937 survey in Mezökövesd district with the data collected in 1927 in the same district by the Rockefeller Foundation. 'Particularly anxious to have indices which could prove and measure the utility of [his] work',[189] Johan came to the conclusion that an annual expenditure of ten cents per capita for a few years would reduce mortality in this poor, backward farming area, by a third: 'It costs about $12.20 to save a life in Mezökövesd.'[190] This sort of conclusion suited the Far East Rural Hygiene Conference held in Bandung (1937), which called for convincing the masses that the funds devoted to health amounted to a 'wise and profitable investment of public money'.[191]

We would be mistaken to think that the indices were used only in 'horse-power Europe': Hungary, Poland, Finland, Cluj and Jassy in Romania, – or even in steam-powered Belgium and France, where Hazemann presented the Conseil Supérieur de Statistique with a list of eighty indices for 'annual reports from local inspectors of hygiene'.[192] The trend was tricontinental, the LN's medical director pointed out in the summer of 1938. As the Bandung Rural Hygiene Conference was slipping into the past and the pan-American one (requested in 1936 by thirteen Latin American delegations, joined by Spain and the Netherlands) was being planned in Mexico City, the time had come to finalise standards for reporting on the population's state of health, which was to be seen not from the European countryside but, instead, from the viewpoint of 'all the countries that have reached a certain degree of health civilization'.[193] Despite the International Labor Organization's hesitation before the scope of such an undertaking, the LNHO had the duty, according to Rajchman, 'today of orienting rural life in Europe, but also yesterday in Asia, and tomorrow in America'.[194]

Ten years of encyclopedic surveys on the methods to 'determine the dietary state of a population',[195] 'identify fundamental data on healthy, low-cost housing', and measure and improve 'existing standards of living'[196] were converging towards the aforementioned 'Skeleton of a standard report'.[197] This outline, along with Stouman and Falk's studies 'which were not to be continued',[198] seemed, by early 1939, to be a document 'still too complicated – but an already well ripened fruit'.[199]

This was quite definitely a tropical fruit, judging by the ultimate attempts to apply the indices in Ceylon,[200] India (at Henry Sigerist's prompting),[201] and later in Malaya, Singapore, Panama and the Canal Zone (at Falk's prompting).[202] These futureless episodes paid heed to the silent links between poverty, illness and malgovernance. They made a big step toward the Bhore Report (1944), the Manitoba Health Plan (1945) and, above all, the joint WHO–UNICEF Conference that would take place in Alma-Ata in 1978. Regardless of how clumsy they might have been, the indices as adapted in 1938 to tropical areas[203] anticipated the all-inclusive conception of rural rehabilitation that would be tried out most extensively not in Southern Europe or Latin America but in the Far East, in plans there for an integrated, village-based system designed to meet the community's full needs from its own resources rather than a single need such as public health.

This is the point where, in my opinion, the Atlantic rift widens. A national health plan for India on the eve of independence? 'Rural electrification,' Sigerist suggested.[204] We might also quote Stampar telling Harvard's medical students about the usefulness of 'drying up social griefs'[205] thanks to agrarian reform, the *sine qua non* for obtaining the population's co-operation in health matters. Social medicine was nothing other than this illicit mixture of series thought to be allergic to each other. By bringing heterogeneous information into a single place, the Geneva index intended to formalise this general interconnection of factors affecting a population's health and wealth. When, in New Haven, it was applied for the first time, Winslow had insisted on developing the 'section concerning the social background of health, notably housing and nutrition' and suggested finding items for the population's 'cultural level'.[206] Rajchman, during his frequents stays in China, paid attention to questions about the civil service, questions so important that they required sending there an expert well versed in the mysteries of the British administration and another on the German municipal system.[207] John Grant, the Rockefeller Foundation's 'medical Bolshevik', had, in the mid-1930s, declared from the Peking Union Medical College, and repeated, in the mid-1940s, from the All-India Institute of Hygiene and Public Health in Calcutta, 'The lower economic levels are, the more does the use of medical knowledge depend upon organization.'[208]

Social, socialised, socialist medicine: this route with its many bifurcations was not the one that the USA was willing to take. The Americanness of the appraisal form could be seen in this drift away from the ongoing transnational trend to style food, housing and income as 'currencies of health'. Welding them into a single block corresponded so little to the views of Surgeon General Hugh Cumming that he spoke out against 'an attempt of the League to intrude itself into national problems, such as nutrition and housing'.[209] But, as already pointed out, the experts designing the indices countered by referring to John Billings, who, in 1875, had pointed to the 'influence of urbanism, housing and overpopulation on public health, factors that in his own country are still hardly considered to be facts of public interest', and concluded sarcastically about the CAP's work: 'We apparently cannot see there a direct continuation of Dr Billings' original idea to gather information which could be used for planning instead of organizing contests.'[210] Stouman and Falk's mockery was in vain, given that 'the struggle within APHA' was turning to the disadvantage of 'doctor-sociologists'.[211]

Nonetheless, prevailing ideas were not at odds on the respective places of politics and expertise. The Rockefeller Foundation's first president, George Vincent, a rural social scientist, had no doubts that public health 'lends itself to objective measurement'.[212] But it should not be the 'football of politicians'.[213] The CAP endeavoured to keep this from happening. The title of the article published in the early 1920s by W.S. Rankin, its first field director, 'Elimination of politics from public health work', is evidence of this: standardisation 'means lifting public health work from a political to a professional plane'.[214] Political decision was as naïvely disparaged on the shores of Lake Geneva, where it was asserted that a rational consensus should be based on objective laws backed up by data produced by experts, that it was not the arbitrary expression of the majority's will. On the eve of totally divorcing 'all its technical and humanitarian activities from its political status',[215] an 'economic League' could not long withstand the rising trend, which inflated the role of expertise and hollowed out the practice of politics.[216] Seen from this angle, both the APHA's and the LNHO's assessment instruments were an attempt to evade the difficulties of political judgement.

In conclusion, the Atlantic was more a barrier than a connective lifeline. The differences are not slight between measuring health practice and improving the population's health. The US form, a tool of microefficiency, was limited to gauging 'actual administrative achievement by a quantitative objective scoring procedure'.[217] Compelled to become a global planning agency, Geneva was dreaming of tools whereby a society could foresee and plan its needs instead of just recording them.[218] Assessing the extent to which local health departments achieve their assignment did not suffice. Imbued with the potency of a 'Keynesian medicine' as the soothing balm of international strife, the LNHO's collection of indices differed 'considerably'[219] from the appraisal form in that it was intended to provide leverage for economic and social change. This intention did not guide the behaviour of health officers who were not trying to engineer welfare but, instead, to assess the urgency of their actions.

As we move from evidence-based medicine to evidence-based health policy,[220] few would argue with the observation made in the November–December 2003 issue of *Public Health Reports*, 'At this time, no gold standard measure of public health system performance exists.'[221] After eighty years of measurement, two US specialists stated, 'we have neither a clear nor a complete picture of the status of public health practice at the end of the twentieth century'.[222] Even though there is no nationally agreed upon tool or instrument, inferences from the 'Assessment Protocol for Excellence in Public Health' and from the practice performance studies by the Centers for Disease Control and Prevention (CDC) suggest that the current level of performance is 50–70 per cent of what might be considered 'fully' effective. Along with the 1988 report by the US Institute of Medicine, which described public health as in disarray, such observations can but relaunch the unended quest for performance assessment instruments. The CDC's National Public Health Performance Standards Program is now striving to test in several states a set of indicators for the '10 Essential Public Health Services' and a model standard for each indicator.[223] The European Community has also just proposed a comprehensive list of generic indicators as part of its Health Monitoring Program.[224]

Epidemiological, standard-of-living and health status indicators have proliferated in the dispersed efforts by the United Nations, World Bank and OECD, and in a multitude of bone-dry journals.[225] But this very disparity reflects a disenchantment with the quest for a single-number index. The many indicators actually produced were, as the WHO itself admitted in the 1970s, 'all measures of ill-health, none can be regarded as a measure of health'.[226] Even today, as data are piling up on the body's mass index, height and birth weight, it is still hard to propose an unambiguous measure of health betterment.[227] The agenda adopted by Sydenstricker for his famous early 1920s Hagerstown morbidity studies is still pertinent, namely, to catch 'glimpses of what the sanitarian has long wanted to see – a picture of the public-health situation as a whole, drawn in proper perspective and painted in true colors'.[228]

Notes

1 J. Farley, *To Cast out Disease: a History of the International Health Division of Rockefeller Foundation, 1913–1951*, Oxford: Oxford University Press, 2004; P. Baldwin, *Contagion and the State in Europe, 1830–1930*, Cambridge: Cambridge University Press, 1999; P. Weindling (ed.), *International Health Organisations and*

Movements, 1918–1939, Cambridge: Cambridge University Press, 1995; Milton I. Roemer, 'Internationalism in medicine and public health', in W. Bynum and R. Porter, *Companion Encyclopedia of the History of Medicine*, London: Routledge, 1993, II, pp. 1417–35.

2 E. Condliffe Lagemann (ed.), *Philanthropic Foundations: New Scholarship, New Possibilities*, Bloomington: Indiana University Press, 1999; A. McGehee Harvey and Susan L. Abrams, *'For the Welfare of Mankind': the Commonwealth Fund and American Medicine*, Baltimore: Johns Hopkins University Press, 1986; Clyde V. Kiser, *The Milbank Memorial Fund. Its Leaders and Its Work*, New York: Milbank, 1975.

3 W. Rose, quoted by R.B. Fosdick, *The Story of the Rockefeller Foundation*, New Brunswick, NJ: Transaction, 1989 [1958], p. 266.

4 L. Farrand, quoted by Charles Hastings in his presidential address, 'Democracy and public health administration', American Public Health Association, 9 December 1918, *American Journal of Public Health* [henceforth *AJPH*] 9(2), 1919: 86.

5 For a case-study of the hookworm campaign, which launched the Rockefeller public health programmes, see J. Ettling, *The Germ of Laziness: Rockefeller Philanthropy and Public Health in the New South*, Cambridge, MA: Harvard University Press, 1981. See also, J. Sealander, *Private Wealth and Public Life. Foundation Philanthropy and the Reshaping of American Social Policy from the Progressive Era to the New Deal*, Baltimore and London: The Johns Hopkins University Press, 1997.

6 W.H. Schneider (ed.), *Rockefeller Philanthropy and Modern Biomedicine. International Initiatives from World War I to the Cold War*, Bloomington: Indiana University Press, 2002; S. Gross Solomon and N. Krementsov, 'Giving and taking across borders: the Rockefeller Foundation and Russia, 1919–1928', *Minerva* 39, 2001: 265–98; I. Lowy and P. Zylberman (eds), 'The Rockefeller Foundation and the biomedical sciences', *Studies in History and Philosophy of Biological and Biomedical Sciences* 31(3), 2000: 365–510; G. Gemelli, J.-F. Picard and W.H. Schneider (eds), *Managing Medical Research in Europe. The Role of the Rockefeller Foundation, 1920s–1950s*, Bologna: CLUEB, 1999; M. Cueto (ed.), *Missionaries of Science: The Rockefeller Foundation and Latin America*, Bloomington: Indiana University Press, 1994; P. Weindling, 'Public health and political stabilisation: Rockefeller funding in interwar Central/Eastern Europe', *Minerva* 31, 1993: 253–67.

7 J.F. Hutchinson, *Champions of Charity. War and the Rise of the Red Cross*, Boulder, Colorado, and Oxford: Westview Press, 1996.

8 M. Dubin, 'The League of Nations Health Organisation', in P. Weindling (ed.), *International Organisations*, 1995, pp. 56–80. On the League itself, see F.P. Walters, *A History of the League of Nations* (1952), London, New York and Toronto: Oxford University Press.

9 P. Weindling, 'Philanthropy and world health: the Rockefeller Foundation and the League of Nations Health Organisation', *Minerva* 35, 1997: 269.

10 G.E. Vincent, 25 April 1928, quoted in G.K. Strode, 'Memorandum on the Health Organisation of the League of Nations and the relationship thereto of the International Health Division of the Rockefeller Foundation', 10 July 1928, Rockefeller Archive Center [henceforth RAC], RG 1.1., 100, 22, 184.

11 E.H. Ranshofen-Wertheimer, *The International Secretariat. A Great Experiment in International Administration*, Washington, Carnegie Endowment for International Peace: Rumford Press, 1945, p. 159.

12 H.F. Vaughan, 'Local health services in the United States: the story of the CAP', *AJPH* 62(1), 1972: 95–111.

13 P. Weindling, 'From moral exhortation to the new public health, 1918–45', in E. Rodriguez-Ocana (ed.), *The Politics of the Healthy Life: an International Perspective*, Sheffield: European Association for the History of Medicine and Health Publications, 2002, pp. 113–30.

14 I.S. Falk to L. Rajchman, 26 February 1936, League of Nations Archives [henceforth LNA], 8A/20615/20615, R6121.
15 W.G. Smillie, *Public Health Administration in the United States*, New York: Macmillan, 1949 [1935], p. 422.
16 R.-H. Hazemann, 'Living standards and health' [typescript, 14p.], WHO Study Group on the Measurement of Levels of Health, Geneva, 24–8 October 1955, WHO/PHA/Lev. Hlth/13.
17 K. Stouman and I.S. Falk, 'An international system of health indices: a preliminary report', *AJPH* 27(4), 1937: 364.
18 Hazemann, 'Le Recueil d'indices sanitaires, instrument d'administration', *Annales d'Hygiène Publique, Industrielle et Sociale* 18(3), 1940: 90.
19 Stouman and Falk, 'International System', 1937, p. 363.
20 C.-E.A. Winslow, 'The international appraisal of local health programs', *Milbank Memorial Fund Quarterly* 15(1), 1937: 5.
21 D.T. Rodgers, *Atlantic Crossings. Social Politics in a Progressive Age*, Cambridge, MA, and London: Belknap Press, Harvard University Press, 1998.
22 Quoted by G. Rosen, 'The committee of one hundred on national health and the campaign for a national health department, 1906–1912', *AJPH* 62(2), 1972: 261–2.
23 H. Biggs, 'The administrative control of tuberculosis', *Medical News* 84(8), 20 February 1904: 345; and 'Preventive medicine: its achievements, scopes, and possibilities', *Medical Record* 65(2), 11 June 1904: 955.
24 M.J. Schiesl, *The Politics of Efficiency: Municipal Administration and Reform in America, 1880–1920*, Berkeley: UCLA, 1977, p. 125; S. Haber, *Efficiency and Uplift: Scientific Management in the Progressive Era, 1890–1920*, Chicago: University of Chicago Press, 1964, pp. 51, 61–2.
25 C.V. Chapin, *A Report on State Public Health Work Based on a Survey of State Boards of Health* [1915], quoted by Vaughan, 'Local health services', 1972: 96.
26 Smillie, *Public Health Administration*, 1949, p. 420.
27 L. Veiller, 'Housing and health', in 'The public health movement', *The Annals of the American Academy of Political and Social Science*, Philadelphia, 37(2), March 1911: 269: 'We are rapidly ceasing to be "barbarous America".'
28 D.T. Rodgers, *Atlantic Crossings*, 1998, pp. 248, 262–4.
29 L.K. Frankel, 'Insurance companies and public health activities', *AJPH* 4(1), 1914: 5.
30 L.I. Dublin, *After Eighty Years, the Impact of Life Insurance on Public Health*, Gainesville: University of Florida Press, 1966, p. 38.
31 L.I. Dublin, *A Family of Thirty Million: The Story of the Metropolitan Life Insurance Company*, New York: Metropolitan, 1943, p. 439.
32 Unsigned editorial [Winslow, editor], 'From health honor roll to national reporting area', *AJPH* 34(10), 1944: 1099.
33 According to his student I.S. Falk, in L.E. Weeks (ed.), *I.S. Falk in First Person: an Oral History*, Chicago: American Hospital Association, 1983, p. 12.
34 L.I. Dublin, 'The statistician and institutional policy', *AJPH* 54(5), 1964: 876.
35 C.-E.A. Winslow, 'Administrative practice', *American Public Health Association Yearbook, 1930–1931*, Supplement to *AJPH* 21, 1931: 63.
36 C.-.E.A.Winslow, 'Fifteen years of the CAP, II. The evolution of the program', *AJPH* 25(12), 1935: 1308.
37 Anon., 'Moyens employés aux États-Unis pour apprécier numériquement les services d'hygiène publique', *Revue internationale des sciences administratives* 4, 1931: 625.
38 K. Stouman and I.S. Falk, 'Indices de santé. Leurs rapports avec le milieu et l'action sanitaire', *Bulletin trimestriel de l'Organisation d'Hygiène de la Société des Nations* [henceforth BOH] 5(4), 1936: 1003.

39 The standards in general represent 'the median result achieved by the upper third of the cities surveyed', C.-E.A. Winslow, 'The appraisal of administrative health practice', *Journal of the Royal Sanitary Institute* 47(2), 1926: 133–51.

40 'Always in an upward direction', Winslow, 'Administrative practice', p. 66.

41 R.-H. Hazemann, 'Application de la méthode des indices en vue de l'établissement, de l'exécution et du financement des programmes sanitaires', *Bulletin de la Statistique Générale de la France* 28(4), 1939: 675–6.

42 Winslow, 'Appraisal', pp. 133–51.

43 Anon., 'L'appréciation des services d'hygiène au moyen de l'*Appraisal Form*, APHA, 1929', *Bulletin mensuel de l'Office International d'Hygiène Publique* 23(6), 1931: 1115.

44 R.-H. Hazemann, 'Du planisme au civisme par la technique', *Le Mouvement Sanitaire*, January 1936: 15.

45 I.D. Rawlings, *The Rise and Fall of Disease in Illinois*, Springfield, IL: State Department of Public Health, 1927, quoted by B.T. Turnock and A.S. Handler, 'From measuring to improving health practice', *Annual Review of Public Health* 18, 1997: 264.

46 G.T. Palmer, P.S. Platt and W.F. Walker, 'Eighty-six cities studied by objective standards', *AJPH* 15(5), 1925: 392.

47 Stouman and Falk, 'Indices de santé', p. 1003.

48 L.D. Bristol, 'An appraisal form for industrial health service', *AJPH* 22(12), 1932: 1263.

49 J.A. Tooze, *Statistics and the German State, 1900–1945: The Making of Modern Economic Knowledge*, Cambridge: Cambridge University Press, 2001.

50 Palmer, Platt and Walker, 'Eighty-six cities', p. 390.

51 H.W. Acland [1872] quoted by J.M. Eyler, 'Mortality statistics and Victorian health policy: program and criticism', *Bulletin of the History of Medicine* 50(3), 1976: 343.

52 A formula from K. Baker, *Condorcet. From Natural Philosophy to Social Mathematics*, Chicago: Chicago University Press, 1975, pp. 56–7, 75, 209–14.

53 W. Hampden Frost, 'Rendering account in public health', *AJPH* 15(5), 1925: 394.

54 C. Hamlin, *Public Health and Social Justice in the Age of Chadwick. Britain, 1800–1854*, Cambridge: Cambridge University Press, 1998, p. 246.

55 L.I. Dublin and A.J. Lotka, *The Money Value of a Man*, New York: Ronald Press, 1930, pp. 131, 135.

56 C.-E.A. Winslow, *A City Set on a Hill: the Significance of the Health Demonstration at Syracuse*, New York: Doubleday, Doran & Company, 1934, pp. 356–8.

57 J.W. Mountin, 'Methods for increasing the return on public health expenditures' [1932], in *Selected Papers of Joseph W. Mountin*, J.W. Mountin Memorial Committee, 1956, p. 266.

58 J.A. Ferrell, 'Economics of public health', *Journal of the American Medical Association* [henceforth *JAMA*], 89(2), 9 July 1927: 77.

59 Committee on Administrative Practice, Appraisal Form for City Health Work, New York: APHA, 1929, p. 3.

60 Winslow to J. Kingsbury, 24 October 1928, Yale University Library, Manuscript Collections, C.-E.A. Winslow Papers, Group 749, Series 111, Box 81, f.1283.

61 Winslow to Kingsbury, same letter.

62 Winslow to Kingsbury, 30 November 1928, same reference.

63 L.I. Dublin, 'Public health service – a sound economic investment', *AJPH* 21(5), 1931: 489.

64 Dublin, *Eighty Years*, pp. 55–6.

65 E.R. May, 'Comment', *American Historical Review* 82, 1977: 603, quoted by D. Reynolds, *Rich Relations. The American Occupation of Britain 1942–1945*, London: Phoenix Press, 2000 [1996], p. 26.

66 Winslow, 'Fifteen years', p. 1315. Likewise in a 1944 private correspondence: 'The structure of public health administration in this country is largely based on work of the CAP, of which I was, for fifteen years, chairman', quoted by A.J. Viseltear, 'C.-E.A. Winslow and the later years of public health at Yale, 1940–1945', *Yale Journal of Biology and Medicine* 60, 1987: 460.

67 E. Sydenstricker, 'Economy in public health' [1936], in R.V. Kasius (ed.), *The Challenge of Facts: Selected Public Health Papers of Edgar Sydenstricker*, New York: Prodist, 1974, pp. 88–9.

68 Sydenstricker, ibid.

69 I.S. Falk, 'Preliminary memorandum on sanitary indices' [typescript, 62p.], 7 August 1935, LNA, 8A/10407/403, R6033.

70 J. Mountin, 'Measurements of efficiency and adequacy of rural health service' [1929], in *Selected Papers*, 1956, p. 299.

71 W. Schonick, Government and Health Services. Government's Role in the Development of US Health Services 1930–1980, Oxford: Oxford University Press, 1995, p. 24.

72 Stouman and Falk, 'Indices de santé', pp. 1003–4.

73 'Report of the General Director [Barry C. Smith] to the Directors of the Commonwealth Fund presented at the April 8, 1943 meeting of the Commonwealth Fund's Board of Directors', RAC, CF, Series 18.1, f.105, p. 3546.

74 Winslow, 'Health honor roll', p. 1100.

75 N. Krieger and E. Fee, 'Measuring social inequalities in health in the United States, a historical review, 1900–1950', *International Journal of Health Services* 26(3), 1996: 407.

76 E. Sydenstricker, 'Health in the New Deal', *Annals of the American Academy of Political and Social Science* 176, November 1934: 131.

77 Ibid., p. 135.

78 K. Stouman's formula, 'Lecture given at the Yale Medical School, January 17, 1936', addressed to I.S. Falk, 24 January 1936, Yale University Library Manuscript Collections, Falk Papers, Series I, General Correspondence, Box 25, f. 522.

79 Winslow, 'Administrative practice', p. 66.

80 In a speech to the Jubilee Congress of the Royal Sanitary Institute, 'Appraisal', 1926: 133–51, and six years later in a lecture to British sanitarians about the CAP, Winslow emphasised: 'I doubt if any single force has had so marked an influence in raising the general level of health service on our side of Atlantic'. Winslow, 'Current tendencies in American public health', *Journal of the Royal Sanitary Institute* 53(1), 1932: 63.

81 C.-E.A. Winslow, 'When is public health?' *Survey Graphic*, June 1936: 373–5, 389–90, Falk Papers, 25, 522.

82 Stouman and Falk, 'International system', p. 364.

83 Falk, 'Preliminary memorandum', 1935, LNA, R6033.

84 R.-H. Hazemann and R.M. Taylor, 'Les inventaires sanitaires', *Revue d'hygiène et de médecine préventive* 45(2), 1933: 82. Likewise R.-H. Hazemann, 'Inventaires et bilans sanitaires', *Revue d'hygiène et de médecine sociales* [Nancy], 18(3), 1939: 79–87.

85 Winslow, 'Health honor roll', p. 1102.

86 Stouman and Falk, 'International System', p. 369.

87 Sydenstricker, 'The measurement of results of public health work' [1926], in Kasius, *Challenge*, 1974, p. 42.

88 Winslow, 'International appraisal', p. 5.

89 E. Sydenstricker, 'The outlook for international vital statistics', *AJPH* 14(10), 1924: 832.

90 F.G. Boudreau to G.K. Strode, 21 October 1932, LNA, 8A/39674/39674, R5936.
91 Boudreau to H.S. Cumming, 28 October 1932, ibid.
92 'Note sur les travaux relatifs aux indices sanitaires', Geneva, 15 June 1938, LNA, CH1346.
93 Winslow, 'Fifteen years', pp. 1303–4; G. Rosen, 'John Shaw Billings and the plan for a sanitary survey of the United States', AJPH 66(5), 1976: 494.
94 Stouman and Falk, 'Indices', pp. 990–1089; *Milbank Memorial Fund Quarterly* 15(1), 1937, with the preface by Winslow, 'International appraisal of local health programs'.
95 Falk to J.P. Koehler, Chairman, Health Officer Section, APHA, 10 June 1936, Falk Papers, 25, 522.
96 Stouman and Falk, 'Indices', p. 994; also Hazemann, 'Application', p. 684: 'We owe the idea of such a method to Dr L. Rajchman.'
97 L. Hersch, L'Inégalité devant la mort d'après les statistiques de la Ville de Paris. Effets de la situation sociale sur la mortalité, Paris: Sirey, 1920, quoted by A. Fagot-Largeault, Les Causes de la mort. Histoire naturelle et facteurs de risque, Paris: Vrin, 1989, p. 154.
98 According to a 'Note du directeur médical', 24 October 1933, LNA, CH 1124.
99 Preceded by *La misura della vita* (1919), A. Niceforo's *Indices Numériques de la civilisation du progrès* (1921) attracted the attention of P. Lazarsfeld, 'Notes on the history of quantification in sociology: trends, sources and problems', *Isis* 52, 1961: 277ff.
100 R.-H. Hazemann, 'Commentaires concernant les indices sanitaires des districts ruraux', Geneva, 5 May 1938, LNA, CH 1331.
101 Boudreau on Rajchman to Winslow, 22 February 1929, Winslow Papers, Box 79, f.1226.
102 M.I. Roemer, 'I.S. Falk, the committee on the costs of medical care, and the drive for national health insurance', *AJPH* 75(8), 1985: 841–8. On Falk's 'outright demonisation' during the McCarthy period, A. Derickson, 'The house of Falk: the paranoid style in American health politics', *AJPH* 87(11), 1997: 1836–43.
103 J.F. Jekel, 'Health departments in the US, 1920–1988: statements of mission with special reference to the role of C.-E.A. Winslow', *Yale Journal of Biology and Medicine* 64, 1991: 468.
104 Stouman to Rajchman, 'Preliminary memorandum on the establishment of sanitary indices' [typescript, 7p.]., 19 September 1935, LNA, 8A/20615/20615, R6121.
105 Stouman and Falk, 'International system', p. 364.
106 As Stouman and Falk pointed out in 'Indices', this was following the model of Philip S. Platt's correlations factors. For frequent surveys to measure change or progress in a community, Platt had, in 1928, shrunk the 131 items of the American Appraisal Form down to eleven by choosing a single item for each group of activities. For instance, immunisation of pupils against diphtheria was taken to be the most typical indicator of the fight against contagious diseases. 'His procedure is valid,' Falk wrote to Stouman on 24 March 1936, while asking him to refer to Platt's article, 'The validity of the appraisal form as a measure of administrative practice', APHA, 1928.
107 Falk to Sydenstricker, 2 October 1935, Falk Papers, 25, 521.
108 Falk to Sydenstricker, 5 December 1935, same reference.
109 C.-E.A. Winslow, *Health Survey of New Haven*, New Haven, CT: Quinnipiack Press, 1928.
110 Falk to Stouman, 31 October 1935, Falk Papers, 25, 521.
111 Falk to Rajchman, 26 February 1936, LNA, 8A/20615/20615, R6121.
112 Stouman, a Dane, was a volunteer in the US Expeditionary Forces and Dublin's assistant in the American Red Cross unit in Italy. After the war, he stayed on in

Rome till recruited by the League of Red Cross Societies as chief of the Vital Statistics Department. He kept this position after his 1 September 1921 transfer, on Winslow's recommendation, to the LN. This transfer delayed the revision of the nosological nomenclature for ten years, a task that an ailing Jacques Bertillon had asked Stouman to undertake that same year. See T.D. Tuttle, 'Theory vs. practice in vital statistics', *AJPH* 8(2), 1918: 153; Dublin, *Eighty Years*, p. 72.

113 Stouman, 'Lecture', 1936, Falk Papers, 25, 522. A recurrent temptation: Martin Kacprzak, director of the Warsaw Institute of Hygiene, suggested during a meeting of the subcommittee on health indices in Geneva on 26 November 1937 identifying a 'nomenclature of true health indices, as Dr Bertillon did for the causes of death', LNA, CH 1297.

114 From G.G. Granger, *La Science et les sciences*, Paris: Presses Universitaires de France, 1995, p. 94.

115 Falk to Sydenstricker, 18 October 1935, Falk Papers, 25, 521.

116 Falk to Stouman, 24 March 1936, Falk Papers, 25, 522; Falk to Rajchman, 9 April 1936, ibid., 25, 421.

117 P. Weindling, 'From moral exhortation', p. 124.

118 E. Burnet to the LN Health Committee, Minutes of the 22nd session [mimeo], Geneva, 7–14 October 1935, Archives J. Parisot [henceforth AJP], Vandoeuvre-les-Nancy, p. 52.

119 W. Aykroyd, 'International health; a retrospective memoir', *Perspectives in Biology and Medicine* 11(1), 1967: 279. Compare J.B. Orr's *Food, Health and Income*, 1936, with F.L. McDougall's *Food and Welfare*, 1938.

120 F.L. McDougall, 'The agricultural and the health problems', 1934, FAO Archives [Rome], RG 3.1, Series D1, p. 4.

121 S.M. Bruce on 11 September 1935, Société des Nations, Journal Officiel, Supplement 138, Actes de la Seizième Session Ordinaire, p. 53.

122 J. Avenol, LN secretary-general, Note of 19 January 1938, LNA, 8A/31762/8855, R6103.

123 M. Mazower, *Dark Continent: Europe's Twentieth Century*, London: Penguin, 1998, p. 79.

124 W. Bronner (USSR), M. Kacprzak (Poland), N.M.J. Jitta (Netherlands), M.T. Morgan (UK), J. Parisot (France) and G. Pittaluga (Spain). A. Stampar in Moscow (after three long trips to China) represented, along with Rajchman, the Health Section.

125 Rajchman to Falk, 2 October 1936, Falk Papers, 25, 421.

126 J. Parisot, 'Procès-verbal de la session du Bureau du Comité d'Hygiène, tenue à Moscou du 22 au 28 juin 1936' [typescript, 34p.], LNA, CH/Bureau/IV/Procès-Verbal, p. 3.

127 J. Parisot, 'L'Œuvre poursuivie et à poursuivre dans le domaine de l'hygiène rurale par l'Organisation d'Hygiène de la Société des Nations', a report to the Health Committee's Bureau during the June 1936 session in Moscow, LNA, CH 1218, pp. 14–15.

128 'Note du Pr Parisot et du Directeur Médical au sujet des études ultérieures sur l'hygiène rurale, cinquième réunion du Bureau d'Hygiène, Paris, 29 octobre 1936', Geneva, 8 October 1936, LNA, CH/Bureau/6.

129 Hazemann to Sand, 24 January 1938, LNA, R6121.

130 'Aide-mémoire à l'intention des membres de la commission préparatoire de la conférence européenne sur la vie rurale, juillet 1939', Geneva, 28 March 1938, LNA, CH 1321, R6103.

131 Rajchman to R. Sand, 25 October 1938, LNA, 8A/34605/8855, R6106.

132 B. Johan to Boudreau [now director of the Milbank], 3 February 1937, LNA, 8A/20615/20615, R6121.

133 B. Johan, 'Commission pour l'étude des centres de santé ruraux' [typescript of the minutes], Geneva, 28–30 April 1931, LNA, R5927.

134 J. Parisot, revised minutes of the Hygiene Committee's 26th session [mimeo], Geneva, 1–5 November 1937, AJP.

135 Falk to Stouman, 14 September 1937, Falk Papers, 25, 523.

136 K. Stouman, 'Indices de santé établis au cours d'une étude expérimentale de la ville de Bruxelles', BOH 7(1), 1938: 127–77.

137 Anon., 'Rapport sur la réunion des directeurs d'instituts et d'écoles d'hygiène tenue à Genève du 22 au 27 novembre 1937', BOH 7(2), 1938: 184.

138 Minutes of the Health Committee's 25th session, Geneva, 26 April–1 May 1937, AJP, p. 8.

139 According to M.T. Morgan, Health Committee's 25th session, p. 10. Yves Biraud replied in the Health Section's name, 'Since Great Britain has quite complete epidemiological statistics, Greenwood might not be very aware of the needs of other countries. Stouman and Falk's system has the advantage of showing health authorities the shortcomings in their statistics for determining the population's state of health. This has an educational benefit.'

140 W. Jameson to A. Stampar, 9 October 1937, LNA, 8A/25954/587, R6048.

141 Y. Biraud and R.-H. Hazemann, 'Les Recueils d'indices de santé' [typescript, 5p.], 17 November 1937, AJP.

142 Stouman to Gautier, 2 March 1938, LNA, 8A/20615/20615, R6121; the same letter to Hazemann, 3 March 1938.

143 Anon., 'Rapport sur la réunion', p. 185.

144 [M. Kacprzak, R. Sand], 'Aperçu général sur la politique médico-sociale à la campagne', BOH 7(6), 1938: 983. This overview was 'naturally prepared by Hazemann', according to a letter from Rajchman to Parisot, 24 November 1938, R6105.

145 [Y. Biraud], 'Les indices sanitaires. Leur place dans les rapports sur la santé publique', BOH 8(1–2), 1939: 63.

146 'Premier voyage d'études du Dr R.-H. Hazemann [Danemark, Suède, Lettonie, Meurthe-et-Moselle] concernant la politique médico-sociale dans les campagnes' [typescript], June 1938, LNA, 8A/34168/8855, R6104.

147 L. Febvre quoted in G. Baudelle, M.V. Ozouf-Marignier and M.C. Robic, *Géographes en pratiques (1870–1945). Le terrain, le livre, la cité*, Rennes: Presses Universitaires de Rennes, 2001, p. 18.

148 Hazemann, 'Application', p. 668.

149 Hazemann and Taylor, 'Inventaires', p. 82.

150 'A means of promoting community consciousness', as M. Bulmer emphasised in 'The decline of the social survey movement and the rise of American empirical sociology', in M. Bulmer, K. Bales and K.K. Sklar (eds), *The Social Survey in Perspective, 1880–1940*, Cambridge: Cambridge University Press, 1991, p. 303.

151 Oral History Research Office, Columbia University, *The Reminiscences of Doctor John B. Grant* [1961], Glen Rock, NJ: Microfilm, 1976, p. 522.

152 For instance the dissertations by L. Amidieu du Clos, 'L'amélioration des conditions sanitaires et sociales de la vie rurale. L'effort réalisé en Meurthe-et-Moselle', Nancy, 1935; and J. Bichat, 'La vie et la santé dans une cité lorraine à travers les siècles. Lunéville, 1034–1936', Nancy, 1936.

153 P. Weindling, *Epidemics and Genocide in Eastern Europe, 1890–1945*, Oxford: Oxford University Press, 2000.

154 G. Pittaluga, 'Sur l'établissement des services de santé rurale dans certains pays d'Amérique et en général dans les pays à faible densité de population', *Revue d'Hygiène* 61(1–2–3), 1939: 5–23, 95–124, 179–207.

155 D. Gusti, *La Monographie et l'action monographique en Roumanie*, Paris: Domat-Montchrestien, 1937, p. 52.

156 A. Blum and M. Mespoulet, *L'Anarchie bureaucratique. Statistique et pouvoir sous Staline*, Paris: La Découverte, 2003, pp. 316–18.
157 [Y. Biraud], 'Note sur les travaux relatifs aux Indices de santé', 2 July 1938, LNA, R6121.
158 M. Sorre, *Les Fondements de la géographie humaine*, Vol. 1, *Les Fondements biologiques*, Paris: A. Colin, 1947, pp. 379–80.
159 R.-H. Hazemann, 'Méthodes facilitant la planification de la politique médico-sociale dans les collectivités', *Vie urbaine* 51, 1939: 70.
160 Stouman and Falk, 'Indices', pp. 1003–4.
161 E.L. Bishop, 'The TVA's new deal in health', *AJPH* 24(12), 1934: 1023–7; and 'The health programme of the Tennessee Valley Authority', *Canadian Public Health Journal* 27(1), 1936: 1–5.
162 Falk to Rajchman, 17 December 1937, LNA 8A/20615/20615, R6121.
163 Atwater to Hazemann, 13 April 1938, LNA, R6121.
164 Smillie, *Public Health Administration*, pp. 420–1.
165 Winslow, 'From health honor roll', 1944: 1102; Winslow expressed the same idea in another way: 'on measurement of results rather than mere activity'.
166 W.F. Walker, 'The new appraisal form for local health work', *AJPH* 29(5), 1939: 500.
167 Stouman to Falk, 30 December 1938, Falk Papers, 25, 523.
168 Walker to Falk, 2 February 1937, Falk Papers, 25, 523.
169 Boudreau to Winslow, 3 March 1937, Winslow Papers, 80, 1230.
170 Falk to Stouman, 9 February 1937, Falk Papers, 25, 523.
171 [R.-H. Hazemann], 'Indices sanitaires. Commentaires concernant les indices sanitaires des districts ruraux', 5 May 1938, LNA, CH 1331.
172 R.M. Atwater to Hazemann, 13 April 1938, LNA, 8A/20615/20615, R6121.
173 Winslow to G. Vincent, 6 June 1918, Winslow Papers, 97, 1691.
174 B. Borcic, in 'Consultation sur la politique médico-sociale à la campagne, Octobre 10–14, 1938, PV provisoires' [typescript], LNA, CH 1374, R6104.
175 Falk to Rajchman, 26 February 1936, Falk Papers, 25, 421; also in LNA, R6121.
176 J. Tomcsik to Hazemann, 14 February 1938, LNA, 8A/29930/8855, R6100. B. Johan, in Health Committee's 28th session, Geneva, 30 June–2 July 1938, revised minutes, AJP, p. 42, where he added that the Stouman report had been translated and 'on 1 June [1938], all public health officers and doctors of communes had the text in their hands. Moreover, a large number of copies will be distributed to MPs.'
177 [Y. Biraud], 'Indices sanitaires', p. 64.
178 M. Kacprzak, in 'Sub-committee of experts on rural hygiene, 25–27 April 1938, summary of proceedings', LNA, 8A/3176/8855, R6103.
179 'Conférence européenne sur la vie rurale. Rapport de la Commission préparatoire sur les travaux de sa première session, 4–7 April 1938', LNA, C161.M101.
180 Hazemann, 'Recueil', p. 88.
181 Winslow, 'International appraisal', p. 5.
182 Kacprzak to Rajchman, 2 April 1938, LNA, 8A/20615/20615, R6121; and 'Indices de santé. Essai d'application sur le territoire de Plock', 25 April 1938, CH 1325.
183 Grant, *Reminiscences* [1961], p. 159.
184 J. Mountin, 'The evaluation of health services' [1936], in *Selected Papers*, pp. 312–13.
185 R.-H. Hazemann, 'Les tendances récentes de la politique médico-sociale en Europe' [September 1938], BOH 8(4–5), 1939: 759; the correspondence exchanged in the spring of 1938 between Hazemann and Atwater provides evidence of their joint interest in J. Mountin's efforts, for example, to calculate

'expenditures by type of service (administration, vital statistics, cost of maintenance, cost of personnel)', LNA, R6121.

186 Grant, *Reminiscences* [1961], pp. 86, 511.

187 B. Johan, in 'Consultation sur la politique médico-sociale à la campagne', Geneva, 10–14 October 1938, LNA, CH 1374, R6104.

188 B. Johan, in Health Committee's 30th session, Geneva, 4–6 May 1939, Minutes, AJP.

189 Stouman to Rajchman, 1 July 1937, LNA, 8A/20615/20615, R6121.

190 B. Johan, Rural Health Work in Hungary, Budapest: State Hygienic Institute of Hungary, 9, 1939, pp. 225–6.

191 'Première Commission de la Conférence intergouvernementale des pays d'Orient sur l'hygiène rurale', Bandoeng (Java), 3–17 August 1937, LNA, A.19.1937.III, p. 1311.

192 Hazemann, 'Application', p. 688.

193 Rajchman, revised minutes of the Health Committee's 28th session, Geneva, 30 June–2 July 1938, AJP, pp. 40–1.

194 Ibid.

195 'Aide-mémoire', 28 March 1938, LNA, CH 1321, R6103.

196 M.N.F. Hall, 'Enquête préliminaire sur les mesures d'ordre national et international visant à relever le niveau d'existence', Geneva, 13 June 1938, A.18.1938.II.B.

197 LNA, CH1382, 31 October 1938, with pencilled notation on the typescript: 'Note by Dr Biraud, 10 June 1938', R6104.

198 Rajchman, in Health Committee's 28th session, Geneva, 30 June–2 July 1938, minutes, AJP, pp. 40–1.

199 M. Kacprzak to Biraud, 11 February 1939, LNA, 8A/34592/8855, R6104.

200 S.F. Chellapal and W.P. Jacoks, *A Guide to Health Unit Procedure in Ceylon*, Colombo: Government Press, 1937.

201 W.L. Halverston, 'A twenty-five year review of the work of the Committee on Administrative Practice', *AJPH* 35(12), 1945: 1256.

202 I.S. Falk, *Health in Panama, a Survey and a Program*, 1957; and *Survey of Health Services and Facilities in the Canal Zone*, 1958; M.I. Roemer, 'I.S. Falk', pp. 841–8.

203 'Adaptation of the forms of health indices to tropical areas: note by Dr Y. Biraud, 10 June 1938', LNA, CH 1387.

204 H. Sigerist, 'Report on India' [1944], in Roemer (ed.), *Henry E. Sigerist on the Sociology of Medicine*, New York: MD Publications, 1960, p. 292.

205 A. Stampar, 'Observations of a rural health worker', *New England Journal of Medicine* 218(4), 16 June 1938: 994.

206 Stouman to Rajchman, 6 December 1935, LNA, 8A/20615/20615, R6121.

207 Note from Rajchman to the Secretary-General and J. Avenol, 5 December 1932, Paris, Archives of the Ministry of Foreign Affairs, Avenol Papers, vol. 25, Cooperation with China.

208 J.B. Grant, 'Principles for medicine and public health in the China experiment' [1934], in C. Seipp (ed.), *Selected Papers of Dr John B. Grant*, Baltimore: Johns Hopkins, 1963, p. 8.

209 *The Memoirs of Dr Hugh Smith Cumming, Sr*, Cumming Family Papers, University of Virginia Library, Special Collections Department, II [1926–35], p. 565.

210 Stouman and Falk, 'Indices', pp. 1003–4.

211 A.J. Viseltear, 'Emergence of the medical care section of the American Public Health Association, 1926–1948', *AJPH* 63(11), 1973: 992.

212 G.E. Vincent quoted in Lewis Hackett Manuscript, 'History of the International Health Division', RAC, 3, 908, 5, 28, p. 1.

213 L.K. Frankel, 'The future of the American Public Health Association', *AJPH* 9(2), 1919: 89–90.

214 W.S. Rankin, 'Elimination of politics from public health work', *JAMA* 83(17), 25 October 1924: 1287, 1285. Likewise Winslow referring to a shift 'from a haphazard political experiment to a standardized scientific procedure', 'Administrative practice', p. 66.
215 M.D. Dubin, 'Toward the Bruce Report: the economic and social programs of the League of Nations in the Avenol era', in *The League of Nations in Retrospect*, Berlin and New York: W. de Gruyter, 1983, p. 47; and V.Y. Ghebali, *La Société des nations et la réforme Bruce, 1939–1940*, Geneva: Centre Européen de la Dotation Carnegie, 1970.
216 J. Gray, *Two Faces of Liberalism*, Cambridge: Polity Press, 2000, p. 116.
217 Winslow, 'Fifteen years', p. 1305.
218 G. Canguilhem, *Le Normal et le pathologique*, Paris: Presses Universitaires de France, 1975, p. 184.
219 Winslow, 'From health honor roll', p. 1001.
220 M.J. Dobrow, V. Goel and R.E.G. Upshur, 'Evidence-based health policy: context and utilisation', *Social Science and Medicine* 58, 2004: 207–17; N. Black, 'Evidence-based policy: proceed with care', *British Medical Journal* 323, 4 August 2001: 275–8.
221 J. Beaulieu, D. Scutchfield and A. Kelly, 'Content and criterion validity evaluation of national public health performance standards measurement instruments', *Public Health Reports* 118, November–December 2003: 517. On the topic, A. Handler, M. Issel and B. Turnock, 'A conceptual framework to measure performance of the public health system', *AJPH* 91(8), 2001: 1235–9.
222 Turnock and Handler, 'Measuring', p. 264.
223 Beaulieu, Scutchfield and Kelly, 'Content and criterion', pp. 508–17; J. Beaulieu and D. Scutchfield, 'Assessment of validity of the national public health performance standards: the local public health performance assessment instrument', *Public Health Reports* 117, January–February 2002: 28–36.
224 P.G. Kramers, 'The ECHI project: health indicators for the European Community', *European Journal of Public Health* 13(3), September 2003: 101–6.
225 *International Journal of Health Indicators, Journal of Public Health Management and Practice, International Journal of Technology Assessment in Health Care, Journal of Evidence Based Health Policy and Management, Social Indicators Research*, etc.
226 WHO, *Statistical Indicators for the Planning and Evaluation of Public Health Programs*, 14th report of the WHO Expert Committee on Health Statistics, Technical Report Series 472, Geneva, 1971, p. 18.
227 S.L. Engerman, 'The standard of living debate in international perspective: measures and indicators', in R.H. Steckel and R. Floud (eds), *Health and Welfare during Industrialisation*, Chicago: Chicago University Press, 1997, pp. 34–9; R.H. Steckel and J.C. Rose, *The Backbone of History. Health and Nutrition in the Western Hemisphere*, Cambridge, New York: Cambridge University Press, 2002.
228 Quoted by Krieger and Fee, 'Measuring' pp. 397–8 (note 75).

Recommended further reading

D.T. Rodgers, *Atlantic Crossings. Social Politics in a Progressive Age*, Cambridge, MA, and London: Belknap Press, Harvard University Press, 1998.

E. Rodriguez-Ocana (ed.), *The Politics of the Healthy Life: an International Perspective*, Sheffield: European Association for the History of Medicine and Health Publications, 2002, pp. 113–30.

B.T. Turnock and A.S. Handler, 'From measuring to improving health practice', *Annual Review of Public Health* 18, 1997: 261–81.

H.F. Vaughan, 'Local health services in the United States: the story of the CAP', *American Journal of Public Health* 62(1), 1972: 95–111.

P. Weindling (ed.), *International Health Organisations and Movements, 1918–1939*, Cambridge: Cambridge University Press, 1995.

2 Between war propaganda and advertising

The visual style of accident prevention as a precursor to postwar health education in Switzerland

Martin Lengwiler

In the following chapter, I will analyse the changing styles of accident prevention in Switzerland from the end of the nineteenth century to the 1960s. Embedding the Swiss case into a comparative perspective including Germany, Britain and the USA, I will argue that the methodological innovations introduced into accident prevention before and during the Second World War had an important methodological influence on the styles of postwar health education undertaken by institutions of public health. Particularly, the strategies of visualisation in postwar health education have profited a lot, at least in the case of Switzerland, from the distinct professional experiences that institutions of occupational safety had acquired before 1945. Although we only know very little about the early history of the use of modern media in public health, it seems that, in European countries, institutions of public health have used the audio and visual opportunities of modern media since their early days in the 1930s.[1] The national socialist regime in Germany was presumably the first to lead innovative, media-based campaigns in public health, notably with their anti-tobacco campaign for the prevention of cancer.[2] However, the Nazis' innovations in public health did not survive the collapse of the regime in 1945, and most European countries developed their media-based approaches in public health in the 1950s and 1960s without referring to German policies. In Britain, the use of modern media was partly motivated by domestic purposes, as with the vaccination programmes of the 1950s, the need to promote the newly implemented National Health Service through television, or, after the 'great London smog' of 1952, by the question of industrial air pollution.[3] Other countries like Switzerland or Germany, as I will point out below, also learned from public health in the USA and its methodological experiences during and immediately after the Second World War.

The chapter argues that the styles of visualisation and the uses of media in health education after 1945 had important predecessors in the area of occupational safety. Since the 1890s, in a period of rapid industrialisation, occupational hygiene was gradually established as an independent medical discipline, whereas occupational safety became an important issue in public health. Consequently, since the 1920s most institutions engaged in occupational safety experimented with innovative approaches in public health. These methodological innovations in accident prevention, both in the interwar period and during the Second World War, were later partly adopted by other institutions of public health. Because of its relatively small system of public health institutions and its interrelated expert communities, Switzerland offers a particularly rich case study to examine how occupational safety acted as a methodological laboratory for innovative media-based strategies of prevention, particularly strategies of visualisation, thus predetermining the professionalisation and institutionalisation of media-oriented approaches in public health. In Switzerland, the most important organisation of occupational safety was the Swiss Institute for Accident Insurance, founded in 1918 and representing the main social insurance institution for occupational accidents. Focusing on this institution, I will analyse the reasons for the early uses of visualisations, the professionalisation of media-based methodologies in accident prevention, and the institutionalisation of accident prevention until the 1960s. Also, I will examine how these experiences in accident prevention, after the Second World War, were taken up by other areas of public health. As international networks of scientific expertise played a crucial part in the development of media-based approaches in accident prevention, the case of Switzerland has to be embedded into the international context. The article will therefore briefly discuss how Switzerland relates to important precursors in the history of occupational safety, most importantly to institutions in the USA, in Germany and partly also in Britain.

The article distinguishes three periods in the development of media-based approaches in occupational safety, each discussed in one of the following sections. The first period, the pre-professional era, lasted from the 1880s, when the first associations and institutions specific to accident prevention were established, until the eve of the First World War. In the first period, two legal systems for accident prevention emerged. The first, liberal system, prevalent in the USA and France, was based upon industrial liability legislation, with a style of accident prevention that appealed primarily to the responsibility of the individual worker. The second, corporatist system was based upon centralised, national institutions of social insurance. Germany, in 1884, was first to switch from the liability to the insurance legislation, followed by other European countries like Austria, the Netherlands and Switzerland.[4] Great Britain, after the introduction of the German-inspired 1897 Workmen's Compensation Act, represented a mixture of the two systems. The law stipulated compulsory insurance against industrial accidents, offered by employers for their employees, but insurance still remained in the hands of private organisations without a centralised national institution like social insurance in Germany or Switzerland.[5] The second period, spanning the First World War and the interwar period, was marked by the institutionalisation of accident prevention within social insurance schemes or in private sector organisations. As will be argued below based upon the case of Switzerland, accident prevention became the focus of an international network of safety experts. This period also gave rise to the first methodological debates, focusing on the visualisation of occupational risks by accident posters. The third period, starting with the Second World War and including the post-war decades, saw the professionalisation of accident prevention, based upon the professional use of media and guided by scientific research into the effects of media messages. In this third period, the methodological experiences gained in occupational safety were generalised and adopted, at least in Switzerland, for the purposes of health education and for the prevention of chronic diseases.

The origins of accident prevention: the 'Safety First' movement and technical approaches

The use of media in modern accident prevention has been shaped by two distinct approaches to occupational safety: a visualising, *psychological* approach, epitomised by the prevention campaigns of the US 'Safety First' movement, and a *technical* approach, focused on technological design and originally more prevalent in European states with a social insurance system like Germany or Switzerland. Both styles of prevention originated before the First World War, and each is related to an institutional model of occupational safety. To understand the methodological debates in Switzerland in the interwar period and afterwards, it is necessary to discuss the emergence of both approaches within the institutional context of their main national background: the USA for the psychological and Germany for the technical approach.

In the USA, the history of occupational safety at the national level began in the 1890s with legislation for specific professions, namely with the introduction of compulsory accident insurance ('Workers' Compensation') for the mining industry in 1891 and for the railway industry in 1893. After 1911, several federal states followed with similar legislation for other branches of industry. Some even shifted from mere liability legislation, in which the injured person had to claim payments, to insurance legislation with automatic payments in case of accidents.[6] But in contrast to the German model of social insurance, the USA never established a public, centralised insurance fund at the national level. This meant that industrial employers generally provided insurance by contracting with private insurance companies. Also, the liberal system of occupational safety in the USA lacked a central authority from the government with a mandatory power over industrial corporations.

The strong position of private insurance corporations in the USA helped to determine the characteristic features of American accident prevention. In the USA, the principles of accident prevention centred on entrepreneurial self-organisation and the individual responsibility of workers. The most prominent actor in the US history of accident prevention was the National Safety Council (NSC) in Chicago, founded 1913. The NSC was initiated by the steel and the electrical industry. As a non-governmental organisation supported by the insurance industry, by employers' associations and by trade unions, it quickly became the institutional motor for the professionalisation of accident prevention. The NSC was an instant success, boosted by the combination of emerging liability legislation after 1911 and the need for industrial safety during the First World War. By 1920, the NSC counted over 4,000 institutional members, representing over 6 million workers.[7]

As the dominant institution for accident prevention, the NSC became the flagship for the 'Safety First' movement, the American way of occupational safety.[8] The 'Safety First' approach emphasised the responsibility of individual workers and stressed the need for professional advertising in accident prevention. The individuals' responsibility mirrors the liability laws that forced workers and employers to argue before court over whose individual faults were responsible for an accident. Under these premises, pointing at the responsibility of workers was part of the strategy of employers to distract from their own liabilities. Among the characteristics of the 'Safety First' style of prevention, the significant role of advertising and graphic messages was internationally the most influential, as we will see when discussing the cases of Switzerland and Germany. Visual advertising had a particular appeal in the USA, as its working class around 1900 was particularly heterogeneous, both in social and cultural terms. Thus, the main instruments of accident prevention were illustrations and posters put up in the workplace, which seemed to be more promising than written guidelines or investment in technical facilities. After the First World War, the 'Safety First' movement began to reach out, particularly to Britain. In reaction to soaring rates of accidents in industrial workplace and on the roads (as an effect of lighting restrictions), representatives from industrial corporations and the government jointly founded the Royal Society for the Prevention of Accidents (RoSPA) in 1923. The RoSPA was modelled on the US National Safety Council (NSC) with the same emphasis on professional advertisements.[9]

The organisation of accident prevention in the USA through the private sector differed clearly from the European countries with a social insurance system like the German one. The difference was not only institutional (the public authorities of social insurance versus private organisations in the US system), but it also affected the methodologies of accident prevention. After 1900 within the circles of insurance experts, this methodological difference was commonly referred to as the choice between the German 'technical' and the American 'psychological' approach to accident prevention. The technical approach favoured technical investments into the safety of industrial machinery with little or no interest in media-based advertising, whereas the psychological approach favoured the use of media-based educational campaigns addressed to the industrial workers.[10]

There were two reasons for the technical focus of accident insurance in Germany and other European nations with a social insurance system. First, by comparison with private organisations like the NSC or the RoSPA, social insurance organisations were constituted as institutions of public law, a status that was traditionally combined with special mandatory authority over workers and particularly over employers. In Switzerland, for example, the national institution for accident insurance was authorised to stipulate and enforce the use of preventive technical installations even against the opposition of factory owners. If the employer did not follow the instructions, the insurer was vested with the penal power to impose fines or to raise the insurance premium.[11] In other words: the prevention policies of social insurance were based upon means of state intervention, whereas private organisations had to rely on entrepreneurial self-organisation and the initiative of individuals. The second reason for the technical focus is that social insurance in the Bismarckian tradition had a corporatist organisational structure. In Germany as in Switzerland, the leading boards of the national accident insurers were composed on the principle of parity, with equal representation for trade union and employers' associations.[12] As we will see below, corporatist organisation prevented European social insurance from stressing prevention strategies which focussed primarily on the faults of workers. This was the prevention style of the 'Safety First' approach.

The technical approach to accident prevention originated in Germany in the 1880s after Bismarck established national accident insurance as the first branch of the social insurance system in 1884. The prevention of occupational accidents was mainly in the hands of technical experts. In 1914, for example, nearly all of the 500 German factory inspectors were engineers and architects (the professional term was '*Revisionsingenieure*') with only a handful of lawyers and five physicians among them, and no psychologists or advertising professionals.[13] They founded a new scientific discipline, 'technical accident protection' ('*technischer Unfallschutz*') with its own university courses, its associations and congresses, and its journals like the *Gewerblich-technischer Ratgeber* ('Industrial-technological adviser') or the *Revisions-Ingenieur*.[14] The advocates for technical prevention were also engaged at the international level, dominating both the Congresses for Social Insurance and the Congresses for Accident Medicine.[15] Finally, national governments built up museums and exhibitions to popularise the message of technical prevention by exhibiting machines designed or converted after the instructions of prevention engineers. Almost every major city in Europe, like Berlin, Amsterdam, Vienna, Munich and Zurich, established its own museum for accident prevention.[16] For the prevention experts in social insurance, the notion of industrial risk came down to dangerous technology and their preventive remedy was simply better technology.

Psychological approaches to accident prevention in interwar Germany and Switzerland

The split between the US and European regimes of accident prevention dominated the interwar period and even reached out into the postwar era. Even in the 1950s, European prevention experts were stunned by the difference between their technical approach and the preventive practices in US factories. In 1956, the Swiss national insurer for accident prevention sent one of their senior staff members on an educational journey to the USA to report on the US methods of accident prevention. Stanislaus Nicolet, the director of the department of prevention of the Swiss Institute for Accident Insurance ('*Schweizerische Unfallversicherungsanstalt*' or abbreviated: Suva), participated in the yearly safety congress of the National Safety Council in Chicago, and visited two research institutions, Harvard University's School of Public Health and the Center for Safety Education at New York University, which was funded by the insurance industry.[17] Crucially, he also visited a few industrial factories. Nicolet was impressed by the amount of educational advertising and propaganda. In his report he clearly recommended learning from the USA and increased spending on psychological prevention, which the Suva eventually did.[18] More interestingly, Nicolet also pointed at the striking differences in practical prevention styles between Europe and the USA, literally visible in the industrial production facilities he visited. On the US factories he wrote:

> The main focus is to teach the workers and the management in occupational safety that means psychological accident prevention....However, the security of the machines is less looked after. Even in well organized factories, one can discover numerous machines that are not equipped with any safety facilities, and those facilities present are often more primitive than our facilities. In Switzerland, technical accident prevention is more advanced than in the United States.[19]

Although the difference between the psychological approach in the USA and the technical approach in Europe was still feasible in the postwar period, countries like Germany or Switzerland started to discuss the uses of educational propaganda and of the US way of accident prevention as early as the 1920s. In both countries, the limitations of the technical approach to accident prevention gradually led to calls for more educational and psychological approaches. Although machines became safer, their operation remained a constant source of accidents. As early as the 1890s, critics demanded a psychological approach supporting the workers' 'courage to fear', as the German factory inspector Georg von Mayr put it.[20] After the experiences of the First World War, with soaring rates of industrial accidents caused by the war economy, and with the rise of the 'Safety First' movement in the USA and its adoption in Britain, the psychological way of accident prevention became an international phenomenon. Since the 1920s it was widely debated in countries with corporatist social insurance systems like Germany or Switzerland, with long-term consequences into the postwar era.

Before the 'Safety First' approach gained momentum, the national institutions for accident insurance in Switzerland and in Germany used crude, mainly textual posters, which corresponded to the general trends of the advertising profession.[21] Trying to transmit as much information as possible, these traditional accident posters were full of written explications, exhortations and instructions. The posters for the printing industries in Switzerland for example included text-laden warnings for workers about the dangers of lead poisoning and the latency period of the disease, giving four precise instructions on how to avoid poisoning, like regular washing of hands or keeping food away from workplaces (see Figure 2.1).[22]

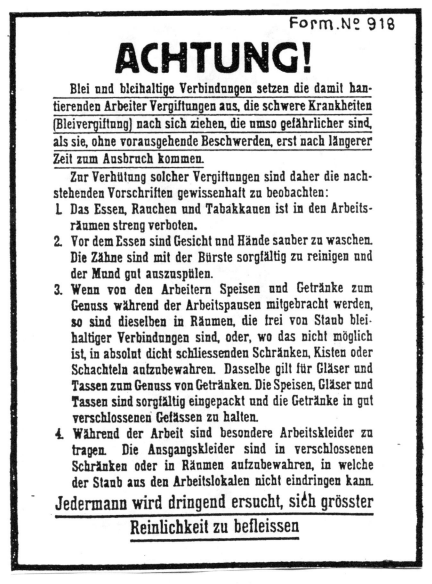

Figure 2.1 Before the arrival of the 'Safety First' approach

From the 1920s, however, under the growing influence of the 'Safety First' movement, the national accident insurers changed their methodological approaches to accident prevention. Among the earliest European innovators which promoted a psychological emphasis was the German Professional Association for Civil Engineering ('Tiefbau-Berufsgenossenschaft'), one of the institutional branches of the national accident insurance scheme. In the

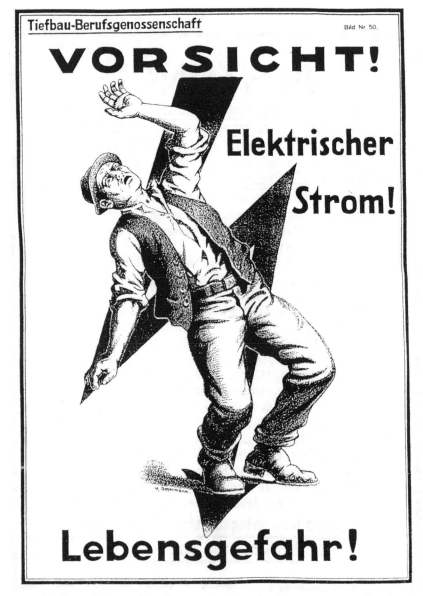

Figure 2.2 One of the earliest illustrated posters in European occupational safety using the style of the US 'Safety First' movement

early 1920s, the civil engineering association commissioned a professional graphic designer to revise their poster campaigns. The result was a series of new posters published in 1923 and designed after the US example with illustrations replacing written messages (see Figure 2.2).[23]

However, the case of Switzerland shows that the authorities of the national accident insurance scheme still trusted more in their established technical prevention and remained sceptical about the 'Safety First' approach. Gradually, the Suva gave way to the psychological turn and introduced a few innovative measures in the 1920s. In particular, it designed and distributed two illustrated posters, one particularly for the textile industries, the other appealing to workers in general. The second poster was drawn by the graphic artist Emil Cardinaux and showed the picture of a dead worker and his mourning wife, with the admonitory caption: 'Negligence brings misery into your home.'[24] Apart from these posters, the Suva's psychological measures also included a couple of propaganda stickers to be put on the envelopes of outgoing mail with mottos like 'Do you want to pay lower premiums? Try to prevent accidents! The Institute for Accident Insurance pays the accidents with YOUR money!' or 'No accident prevention without the will of the employers and rigorous surveillance.'[25] But that was all the Suva did to adopt the psychological approach.

The messages on the stickers also indicate why the Suva was cautious about fully adopting the 'Safety First' approach. The Suva was careful not to shift the responsibility for accident prevention from the employers, where the social insurance regime traditionally put it, to the workers, as in the US regime. 'Technical measures,' asserted the director of the Suva's Department of Prevention, Max Helfenstein, in a summarising report in 1940, 'play a decisive role in accident prevention.'[26] Psychological prevention however, he continued, would blame the wrong people.

> [The psychological approach] tries with all possible arguments to make accident prevention look like a matter of the worker's caution....Why don't they [those arguing for a psychological perspective] abandon the illustrations? Because it is a comfortable way for employers and directory boards to shift the responsibility for accidents on to the workers.[27]

In addition, Helfenstein reminded the board of directors of his sobering practical experiences with psychological accident prevention. Once displayed, Helfenstein argued, accident posters would lose their attraction within days, most films available would moralise about the behaviours of workers, most lectures would be too superficial, and accident prevention contests among workers, a popular strategy in the USA, would just push workers to hide accidents.[28]

For the Suva, the main responsibility for accident prevention had to be on the employers' side. In 1929, the director of the Suva, Arnold Bohren, a social democrat, claimed before a meeting of the directory committee:

> The employers have to be brought to accept the prevention of industrial accidents as their own duty. If the Suva addresses the workers directly by editing calendars, posters etc, it would support the opinion that it was primarily the workers' business to prevent accidents and that the employer would fulfil his duty by hanging up the posters and passing on the publications to the workers.[29]

The main support for psychological approaches in accident prevention came from the employers' associations. Since the late 1920s, the journal of the Swiss Employers' Association repeatedly praised the successes of the American 'Safety First' movement. This entrepreneurial support was hardly idealistic: poster campaigns pointing out the responsibility of workers were much cheaper than investments into preventive technical facilities.[30] The Suva ridiculed the symbolic activism of the employers' association as mere 'accident prevention fever' consisting of a flood of publications with no practical impact.[31] With the economic depression of the 1930s and the overheated wartime economy during the Second World War, the issue of accident prevention lost its significance. Moreover, after the mobilisation of the army in 1939, a major part of the Suva's workforce was called up for military service. All activities that went beyond the core insurance business were reduced to a minimum. The Department for Prevention was one of the first victims. It was shut down in 1939 and did not reopen until the war was over.[32]

The Second World War is a revealing period to compare the impact of prevention between the two institutional approaches, the centralised and corporatist system of social insurance in Europe and the liberal system based upon private sector organisations in the USA. Before the war, the system of social insurance offered the advantage of a strong interventionist power held by public authorities, whereas in the liberal system the self-organising bodies and associations responsible for accident prevention were comparably weak and ineffective. However, under the conditions of a wartime economy, the US system showed some of its advantages. Organised by independent organisations like the NSC, decentralised 'Safety First' committees, or by the initiative of individual employers, activities in accident prevention were not fundamentally disrupted but continued throughout the war. In Switzerland, however, the centralised system was more vulnerable as it depended on one single institution. As soon as the central institution responsible for accident prevention, the Suva, had to shut down its Department of Prevention, accident prevention was practically suspended as an activity of public health. The impact of this institutional difference is reflected in the national accident statistics. Whereas, in the USA, accident rates remained generally stable during the Second World War, with rates even decreasing in the manufacturing sector, overall accident rates in Switzerland increased significantly.[33] In the US mining industry, for example, the mortality rate remained practically unchanged during wartime. In

Switzerland, however, the accident rate (including fatal accidents) rose by over 100 per cent.[34]

The Second World War and beyond: professionalised accident prevention as the model for health education

In the history of social insurance in Switzerland, the postwar period is marked by a steep rise of both technical and psychological accident prevention. Paralleling this development, the psychological branch of accident prevention was professionalised. In the postwar era, the influence of the psychological approach, based upon its long-term methodological experience, went beyond the scope of occupational safety, institutionally and methodologically. Accident prevention, at least in Switzerland, prepared the methodological ground for some of the postwar campaigns in health education and for some of the methodological approaches of social and preventive medicine.

The rise of the psychological approach was only one feature of a general boom in accident prevention after the Second World War. This expansion followed, more or less, the expansion of the economy in general. Accordingly, the Suva's Department for Accident Prevention grew alongside the prospering economy. In 1950, the department's budget was 690,000 Swiss Francs, in 1955 1.98 million, at which point the budget doubled approximately with every decade. By 1980 the expenses for accident prevention were at 22 million per year.[35] Moreover, with the booming productivity a number of industrial firms established or consolidated their own departments for accident prevention. The first foundations, in the metal and engineering industry, date back to the 1930s.[36] In the postwar era, the chemical industry was also particularly active.[37] As in the interwar period, these employers favoured a psychological approach to accident prevention. Thus, most entrepreneurial campaigns for accident prevention addressed the responsibility of the individual worker with slogans like 'Caution is no cowardice, rashness is no courage!' as in the example of an accident prevention week with the chemical firm Geigy AG in 1954.[38]

More surprising was the growing support within the Suva for a psychological approach, particularly as in the interwar period the Suva's authorities took a decidedly critical stand against mere educational propaganda. To understand the reasons for this change, a change that established accident prevention as a precursor for other activities in health education, I will analyse more closely the course of the methodological debates around the psychological approach to prevention. One of the crucial elements of the professionalisation of accident prevention after 1945 was the growing impact of scientific expertise, often on an international level, on the policies of accident prevention.

As mentioned above, the main instrument of psychological prevention from the 1920s was the accident poster, promoted by the Safety First movement and its European imitators. In the interwar period, new posters were designed to replace the old text-laden posters by a simplistic iconography, appealing to negative emotional responses. The new generation of illustrative posters bore shocking, repulsive or fear-arousing messages addressed at the emotions of the spectator.[39] In the USA, illustrative posters were first used in accident prevention under the influence of early business advertisement.[40] The first illustrative prevention campaigns in Europe set up in the early 1920s were also inspired by the methodology of printed advertising and of early movie theatres.[41] Apart from accident prevention, the fear-arousing method had also been common with prevention of traffic accidents since the 1930s.[42]

Professionally, before the Second World War, the methods used in accident prevention mainly relied upon a non-academic, trial-and-error approach. In Switzerland, those responsible for designing prevention campaigns were the safety engineers themselves. Only rarely were they joined by graphic designers.[43] The development of social sciences during the Second World War changed this situation fundamentally. The disciplines of communication studies and of social psychology profited from the political interest in studying the effects of propaganda, not only in the USA but also in European countries.[44] Research into the effects of mass communication and advertising dates back to the beginning of the century, to Gustave Le Bon's mass psychology for example or to Hugo Münsterberg's psycho-technology.[45] However until the Second World War, this research was mainly limited to business advertising with no effects on the use of media in public health. The situation changed with the US and British propaganda studies during the Second World War, when psychological research began influencing educational methodologies in accident prevention and in health education.[46] Thus, the wartime research in psycho-technology and early social psychology became an important precondition for the professionalisation of psychological accident prevention after the Second World War.

Particularly influential for the postwar era, also in the European context, was the wartime research of Carl I. Hovland, Irving L. Janis and their group at the Department of Psychology at Yale. Hovland was an experimental psychologist, who worked for the US War Department between 1942 and 1945 studying the effectiveness of training films and information programmes. In the Experimental Section of the War Department's Research Branch, he worked together with Arthur A. Lumsdaine and with Irving Janis. The group was consulted, among others, by Paul F. Lazarsfeld and Robert K. Merton, and their aim was to 'utilize modern socio-psychological research techniques in the evaluation of educational and "indoctrination" films'.[47] After the war, Hovland and Janis continued their co-operation and studied the effects of different teaching and advertising methods, now with examples from health education, such as the effect of fear-arousing appeals in dental hygiene.[48] In their studies, Hovland and Janis concluded that shock messages had a limited if not counterproductive effect in the long run. The study on dental hygiene, which became an instant classic, showed that fear-arousing emotional appeals were less effective than moderate messages. The authors' point was that positive statements and substantial arguments were at least as important as shocking ones to increase the credibility of the message with the audience.[49] These US studies, together with similar British work, for example research on traffic prevention by the British psychologist Eunice Belbin from the Psychological Laboratory at the University of Cambridge, led to critical debates among prevention specialists on the benefits of fear-arousing iconography, which was seen more and more as too moralising and too paternalistic.[50]

The conclusions of the Anglo-Saxon propaganda studies were known in Switzerland in the 1950s; at the beginning this was primarily by the national accident insurance authorities. As mentioned above, in 1956 the board of directors of the Suva sent the director of the Department for Prevention to the USA to study current US approaches in accident prevention. In the following years and by contrast to their reluctance before the war, the Suva started to support educational and propaganda activities in accident prevention. This was not a U-turn in their prevention policy, as the main focus was still on technical investments. With the general rise of accident prevention after the war and following the growth of the economy, the Suva also built up an institutional engagement in psychological prevention, not as a replacement but as a complementary addition to technical prevention.

In 1952, as a first step in institutionalising psychological approaches, the Suva established a 'Section for Information and Instruction' ('Sektion für Auskunft und Aufklärung'), staffed with journalists and responsible for publications and courses or lectures on accident prevention.[51] One of the first products of this section was to found a journal for accident prevention, edited by the Suva and published since 1956 as the *Swiss Papers for Occupational Safety*.[52] By 1960, the activities of the information section included over 200 lectures a year and numerous publications in newspapers, on the radio and on television.[53] In the 1960s and 1970s, on top of its publications, the Suva established a broad network of courses in accident prevention, mainly for the professional education of safety engineers in private sector companies. About 2,000 people were instructed on the courses by 1970, a figure that rose to 4,000 by 1980. Between fifty and one hundred of the attendees took the course to get the formal degree of a 'safety officer' ('Sicherheitsbeauftragter').[54] Thus, in Switzerland, the Suva was directly responsible for the professionalisation of the field of accident prevention by the establishment of the new profession of the safety engineer.[55]

In the 1960s, the Suva specifically aimed at strengthening its activities in advertising and public relations. Between 1960 and 1987, the most important figure for communicating the Suva's messages and designing their prevention campaigns was Harold Potter, an academic with a PhD in German language studies. Potter was familiar with US and British research in social psychology and in propaganda studies, and he recommended learning not only from social psychologists like Hovland and Janis but also from motivational research and its application in market psychology, as epitomised by the work of Ernest Dichter.[56] With his numerous book and article publications, and his radio and TV appearances, he represented postwar accident prevention like nobody else in Switzerland.[57]

Thus, accident prevention in Switzerland has followed the methodological paths of the Anglo-Saxon model since the 1950s.[58] In 1957, the *Illustrated Journal for Occupational Safety* drew on psychoanalysis to argue that shock posters were antiquated.

> If we want to prevent accidents, our advertising should not create or strengthen the moods and affects that have a promotional effect on accidents (like deterrence or fear). Also, the illustration of misdeeds can lead to the assertion of pictorial impressions in the unconscious, which in the crucial moment directly activates Freudian slips. For all these reasons, advertising should raise positive feelings, like self-confidence, joy and interest by depicting the outcome of observing the safety regulations and not the consequences of accidents.[59]

The methodological turn to more positive messages marked a new style of accident prevention in the postwar era and also introduced irony and humour into the language of accident posters.[60] Moreover, accident prevention also started to use pictures of women in its posters. The reason was not that these adverts were addressing a predominantly female public; on the contrary they were designed to speak to men with positive messages on an emotional level. In fact, the focus on positive emotional messages is behind the conspicuous tradition of numerous sexist illustrations that still mark the style of accident prevention in professions with a largely male workforce, like the building or the metal industries.[61]

The methodological innovations in accident prevention of the 1950s and 1960s prepared the ground for similar postwar health education, particularly for the methodological approach of the founding generation of social and preventive medicine. In Switzerland, the responsibility for public health policy was traditionally federalised. After the Second World War, the central powers of the federal state were still very limited. In the postwar years, the power of the Federal Office for Public Health ('Bundesamt für Gesundheitswesen'), the main national authority for public health, was limited to policies against contagious diseases (mainly tuberculosis), medical statistics, the supervision of the pharmaceutical market and the management of sanitary border services.[62] To a small extent, some activities in health education were built up by the Federal Office in the 1960s, mainly focusing on chronic diseases, with 'rheumatism' as the main concern, and alcohol and tobacco prevention.[63] After 1963, based upon a law against rheumatic diseases, the Federal Office supported research into prevention and institutions involved in the treatment of chronic heart diseases.[64] In the 1960s, most health education activities were the responsibility of health leagues. They were organised as private associations, each focusing on a particular illness, but often supported by public funds. Most leagues originated in the period between 1950 and 1980, mirroring the lack of engagement by public authorities both on the federal and the cantonal level. They were usually led by bodies of physicians and politicians, sometimes also including patients and their relatives.[65] Thus, most leagues promoted their preventive goals independently and without co-ordination, as they were not professionalised. This started to change only in the late 1970s with the foundation of the Conference of the Health Leagues in 1978, an association for the national co-ordination and promotion of the leagues' common purpose.[66]

But the driving force behind the professionalisation of health education in Switzerland was not the health leagues but the institutionalisation of social and preventive medicine in the 1960s. As a consequence of the federal structure of the public health system in Switzerland, social and preventive medicine established itself quite late as an academic discipline, compared for example with the foundation of social medicine in Britain in the mid-1940s.[67] The first institute, the Institute for Social Medicine at the University of Zurich, was founded in 1963, followed by the Institute for Social and Preventive Medicine at the University of Geneva in 1968, a similar institute at the University of Lausanne in 1969 and other foundations in Berne and Basle in 1971 and 1972. All institutes were firmly rooted in medical schools, with more relationship to medical disciplines like cardiology or epidemiology than to social sciences.[68]

From the beginning, representatives of social and preventive medicine were engaged in health education and health promotion. For this goal, they made use of the methodological innovations of accident prevention mentioned above. Kurt Biener, a close collaborator of the first professor for social medicine in Zurich, Meinrad Schär, focussed in much of his academic work on occupational health prevention.[69] Following the approach of psychological accident prevention, Biener argued that the principle of health education should be: 'do it positively, not negatively'.[70] Meinrad Schär, who authored the main Swiss textbook on social and preventive medicine, published in 1968, suggested making use of advertising technologies: 'The goal of health education is the motivation for a healthier way of living, or the change of unhealthy habits. Basically, its method is the same as with advertising.'[71] Schär and Biener also preferred the emotional over the informative media. For health promotion they recommended using TV and cinema, radio broadcasts (directly addressing the audience) and face-to-face lectures or teaching in schools. At the same time, they were explicitly critical about the influence of printed information in newspapers, leaflets or exhibitions.[72] Eventually the concern about the power of media-based communication made its way into health legislation in the 1960s and 1970s. Accordingly, the centrepiece of health legislation was the banning of TV and radio adverts for alcohol and tobacco.[73]

Conclusions

This chapter has analysed the changing styles of accident prevention, particularly the use of media, in Switzerland from the end of the nineteenth century to the 1960s. With rapid industrialisation in the latter nineteenth century, occupational safety emerged as an early focus of the modern public health system.[74] Thus, occupational safety also acted as a laboratory for media-based campaigns in public health, long before the arrival of television in postwar public health. In the introduction, I distinguished three periods of accident prevention: the pre-professional period before the First World War, the period of institutionalisation lasting from 1918 to 1945, and the era of professionalisation after the Second World War. Each period, as the article pointed out, is marked by a distinct approach to the use of media in prevention campaigns. Before the First World War accident prevention focused mainly on technical design, at least in countries with a social insurance system like Switzerland or Germany. The use of media was very limited and merely informative, restricted to a few text-laden posters. In Switzerland, the First World War and the rising influence of the US 'Safety First' movement started an important period of transformation, in which the old technical approaches of accident prevention were gradually undermined and complemented by 'psychological' approaches stressing the need to appeal to the individual worker. This second period, particularly the interwar years, is full of methodological debates about the effects of media-based communications, mainly through illustrated posters. It is in these years that occupational safety was most important as a methodological laboratory for the use of media in public health. In the third period, after the Second World War, accident prevention established a set of distinct styles of media-based campaigns, like the use of illustrated posters, newspaper articles, radio and television programmes. Also in the postwar years, occupational safety underwent a process of professionalisation with the establishment of a research tradition examining the effect of media-based communication and the development of institutions specialised in media-based prevention.

The case of Switzerland also shows that the use of media, like visualising posters, has to be interpreted as part of a larger strategy or trend in public health. The comparison between campaigns in accident prevention before and after the Second World War shows a clear shift towards enhancing the responsibility of the individual in matters of personal health. In occupational safety, media-based methods represent an individualistic approach to health education, in contrast for example to a technical approach with investments into technical design that focuses much more on the responsibility of an employer or a corporation. There were several reasons for the individualisation of health responsibilities in occupational safety in Switzerland. An important element was the increasing activity of the private sector in occupational safety, mirrored by the development of accident prevention departments in large corporations. Typically, private companies tended to stress the role of self-organisation in occupational safety and were therefore particularly interested in stressing the individual responsibility of workers. Media-based methodologies also profited from the growing influence of scientific research, notably the propaganda studies of applied psychology during and after the Second World War. In the postwar years, the methodological experiences of occupational safety made their way to public health sectors outside accident prevention, like the prevention of chronic diseases, in which the responsibility of the individual was also seen as an important issue. Thus, the methodological laboratory of occupational safety in the interwar and postwar period helped to shape a more general move to individualistic campaigns in health education from the 1950s.

The case of accident prevention is also a reminder of the limits of media-based styles of prevention. The comparison between the corporatist system of social insurance, as in Germany and Switzerland, and the liberal system of accident prevention, as in the USA, shows that the amount of media-based prevention is not an appropriate measure of the intensity of preventive activities. The amount of propagandistic material for prevention can also be a sign of weakness. In accident prevention, the 'psychological' approach with its focus on propaganda and education was clearly a weaker model of prevention compared to the technological approach. Technological prevention was equipped with mandatory rights for supervisory institutions to force employers to change their machinery, the hardware of accident risks. By comparison, mere psychological prevention, as epitomised in the 'Safety First' movement, had rather limited means of enforcement and ran the risk of being restricted to rhetoric only.

Notes

1 For a methodological survey: K. Loughlin, 'The history of health and medicine in contemporary Britain: reflections on the role of audio-visual sources', *Social History of Medicine* 13, 2000: 131–45.

2 R.N. Proctor, *The Nazi War on Cancer*, Princeton: Princeton University Press, 1999.

3 V. Berridge, *Health and Society in Britain since 1939*, Cambridge: Cambridge University Press, 1999, pp. 48–51; K. Loughlin, '"Your life in their hands": the context of a medical-media controversy', *Media History* 6, 2000: 177–88.

4 The distinction between 'liberal' and 'corporatist' systems of welfare states is inspired by the typology of Gospa Esping-Andersen's typology of welfare 'regimes'. G. Esping-Andersen, *The Three Worlds of Welfare Capitalism*, Cambridge: Polity Press, 1990.

5 P. Bartrip, 'The rise and decline of workmen's compensation', in: P. Weindling, *The Social History of Occupational Health*, Oxford: Croom Helm, 1985, pp. 157–79.

6 M. Aldrich, *Safety First: Technology, Labor and Business in the Building of American Work Safety, 1870–1939*, Baltimore: Johns Hopkins University Press, 1997, pp. 34–40.

7 Aldrich, *Safety First*, pp. 107–10.

8 Aldrich, *Safety First*, pp. 107–8.

9 J. Green, 'From accidents to risk: public health and preventable injury', *Health, Risk and Society* 1, 1999: 27–9; J. Green, *Risk and Misfortune: a Social Construction of Accidents*, London: UCL Press, 1997.

10 See for example the debates at the International Congress for Social Insurance: L. Bernacchi, 'Des mesures législatives et techniques à prendre pour atténuer les suites des accidents du travail et pour hâter la guérison des blessés', in *Congrès international des accidents du travail et des assurances sociales, Quatrième session, Bruxelles 26 au 31 juillet 1897*, Bruxelles, 1897, pp. 337–408; K. Hartmann, 'Die Entwickelung der Unfallverhütungstechnik in Deutschland', in *Internationaler Arbeiter-Versicherungs-Congress, 6. Tagung, Düsseldorf 17. bis 24. Juni 1902*, Breslau-Berlin, 1902, pp. 501–20; K. Hartmann, 'Die Unfallverhütung nach ihrem neusten Stande', in *Congrès international des assurances sociales, Rome, 12–16 Octobre 1908*, vol. 2, Rom, 1909, pp. 175ff.

11 Schweizerische Unfallversicherungsanstalt, *Ergebnisse der Unfallstatistik der fünfjährigen Beobachtungsperiode 1933–1937*, Bern, 1939, p. 28.

12 D. Zöllner, 'Ein Jahrhundert Sozialversicherung in Deutschland', in: P.A. Köhler and H.F. Zacher (eds), *Ein Jahrhundert Sozialversicherung in der Bundesrepublik Deutschland, Frankreich, Grossbritannien, Österreich und der Schweiz*, Berlin: Duncker & Humblot, 1981; A. Maurer, 'Geschichte des schweizerischen Sozialversicherungsrechts', in: Köhler and Zacher, *Ein Jahrhundert Sozialversicherung*, pp. 741–833.

13 W. Ewald, *Soziale Medizin: ein Lehrbuch für Ärzte, Medizinal- und Verwaltungsbeamte, Sozialpolitiker, Behörden und Kommunen*, vol. 2, Berlin: Springer, 1914, p. 661.

14 Hartmann, 'Entwickelung der Unfallverhütungstechnik', pp. 516ff.

15 Hartmann, 'Unfallverhütung nach ihrem neusten Stande'; *International Congress for Accident Medicine and Occupational Diseases, II. Congresso Medico Internazionale per gl'Infortuni del Lavoro, Roma, 23–7. Maggio, 1909*, 2 vols, Rome, 1909.

16 E. Cheysson, 'Le musée social', in *Congrès international des accidents du travail et des assurances sociales, troisième session, Milan 1er au 6 octobre 1894*, vol. 1, Milan, 1894, pp. 510ff.; H. Mamy, 'Le Musée de prévention des accidents du travail et d'hygiène industrielle de Paris', in *7. Internationaler Arbeiter-Versicherungskongress; VIIe Congrès international des accidents du travail et des Assurances sociales, Vienne 17 au 23 Septembre 1905*, 2 vols, Vienna, 1906, vol. 2, pp. 311ff.; Hartmann, 'Unfallverhütung nach ihrem neusten Stande'; for a comparative history of German and Austrian museums: S. Poser, *Museum der Gefahren. Die gesellschaftliche Bedeutung der Sicherheitstechnik: das Beispiel der Hygiene-Ausstellungen und Museen für Arbeitsschutz in Wien, Berlin und Dresden um die Jahrhundertwende*, Münster: Waxmann, 1998.

17 S. Nicolet, 'Die Arbeitssicherheit in den USA', *Gewerkschaftliche Rundschau* 49, 1957: 358–60.

18 S. Nicolet, 'Die Arbeitssicherheit in den USA', *Zeitschrift für Präventivmedizin* 2, 1957: 322–3.

19 Nicolet, 'Arbeitssicherheit' (*Zeitschrift für Präventivmedizin*), pp. 320–1.

20 Remark of Georg von Mayr, a German factory inspector, at the Congress for Social Insurance of 1894 in Milan. G. von Mayr, 'Diskussionsbemerkung', in: *Congrès international des accidents du travail et des assurances sociales, troisième session, Milan 1er au 6 octobre 1894*, Milan, 1894, vol. 2, p. 97.

21 C. Lamberty, *Reklame in Deutschland 1890–1914: Wahrnehmung, Professionalisierung und Kritik der Wirtschaftswerbung*, Berlin: Duncker & Humblot, 2000, p. 187.

22 Schweizerische Unfallversicherungsanstalt, *Jahresbericht und Jahresrechnung für das Jahr 1926*, Bern, 1927, p. 60.

23 Tiefbau-Berufsgenossenschaft, *Die Unfallverhütung im Bilde*, 2nd edn, Berlin: Hobbing, 1925.

24 Schweizerische Unfallversicherungsanstalt, *Jahresbericht und Jahresrechnung für 1928*, Bern, 1929: addendum.

25 Schweizerische Unfallversicherungsanstalt, *75 Jahre: Das Menschenmögliche*, Luzern: Suva, 1993, p. 40; Schweizerische Unfallversicherungsanstalt, *Ergebnisse der Unfallstatistik der fünfjährigen Beobachtungsperiode, 1963–1967*, Bern, 1969, pp. 65–6.

26 M. Helfenstein, 'Zwanzig Jahre Unfallverhütung', in Schweizerische Unfallversicherungsanstalt, *Rückblick und Ausblick*, Bern, 1942, p. 50.

27 Helfenstein, 'Zwanzig Jahre Unfallverhütung', pp. 52, 57.

28 Helfenstein, 'Zwanzig Jahre Unfallverhütung', pp. 53–63.

29 Schweizerische Unfallversicherungsanstalt, archives of the secretary general's office ('Generalsekretariat'), minutes of the board of directors ('Verwaltungsausschuss'), 1929, p. 138.

30 For example: *Schweizerische Arbeitgeber-Zeitung*, 1927, vol. 22, 152, 219, 272ff., 277; 1928, vol. 23, 20, 231, 291; 1929, vol. 24, 150, 259, 261.

31 Schweizerische Unfallversicherungsanstalt, *Jahresbericht 1926*, p. 35.

32 Schweizerische Unfallversicherungsanstalt, archives of the secretary general's office ('Generalsekretariat'), minutes of the conferences of the agencies' directors ('Konferenzen der Chefs der Kreisagenturen'), 20th conference, 15 March 1940, pp. 4–5.

33 Aldrich, *Safety First*, pp. 271–2; Schweizerische Unfallversicherungsanstalt, *Ergebnisse der Unfallstatistik der fünfjährigen Beobachtungsperioden, 1938–1942*, Bern, 1945, pp. 53–9; W. Sulzer, 'Betriebsgefahren bei neuen Arbeitsverfahren und Stoffen: Unfallverhütungsmassnahmen', *Industrielle Organisation* 10, 1941: 102–3.

34 Aldrich, *Safety First*, pp. 271–2; Schweizerische Unfallversicherungsanstalt, *Ergebnisse der Unfallstatistik der fünfjährigen Beobachtungsperioden, 1933–1937*, Bern, 1939, p. 59; Schweizerische Unfallversicherungsanstalt, *Ergebnisse der Unfallstatistik der fünfjährigen Beobachtungsperioden, 1943–1947*, Bern, 1949, p. 81.

35 Schweizerische Unfallversicherungsanstalt, *Jahresbericht und Jahresrechnung für die Jahre 1955–1980*, Bern, 1956–80.

36 *Schweizerische Arbeitgeber-Zeitung*, 1934, vol. 29, 246, 256, 260ff.; 1935, vol. 30, 135ff.; 1938, vol. 33, 173ff.; 1939, vol. 34, 41ff.; E. Bertschi, *Unfallverhütung: Erfolg und Misserfolg*, Thun: Ott Verlag, 1962, pp. 12–19.

37 *Bericht der eidgenössischen Fabrikinspektion über ihre Amtstätigkeit*, Bern, 1955, pp. 71–2.

38 Ibid.

39 Schweizerische Unfallversicherungsanstalt, *Jahresbericht 1926*, pp. 37–9.

40 Tiefbau-Berufsgenossenschaft, *Unfallverhütung*, pp. 1–2.

41 Ibid.

42 P.T. Borer, *Das Problem der Unfälle*, Genf: Roto-Sadag, 1937.

43 O. Keller, *25 Jahre SUVAL*, Wald, 1946, pp. 96–100.

44 R.M. Farr, *The Roots of Modern Social Psychology 1872–1954*, Oxford: Blackwell, 1996, pp. 1ff., 146ff.

45 Lamberty, *Reklame in Deutschland*, pp. 415–29.

46 Farr, *Modern Social Psychology*, pp. 146ff.

47 C.I. Hovland, A.A. Lumsdaine and F.D. Sheffield, *Experiments on Mass Communication*, Princeton: Princeton University Press, 1949, pp. VII, 3.

48 C.I. Hovland, I.L. Janis and H.H. Kelley, *Communication and Persuasion, Psychological Studies of Opinion Change*, New Haven: Yale University Press, 1953; I.L. Janis and S. Feshbach, 'Personality differences associated with responsiveness to fear-arousing communications', *Journal of Personality* 23, 1954: 154–66.

49 Hovland, Janis and Kelley, *Communication and Persuasion*, pp. 270ff.

50   E. Belbin, 'The effects of propaganda on recall, recognition and behaviour', *British Journal of Psychology* 47(3), 1956: 163–74, 259–70.

51   Schweizerische Unfallversicherungsanstalt, *Ergebnisse der Unfallstatistik der fünfjährigen Beobachtungsperioden, 1948–1952*, Bern, 1955, p. 58.

52   Schweizerische Blätter für Arbeitssicherheit; *Schweizerische Unfallversicherungsanstalt, Ergebnisse der Unfallstatistik der fünfjährigen Beobachtungsperioden, 1953–1957*, Bern, 1960, p. 128; Schweizerische Arbeitgeber-Zeitung 51, 1956: 616.

53   Schweizerische Unfallversicherungsanstalt, *Ergebnisse der Unfallstatistik der fünfjährigen Beobachtungsperioden, 1958–1962*, Bern, 1965, p. 61ff.; Schweizerische Unfallversicherungsanstalt, *Ergebnisse der Unfallstatistik der fünfjährigen Beobachtungsperioden, 1963–1967*, Bern, 1969, p. 64ff.

54   Schweizerische Unfallversicherungsanstalt, *Ergebnisse der Unfallstatistik der fünfjährigen Beobachtungsperioden, 1968–1972*, Bern, 1974, pp. 67–8; Schweizerische Unfallversicherungsanstalt, *Ergebnisse der Unfallstatistik der fünfjährigen Beobachtungsperioden, 1978–1982*, Bern, 1984, pp. 90–1.

55   *Industrielle Organisation* 19, 1950: 219–22; *Gewerkschaftliche Rundschau* 50, 1958: 226.

56   H. Potter, 'Unfallverhütung mit Methoden der Werbepsychologie – Möglichkeit und Grenzen', *Illustrierte Zeitschrift für Arbeitssicherheit* 14(4), 1967: 8–10; 15(1–2), 1968: 10–12, 13–14.

57   H. Potter, *Eine Familienchronik*, Luzern: Selbstverlag, 1995, pp. 133, 137ff.

58   Early examples: K. Humbel, *Unfallsicherheit im Werkbetrieb. Eine betriebswirtschaftliche Studie über Unfallverhütung*, Luzern: Vögeli-Buchdruck, 1948, p. 67; Schweizerische Arbeitgeber-Zeitung 30, 1935: 69; Schweizerische Arbeitgeber-Zeitung 33, 1938: 174.

59   Illustrierte Zeitschrift für Arbeitsschutz 3, 1957: 6–7; similarly: Illustrierte Zeitschrift für Arbeitsschutz 4, 1966: 11.

60   *Illustrierte Zeitschrift für Arbeitssicherheit* 3, 1960: 6–7.

61   Examples: *Illustrierte Zeitschrift für Arbeitsschutz* 5, 1968: 6; 5, 1969: 8–9; 6, 1970: 1; 2, 1976: 10–11.

62   *Bericht des schweizerischen Bundesrates an die Bundesversammlung über seine Geschäftsführung im Jahre 1946*, Bern, 1947, pp. 202–7.

63   *Bericht des schweizerischen Bundesrates an die Bundesversammlung über seine Geschäftsführung im Jahre 1959*, Bern, 1960, p. 280; *Bericht des schweizerischen Bundesrates an die Bundesversammlung über seine Geschäftsführung im Jahre 1964*, Bern, 1965, p. 117; *Bericht des schweizerischen Bundesrates an die Bundesversammlung über seine Geschäftsführung im Jahre 1966*, Bern, 1967, p. 108.

64   *Bericht des Bundesrates über Geschäftsführung 1964*, p. 117.

65   D. Stiefel, *Präventivmedizin im Wandel der Zeit*, Muri: Zentralsekretariat SGGP, 1994, pp. 180ff., 206–7.

66   Stiefel, *Präventivmedizin*, pp. 180–3.

67   D. Porter, 'Introduction', in D. Porter (ed.), *Social Medicine and Medical Sociology in the Twentieth Century*, Amsterdam: Rodopi, 1997, pp. 1–31; N. Oswald, 'Training doctors for the National Health Service: social medicine, medical education and the GMC 1936–1948', in: ibid., pp. 59–80. In Switzerland, the disciplines of social and preventive medicine are usually combined in the same university chairs or institutes. Also, since 1972, the previously separated associations for social and for preventive medicine are joining forces in the Swiss Association for Social and Preventive Medicine. O. Jeanneret, 'Trente années de santé publique en Suisse: un aperçu historique', *Sozial- und Präventivmedizin* 39, 1994: 308–10, 315.

68   Jeanneret, 'Trente années', pp. 308–10.

69 K. Biener, *Gesundheitsprobleme im Lehrberuf*, Basel: Karger, 1969; K. Biener, 'Präventivmedizinische Methoden im Dienst der Unfallverhütung', *Schweizerische Arbeitgeber-Zeitung* 67, 1972: 537–9.
70 K. Biener, 'Gesundheitserziehung der Erwachsenen', in: M. Blohmke *et al.* (eds), *Handbuch der Sozialmedizin*, vol. 2, Stuttgart: F. Enke Verlag, 1977, p. 577.
71 M. Schär, *Leitfaden der Sozial- und Präventivmedizin*, 2nd edn, Bern: Huber, 1973, p. 120; similarly: Biener, 'Gesundheitserziehung der Erwachsenen'.
72 Schär, *Leitfaden*, pp. 120–1; K. Biener, *Wirksamkeit der Gesundheitserziehung*, Basel: S. Karger, 1970, pp. 3–12; Biener, 'Gesundheitserziehung der Erwachsenen', pp. 571–2.
73 Schär, *Leitfaden*, pp. 148–51.
74 P. Weindling, 'Linking self help and medical science: the social history of occupational health', in: P. Weindling, *The Social History of Occupational Health*, Oxford: Croom Helm, 1985, pp. 2–31.

Recommended further reading

M. Aldrich, *Safety First: Technology, Labor and Business in the Building of American Work Safety, 1870–1939*, Baltimore: Johns Hopkins University Press, 1997.

R. Cooter and B. Luckin (eds), *Accidents in History: Injuries, Fatalities and Social Relations*, Amsterdam and Atlanta, GA: Rodopi, 1997.

J. Green, *Risk and Misfortune: a Social Construction of Accidents*, London: UCL Press, 1997.

R.N. Proctor, *The Nazi War on Cancer*, Princeton: Princeton University Press, 1999.

Part II

The importance of the media in postwar public health

3 The media and the management of a food crisis

Aberdeen's typhoid outbreak in 1964

Lesley Diack and David Smith

An important feature of the Aberdeen outbreak was the attention that it received from the press, television and radio. That such attention should be focused on the epidemic was the deliberate intention of the Medical Officer of Health so that he could convey to the citizens of Aberdeen the absolute need for the measures that he was advocating. In general we recognise the value of the press and other publicity media in the realm of health education.[1]

(Milne Report, 1964)

When the official inquiry chaired by Sir David Milne reported on the Aberdeen typhoid outbreak at the end of 1964 they were very aware of the use of the media in the outbreak by the Medical Officer of Health and yet went on to criticise his methods, as not 'wholly justified'.[2] The cause of the outbreak appeared to be one can of contaminated corned beef from Argentina, which hospitalised over 500 people during May and June 1964. This chapter seeks to explore the background of the media response to the events in Aberdeen in 1964 and to place it in context. It will be suggested that the media usage could be interpreted as a development of press and policy relations at a time when a 'new' style of public health more concentrated on prevention, i.e. health education, was developing in the United Kingdom.

The media and the management of food safety reporting before 1964

The 1960s was a time of change in society, a change that was reflected in the development of a different style of news reporting and in the advent of a new type of journalism in the British press. Feature writers and specialist reporters were beginning to be employed to provide in-depth study and analysis of issues.[3] The *Sunday Times* had, from the late 1950s, begun to build a strong team of investigative journalists and by the 1960s they were winning a number of prestigious journalism awards. This special projects unit was known as the Insight team and worked on long-term stories and analysis. They became especially well known for their investigation of the Thalidomide scandal.[4] Their coverage of the Aberdeen typhoid outbreak and other related food safety stories was declared a 'fine piece of team reporting'.[5] This period in the early 1960s has been considered as the 'heroic years'[6] for British newspapers, a time when the broadsheet papers began to increase their market share and sell better than the mass-appeal tabloid press. In 1960 the *News Chronicle*, one of the middle-ground newspapers, disappeared and in 1961 the *Daily Herald* was sold to the Mirror Group and its publication stopped. These closures and mergers polarised the divide between the broadsheets and the tabloid newspapers even more than previously, creating a new marketplace for the British press. The *Sunday Times* and the *Observer* launched their colour supplements in 1962 and 1964 respectively. The new and increasing rivalry from television news and current affairs programmes and the fierce competition from other newspapers, allied to the rising costs of production, helped to start a circulation war that, in 1964, the broadsheets seemed to be winning, especially the *Guardian*.

The first outbreak of typhoid to hit the headlines at this period was in 1963 in the popular Swiss skiing resort of Zermatt. On 18 March the story broke in the press that there were cases of typhoid among British tourists, 'Ten British cases after visits to Zermatt'.[7] The Zermatt typhoid story appeared for most of March and April in the press, and often featured on the front page, with small news items. The typhoid in this Swiss resort came from a contaminated water supply and the tourist industry was so badly damaged that the officials in the resort offered free holidays to those who had fallen ill.[8] The Swiss story had barely finished its run in the media when the next outbreak started in Harlow, Essex, and was reported from the end of May. There were three small outbreaks between May and October 1963 in Harlow, South Shields and Bedford, and this time all were associated with canned corned beef from the same factory in Argentina. However, these British outbreaks involved a total of just over sixty cases between the three towns. Stories about these outbreaks appeared intermittently in the press from early summer until the end of 1963. But in comparison with the Aberdeen typhoid outbreak the reporting was very low key and yet, even so, press enquiries seem to have caused problems for local officials. A paper published on the Harlow outbreak in *Municipal Engineering* suggested that 'special arrangements are required from the outset of such an outbreak if chaos is to be avoided'.[9]

If the media was reporting the food safety crises stories in a low-key manner, how were the relevant government departments dealing with the outbreaks? After three outbreaks in five months the Ministry of Health (MH) accepted that the link with corned beef from a particular canning plant was sufficiently strong to merit action.[10] The firm concerned was asked to stop further shipments, and to withdraw stocks in circulation. The government undertook not to release the names of the brands concerned. Once again the reporting was low key and the British press seemed very unconcerned with following up the details of the story. Table 3.1 shows the number of articles published in *The Times* on the typhoid outbreaks in Britain in 1963 and in 1964. It is very apparent that the Aberdeen outbreak received much more media interest than even the other three British

Table 3.1 Items in *The Times* on typhoid outbreaks, 1963–4

Incident	Story	Lead article	Parliament report	1963	1964
Harlow	16	0	0	15	1
South Shields	12	0	0	12	0
Bedford	5	0	0	5	0
Aberdeen	123	2	10	0	123
Other typhoid	16	3	11	3	13

outbreaks put together. Yet it is not often appreciated now that the Aberdeen typhoid outbreak was not a unique event; there had been the three others in the previous year in Britain and one in Switzerland that had also affected a number of British tourists, but none of these outbreaks achieved the level of press reporting of the Aberdeen incident. This chapter poses a number of questions that are relevant to any discussion of the media's representation of a crisis. Was there something different that characterised the reporting of this outbreak? Or did it just happen when the newspapers were ready to run with it as an ongoing feature? Or was it, as was reported at the time, a monster created by the local Medical Officer of Health?

The media and the Aberdeen typhoid outbreak

Aberdeen's typhoid outbreak in 1964 was a unique event in the history of the city and the first food safety crisis in Britain that attracted such media interest. The testimonies of journalists, civil servants, politicians, health professionals and Aberdonians, as well as the evidence in newspaper and other archives, all show that this was an intensely reported story. Every major newspaper in Britain reported this story on its front page for a number of days and the Scottish newspapers reported the story every day for nearly a month. Several newspapers also ran background features and a number ran hygiene campaigns as a result of the problems in Aberdeen. Even in the more specialist press the Aberdeen typhoid outbreak was treated with more interest. Stephen Lock who became editor of the *British Medical Journal* in the 1980s remembers that he was 'a cub editor' in 1964 and was sent to Aberdeen on his first assignment, 'the first external assignment that anyone had done for decades at the BMJ'.[11] Many overseas newspapers especially in the USA, Canada and Argentina also had coverage of the Aberdeen typhoid outbreak. Fiona Milne, a technician at the time at Aberdeen's City Hospital, recalls that, during the outbreak of 1964, journalists and TV crews, including some from Germany, Japan and the USA, besieged her laboratory.[12] Journalist Keith Webster of the *Glasgow Herald* remembers that the press conferences held by the Medical Officer of Health, Dr Ian MacQueen, began to get crowded by the beginning of June. They included 'the Flash Harrys from Fleet Street as well as local reporters, and local representatives of the national dailies and major press agencies, and some foreign journalists'.[13] Webster also recalls sending details of the crisis to the *Chicago Tribune*, communicating with their London bureau by phone. Frank Fraser, a columnist with the *Scotsman* at the time, remembered it was 'a tremendous experience for a newspaperman...because it went on and on. It seemed to go on forever. And the whole world wanted to know what was happening'.[14] Fraser recalled that the story was 'on the front page for three weeks'. There were also numerous feature articles in the daily and Sunday papers, as well as daily television and radio news items. Locally there were often two if not three reports a day about the outbreak and the local independent television channel, Grampian Television, began to broadcast all day rather than closing down in the afternoon. Whereas the three British typhoid outbreaks of 1963 at Harlow, Bedford and South Shields were reported in the press as 'news', none of them generated the level of feature articles or follow-up stories engendered by the Aberdeen outbreak. Another element that characterised the Aberdeen outbreak as different from the outbreaks of 1963 was that there was plenty of scope in this 1964 story for striking photographs that captured the public's interest and sympathy. The most poignant showed a boy looking out of the window at his visitors who were not allowed inside the hospital because of the risk of infection. His father and grandmother were holding a slate with the words written in chalk 'Mummy and Daddy send their love'. The little boy, heartbroken at being separated from his family, had a tear running down his cheek. As one journalist commented, this was 'the pinnacle' of 'the craft of photo journalism'.[15] However, with over 500 people affected by the disease and hospitalised, there were plenty of stories of human suffering to be reported and the newspapers capitalised on these numbers and began to feature stories about individuals gleaned from the visitors standing outside the wards. Besides the fates of the patients and their families, there were articles about the downturn in the fortunes of businesses, and the disruption of social life within the city.

The story first hit the headlines in the local evening paper, the *Evening Express*, on 22 May with the headline 'Typhoid schoolboy is serious'.[16] The Medical Officer of Health had not been responsible for breaking the news, but in response he began daily press conferences at which he initially attempted to reassure the public that the unnamed source of the outbreak had been identified and made safe, that the contacts had been traced and tested, and that the situation was under control. When it became clear, however, that against MacQueen's predictions the number of cases was escalating, and in response to criticism in the local press, he began to use the press conferences to issue much more detailed hygiene advice and to announce a series of measures to control the spread of the infection. By the end of May all the schools, dance halls and cinemas had been closed. Holidays had been cancelled to Aberdeen and even Britain, and Aberdonians going on holiday elsewhere were being advised to cancel or postpone their planned breaks. The hotels and bed and breakfast establishments were empty and the city lost an estimated £7 million in revenue during the outbreak. The Aberdeen Chamber of Commerce was very concerned by the immediate impact and the possible long-term consequences of the adverse publicity that was being created because of the outbreak. Representatives from the Chamber met to discuss this with the Lord Provost[17] and argued for a publicity effort to be slanted 'in a different direction', which would achieve 'a return to sanity and common-sense' and restore the commercial fortunes of the city.[18]

The press reporting of the Aberdeen typhoid outbreak had not only caused concern to local businessmen and the municipal authorities. The story had also taken a new turn on 29 May when Ian MacQueen dropped a media 'bombshell', seven days after the outbreak had first been made public. He made the announcement that the corned beef involved in the outbreak might be part of a 13-year-old consignment recently released from a government defence stockpile. By this point the authorities already knew that the corned beef had come from one of two possible producers in South America. MacQueen had phoned one of the companies to be told that a can with the shape, weight and identification code that he described had been imported in 1951 by the then Ministry of Food to be placed in a food stockpile or 'nuclear reserve', for use in the event of a nuclear war. The government released food from storage for sale on the open market on a regular basis and replenished the stockpile with fresh stocks. After questioning at the press conference, MacQueen admitted that it appeared the government had been involved in distributing the source of infection from this defence stock. He also dramatically suggested that if the typhoid germ had been allowed to multiply inside the tin for thirteen years, a massive outbreak might be the result.[19] MacQueen's comments about the defence stockpile caused a furore. The government was questioned for not only releasing 'bad' stock but also for not admitting that there was a problem. These two serious allegations were especially alarming for a government in an election year. Nevertheless, the press was soon placated by the assurances given by the government that the stockpile was not the source of the corned beef involved, and the announcement on 2 June of the establishment of a committee of inquiry to investigate the source. Yet the media had now become one of the problems associated with the outbreak that the government had to monitor. It soon became clear that this story was not just a local incident but also one that had implications on a wider stage. The press became more intrusive in their quest for information and 'a good story' to such an extent that MacQueen's health education policy of open reporting began to take on a life of its own.

The next day in parliament, Michael Noble, the Secretary of State for Scotland was asked what arrangements were in place for liaising with the media to alert the public 'in the event of any serious epidemic'. He replied that the arrangements 'must vary according to the circumstances'. However,

Noble did recognise 'the importance of enlisting the co-operation of the press, radio and the television in informing and advising the public'.[20] The same question was posed the next day to the Minister of Health, Antony Barber, who replied 'that all appropriate channels of publicity would be used to make a national announcement'.[21]

No matter what was being stated for public consumption in parliament, within Whitehall MacQueen's handling of the media had already been the subject of discussion. At this stage the officials showed a sympathetic attitude towards his position. The Ministry of Agriculture, Fisheries and Food (MAFF) was still concerned not to blame the outbreak categorically upon contaminated corned beef. On MacQueen a memorandum commented 'in fairness the Medical Officer of Health...has never, except under Press pressure put it higher than....There is a distinct possibility of corned beef having been the source of the infection'.[22]

The Scottish Office politicians were also becoming anxious about the publicity that MacQueen was generating and asked their officials for advice. The Under Secretary of State was advised that 'the Medical Officer of Health was not responsible to the Secretary of State for Scotland', and the officials explained the need for press conferences in the same terms as those used by MacQueen. The press conferences were better than having to respond to 'continual questions asked by different sections of the press throughout the 24 hours'.[23]

The outbreak faded from the national news after the 'all clear' was sounded on 17 June, but continued locally every few days until the last patient left hospital in early September. It returned to the national headlines in late November and early December 1964 when the report of the official inquiry, the Milne report, was published, although comment was muted as a publication date immediately before Christmas was chosen. Later, however, there was a prolonged press campaign against the reprocessing and sale for human consumption of withdrawn suspect corned beef, leading the Prime Minister, Harold Wilson, to veto the proposal. This related story stayed in the press sporadically for another year. The story re-emerged in 1968 when one of the typhoid patients tried to sue for damages and eventually settled out of court.[24]

The management of the Aberdeen typhoid outbreak and the Medical Officer of Health

As can be seen from Table 3.1 and from earlier evidence, the reporting of the Aberdeen outbreak was much more intense than in the 1963 outbreaks. One reason for this was that in Aberdeen the typhoid organism affected many more people. This was not because Aberdonians managed to make a can of corned beef go much further, although this quip about the supposed meanness of Aberdonians was made in 1964 at a local variety theatre. Neither was it because there were a significant number of secondary infections. The corned beef was the primary source of the infection, but the typhoid bacillus spread within the shop because of the lack of modern hygienic practices. The consensus that emerged during the proceedings of the Milne inquiry was that it was because other items in the shop, on and beyond the cooked-meat counter of the supermarket concerned, became infected. One patient interviewed was a vegetarian who only ate an apple from the shop, infected, presumably, by handling.[25] By the end of May, there were 199 people hospitalised, 155 confirmed and forty-four suspected. These figures grew to a peak of 438 people hospitalised on 24 June.

The second factor was the character of the Medical Officer of Health, Dr Ian MacQueen. MacQueen had initially taken an MA at Edinburgh University intending to enter journalism, but finding the job prospects poor in the early 1930s, changed his career to medicine. After working in public health in Barnsley, Mansfield and Edinburgh in the 1940s he moved to Aberdeen in 1952.[26] As Aberdeen's Medical Officer of Health, MacQueen was very interested in the use of health education in the prevention of disease and felt that was where his department was able to be the most successful. In 1956 he initiated a health education section within his department. His staff began a programme of talks to clubs and societies, the aim being to deliver 1,000 talks a year, a target that was soon exceeded. As this work progressed, MacQueen began to develop links with the local print media, providing an outlet for his early enthusiasm for journalism, but he also began to be interested in the possibilities of radio and television for health education work. An in-house publication edited by MacQueen called *Health and Welfare* started in 1959 and was to be published quarterly for fourteen years. The pages of this small magazine give an insight into the mind of this Medical Officer of Health who wrote nearly two-thirds of all the text. He was passionately interested in health education and there was hardly an issue that did not have some comment or article on the latest health education research. He visited Scandinavia and North America to study health education and was intrigued by the possibilities offered by the mass media. In his annual report for 1962, MacQueen analysed three types of health education and the relationship between them. These he summarised as individual teaching by a health visitor, group teaching and mass publicity.[27] MacQueen came to the conclusion that while newspaper articles, and television and radio talks, had so far been used to reinforce individual and group methods, mass publicity was also capable of an 'independent and separate existence'.[28] The typhoid outbreak was to provide MacQueen with the opportunity to experiment with the intensive use of all the mass media for delivering health advice to the public. To this end he arranged daily and, for a time, twice-daily press conferences through which he planned to advise citizens of the precautions that needed to be taken to halt the spread of typhoid. However, he soon found that the press conferences would involve much more than the dissemination of messages about personal hygiene to the Aberdeen public.

Journalism and the creation of news

While MacQueen claimed that the press conferences were a health education exercise, the journalists involved in reporting the story saw them as an opportunity for the creation of news, and MacQueen proved very obliging. Robert Smith, of the local *Evening Express*, remembers that,

> Dr MacQueen had a way with him of producing the telling phrase that a newspaper could splash around. He said at one point in the epidemic that we were now a beleaguered city. And of course all the newspapers...grabbed that and plastered it all over.[29]

Keith Webster also commented on the origins of the 'beleaguered city' headline and story:

> There was one occasion that I recall in a news conference and I think it was on a Saturday ... when MacQueen, who doubtless was very good in the medical issues, but in terms of politics and in terms of public performance and public information, could be pretty naïve. You could feed MacQueen a line and I recall someone saying to him – 'Is it fair then Dr. MacQueen to call this a beleaguered city?'[30]

The 'beleaguered city' phrase hit the headlines the following day; at the time it was phrases such as these that created the dramatic reporting in the national and foreign press. One anguished relative phoned Aberdeen because he had heard a report that 'they're dying like flies in the streets and the bodies are being shovelled into the harbour'.[31] As with the 2001 foot and mouth outbreak in the UK, tourism suffered. Tourists not only avoided the northeast of Scotland, but some Americans were even afraid to visit London during their tours of Europe.

MacQueen's media performances, although loved by the journalists, brought the disapproval of some health professionals dealing with the outbreak. The late Sandy Logie, a young house officer who was seconded to the City Hospital in the first few days, felt that MacQueen had mishandled the outbreak and gave out-of-date information to the press. He recalled 'we were at the coal face and we knew that he was talking rubbish'.[32] Other hospital doctors had reservations about MacQueen. Also at the City Hospital was Elizabeth Russell, now Emeritus Professor of Social Medicine at Aberdeen University. She agreed with Logie, and commented on MacQueen's remarks to the press, 'I think there was a point when his daily media conferences were escalating the "beleaguered city effect", and I think that was what concerned us'.[33] This was a reference to MacQueen's statements about the possibility of a series of massive secondary waves of typhoid, and the anxieties caused by his suggestion of voluntary travel restrictions. The late Professor M.G. McEntegart, a bacteriologist at the university in 1964, commented similarly that MacQueen put people off

Aberdeen to such an extent that 'a bunch of navvies refused to handle Aberdeen granite because it had come from Aberdeen'.[34] This is one example of many similar stories that are still told about the effects of the outbreak.

Another newspaper story that had little basis in reality but that caused considerable discussion and confusion at the time was 'The Vulnerable City', the headline that introduced a two-page spread in the *Sunday Times* on 7 June.[35] The article painted a picture of a city with 'poor sanitation and crowded housing – classic allies of typhoid'. MacQueen at the press conference a few days later attacked the *Sunday Times* and the Insight team for their misreporting of the situation, especially when the figures that they used in their analysis had come from the 1951 census and were out of date. MacQueen was vehement in his attack on the newspaper and stated that Aberdeen now had the best hygiene anywhere in Britain.[36]

MacQueen was to make one other media *faux pas* just as the outbreak was slowing down. He warned the public that bathing off a certain part of the beach might be dangerous in case of infection. Again this warning was blown out of all proportion by the press. However, MacQueen had learned his lesson and had informed the Scottish Office immediately of the problem caused by this inadvertent comment to the press.[37] A statement was issued playing down the danger and the incident was quickly forgotten in the euphoria of the 'all clear'.[38] For MacQueen, the outbreak had been contained successfully. It was over in less than a month and there were few, if any, secondary infections. The main problem remaining was to get the city back to normal as quickly as possible. After the 'all clear' the local council spent an extra £15,000 to attract tourists. The Lord Provost wrote to the 25,000 people who had cancelled holidays in Aberdeen in May and June. In this letter he explained the situation in the city and invited them back. The local Chamber of Commerce organised a fortnight of festivities at the end of July called the *Bon Accord* festival and Queen Elizabeth visited the city to be overwhelmed by the citizens' response to her gesture. By the middle of July, Aberdeen was back on course as a tourist centre and many of the hoteliers were recording a very successful period after their losses of the previous two months.[39] Aberdeen's tourist trade had been very successfully turned around from the brink of disaster and suffered no long-lasting effects of the typhoid outbreak.

The official inquiry

Sir David Milne, a retired civil servant, chaired the official committee of inquiry set up at the beginning of June after MacQueen's inopportune comments to the press about the defence stockpile. The other members were James W. Howie of the Public Health Laboratory Service, Andrew B. Semple, the Medical Officer of Health for Liverpool, A.M. Borthwick, a representative of the meat trade, and Gabrielle Pike, of the National Federation of Women's Institutes. The initial task of the committee was to report on the source of the typhoid outbreak, but it was allowed to extend its remit far beyond this, and it heard evidence and reported on the performance of the local and central participants, and the media aspects of the outbreak. As a result, many participants, especially the government departments and MacQueen, began to treat the preparation of their evidence as a damage-limitation exercise. A chapter of the report was devoted to the 'The Medical Officer of Health and the Press', which recognised MacQueen's intentions 'to convey to the citizens of Aberdeen the absolute need for the measures which he was advocating'. They recognised too, 'the value of the Press and other publicity media in the realm of health education'.[40] Nevertheless, the Milne committee censured MacQueen for his over-dramatic approach stating that 'the outbreak and the possible dangers of its spread were exaggerated to such an extent that the incident received publicity out of all proportion to its significance'.[41] The report suggested that a daily press release would have been adequate – rather than the press conferences and the nightly television reports. The local Chamber of Commerce echoed these comments in a memorandum for the Secretary of State for Scotland that they had prepared after the outbreak was over. They felt that although there had been a victory 'there was unquestionably room for criticism of some of the action taken'.[42] The officials at both ministries involved, the MAFF and the MH, were delighted with this line. It deflected much of the criticism from their inaction after the three 1963 outbreaks. Commenting on a draft version of the report Peter Humphreys-Davies, a deputy secretary at MAFF, wrote to Mrs Hauff, assistant secretary at MH that

> There is some severe criticism of the ridiculous antics of Dr MacQueen, springing partly from professional ignorance and partly (though it does not say so in so many words) from a desire for personal aggrandisement. And some pretty strong words are said about the serious social, economic and financial consequences at home and abroad which flowed from his inept handling of the epidemic and its attendant publicity.[43]

The Stationery Office (HMSO) as publishers of the report were concerned whether some of the comments on MacQueen could be considered defamatory and consulted the government solicitor[44] on whose advice the remarks on the over-exaggeration of the numbers likely to be infected were toned down. And when the report was published in December 1964 the headline in the local newspaper was 'It's bouquets and brickbats for Dr MacQueen'.[45] Besides the criticisms over the use of the media, MacQueen was praised for the speed with which the source of the infection had been traced.

In defence of the Medical Officer of Health

Although he was criticised by the official inquiry, MacQueen's strategy was fully understood and appreciated by his professional colleagues. During the outbreak *The Medical Officer*, the journal of the Society of the Medical Officers of Health, reported that

Dr MacQueen has been holding daily press conferences during most of the course of the epidemic with the result that this has probably been the best 'covered' outbreak of its kind. With an infection so difficult to bring under control, it is fortunate that Aberdeen's population has been so accustomed to accepting guidance on health matters, and there must be a firm hope that strict personal hygiene will bring the outbreak to an end.[46]

Similarly the Medical Officer of Health for Stirling wrote to MacQueen on 12 June 1964 congratulating him, stating that he and his colleagues all thought that 'affairs could not have been handled with greater efficiency, both in operations and public relations, and that the latter probably the most difficult'.[47]

In January 1965 MacQueen used the pages of *The Medical Officer* to argue against the criticisms by the Milne Committee in their official report. With reference to the Croydon typhoid outbreak of 1937, which had been caused by contaminated water, MacQueen remarked that although the Committee of Inquiry on that occasion had criticised the Medical Officer of Health for insufficient publicity, it was 'manifest that the Milne Committee hated the use of the publicity media in Aberdeen'. He argued that the Committee's views could be ruled out on the grounds that 'publicity aspects were completely outside its remit' and 'the Committee took no evidence from any health education officer, public relations officer, journalist, television producer or publicity expert of any type'. Finally, he asserted that a committee consisting of 'a retired Civil Servant, a representative of the meat trade, an administrative bacteriologist, a housewife and an MOH of a city with notoriously poor health statistics – was obviously incompetent to consider health education and publicity'.[48]

The Scottish branch of the Society for the Medical Officers of Health, of which MacQueen was a former president, also supported his actions. They set up a subcommittee to investigate the findings of the Milne Committee that concluded the report had treated MacQueen unfairly and commented that 'the Medical Officer of Health did his work well. It should be noted that there were very few secondary cases. Publicity played a part in this and helped to have the cases detected earlier'.[49] At a conference of the Royal Institute for Health on the safety of canned food held in January 1965 there were further signs of sympathy and support for MacQueen. Dr W.R.M. Couper, the Medical Officer of Health for Pickering in Yorkshire, who had found that a small outbreak of typhoid in 1955 was associated with canned tongue, commented that 'if he [Couper] had been as successful as Dr MacQueen in obtaining publicity, this Conference would have been held in 1956 instead of 1965'.[50] He also remarked that because of the lack of publicity the achievement of himself and his collaborators in tracing the infection to contaminated cooling water at an Argentinian canning factory had met with 'official indifference'.[51] Couper had always felt that his research into his typhoid outbreak had been forgotten and not used to help further canned-food safety. Couper gave evidence to the Milne committee about his outbreak and even travelled to Edinburgh to do so.

MacQueen continued the justification of his actions in his report for 1964, published a few months later. The Milne report had claimed that his publicity methods had caused unnecessary alarm. However, MacQueen asserted that one aim of his media strategy had been to allay existing alarm and in his opinion and that of others it had succeeded.[52] His publicity work had sometimes involved three television appearances a day, which 'had entailed considerable strain' but 'in the expressed opinion of public health workers – in Aberdeen and elsewhere – it made a material contribution to the reduction of public alarm, the improvement of personal hygiene and the temporary eradication of potentially dangerous articles of food'.[53] He justified his actions in these terms for the rest of his life in radio interviews and in his writings. He felt that he had used 'a new weapon to cope with an unprecedented situation'.[54] If he had made mistakes using the media they were 'minor ones' that could be forgiven. MacQueen's performance in the Aberdeen typhoid outbreak also appears not to have permanently affected his ambitions to develop his health education work into the electronic media, and after 1964 he frequently mentioned television and radio programmes in which his department participated. Indeed before he retired he was elected chair of the Scottish Health Education Council, and became a member of the Chief Medical Officers' Advisory Committee on Health Education.[55]

Discussion and Conclusions

Aberdeen's Medical Officer of Health, Dr Ian MacQueen, used the media to inform the public in the immediate vicinity of the need for strict personal hygiene but his health education demands backfired and the press created an image of a dirty and besieged city that no tourist would want to visit. However, for the city and for himself there appeared to be little lasting effect and both were able to continue and function virtually normally from July 1964 onwards. Neither would appear to have suffered any long-lasting effects from the typhoid outbreak. As for the government's own public relations and press strategies, there is little sign that the experience of the Aberdeen typhoid outbreak made any difference as far as decision-making was concerned. This continued to be conducted behind closed doors. However, it could be argued that in many ways this outbreak was a watershed in the new press strategy of the media and the government. Officials and ministers were now very aware of the press and the impact that journalists' reporting could have and sometimes decisions were taken largely in order to avoid possible future adverse publicity. This can be seen with the decisions on some of the Milne Committee recommendations such as that on overseas meat inspection.[56]

The reporting of food poisoning episodes and scares has increased dramatically since 1964, and the damage this has caused to public confidence was one of the reasons for the establishment of the Food Standards Agency (FSA) in 1997. There is seldom a month when there is not some discussion of food as a potential source of health problems in the press or on television. More seriously over the last few years there have been a number of deaths linked to new variant CJD, the BSE crisis and the effects of the foot and mouth disease on the food chain. There has been some academic analysis of these issues: Glasgow University's Media Group has written extensively on the effects of the media and have analysed the main food scares during the 1990s including salmonella, listeria and BSE. Hugh Pennington has also written about his own experiences with the media over *E. coli* 0157 and other food poisoning outbreaks.[57] An article by J. Kitzinger and J. Reilly on 'The rise and fall of risk reporting' published in 1997[58] analysed the BSE story and how it fitted the media template of a 'good story', and is especially relevant to the Aberdeen typhoid outbreak. They argued that the criteria of such a story are threefold, suggesting that an already present media interest, a perception that there is 'another reason to distrust government policy', and on a more pragmatic level the availability of human interest stories and good film footage are the key features that ensure widespread coverage of issues. In the case of the Aberdeen typhoid outbreak, as has already been pointed out, there had been the four earlier typhoid outbreaks in 1963. There were also plenty of accounts of personal suffering that could be covered in connection with the hospitalisation of patients, the ostracism of Aberdeen's citizens because of fear of infection, and the financial losses of businesses and employees. The revelation that the South American corned beef, which was allegedly responsible for the outbreak, might have passed through the government's stockpile elevated the story to one of national and international interest, with implications for the security of the state and for a government seeking re-election.

In some ways, another more discrete food poisoning episode – *E. coli* in Wishaw in 1996 – may be a better example for comparison with the Aberdeen typhoid outbreak. The official inquiry reported that 'media demands can distract attention and scarce resources from the main task of outbreak control' and that 'sometimes ill-informed media commentary or speculation can fuel public anxiety'. The report recommended that there was a need for 'a clear and pro-active media management and public relations strategy'.[59] In 1996, of course, there was no Medical Officer of Health, and no equivalent MacQueen-like figure. The Designated Medical Officer was effectively forbidden to speak to the press, and publicity was the responsibility of the health authority's press office. And yet the press appeared to antagonise everybody. The *E. coli* affair was the latest of a series of food poisoning episodes before the establishment of the FSA. The FSA remit was explicitly to restore public confidence in food safety in Britain. It remains to be seen whether the work of the Agency will have any effect on the recurrent PR problems surrounding outbreaks that occurred in Wishaw and also, in very different circumstances, thirty-two years earlier.

This is especially true when the 2001 foot and mouth crisis is considered. There were many similarities to the typhoid outbreak in 1964. The percentage of the population directly affected was very small, yet the financial implications were much larger. The effect on the tourist industry also had a strong resonance with 1964. The press and media again appeared to be able to create the same sort of media circus surrounding the foot and mouth outbreak without the presence of an Ian MacQueen-like figure. It was, perhaps, not just the character or strategy of Ian MacQueen that was the cause of the media problems in 1964 but the beginnings of the new style of media that was more aggressive in its search for the 'good story' and of government who was more determined than ever to make the search more difficult. From this perspective, Ian MacQueen was not the publicity seeker as the Milne report implied, but was, to some extent, another victim of the Aberdeen typhoid outbreak.

Notes

1 Scottish Home and Health Department, *Report of the Milne Committee of Inquiry into the Aberdeen Typhoid Outbreak of 1964*, London: HMSO, 1964 (hereafter SHHD, *Typhoid*), p 68.

2 SHHD, *Typhoid*, p. 7.

3 Further information on the development of the press and medical coverage can be found in K. Loughlin, 'Networks of mass communication: reporting patterns in early post-war coverage of science, health and medicine', in V. Berridge (ed.), *Making Health Policy*, Amsterdam: Rodopi, 2005.

4 M. Rosen, *The 'Sunday Times' Thalidomide Case: Contempt of the Court and Freedom of the Press*, London: Writers & Scholars Educational Trust, 1979.

5 H. Hobson, P. Knightley and L. Russell, *The Pearl of Days: an Intimate Memoir of the Sunday Times*, London: Hamish Hamilton, 1972, p. 409.

6 Ibid., p. 396.

7 'Ten British cases after visits to Zermatt', *Glasgow Herald*, 18 March 1963, p. 1.

8 'Swiss offer typhoid victims free holiday', *Glasgow Herald*, 20 April 1963, p. 1.

9 H.L. Hughes, 'How Harlow tackled its Whitsun typhoid outbreak', *Municipal Engineering*, 2 August 1963, p. 1176.

10 Public Record Office (hereafter PRO), MAF 276/195, MAF 282/75

11 Personal correspondence from Dr Stephen Lock, BMJ editor, to Dr M.G. McEntegart, dated 7 March 1989.

12 Interview: Fiona Milne, lab. technician, 1 June 1999, tape ref. Aberdeen typhoid outbreak (hereafter AT0/) ATO/9. All interviews recorded by L. Diack.

13 Interview: Keith Webster, trainee journalist with the *Glasgow Herald*, 2 June 1999, ATO/10.

14 Frank Fraser in *A City under Siege*, a BBC radio programme transmitted on 13 April 1984 and now archived as MS 3628 in Aberdeen University Library Special Collections (hereafter AULSC).

15 ATO/10.

16 *Evening Express*, 2 May 1964, p. 1.

17 Lord Provost is the person in charge of the administration of a royal burgh in Scotland. The role of a provost would equate to that of a mayor in England.

18 Memorandum on action taken by the Chamber of Commerce since the beginning of the outbreak recorded 25 June 1964 in Minute Book 11, Aberdeen

Chamber of Commerce, p. 83, item 2. (These archives are still held by the local Chamber of Commerce.)

19 William Beattie, 'And City MOH says contaminated meat may be Government issue', *Scottish Daily Express*, Saturday 30 May 1964, p. 1.
20 *Parliamentary Debates (Commons)*, written answers, 3 June 1964, Col. 170.
21 *Parliamentary Debates (Commons)*, 4 June 1964, Col. 206.
22 PRO, MAF 282/87.
23 Notes on meeting with Dr John Smith, Mr Stodart and Mr Hogarth at the Scottish Home and Health Department on 3 June 1964 in National Archives of Scotland (NAS) HH058/00160.
24 Barton versus William Low and Co. Ltd (1968), *Scots Law Times* 27, 1968: 301.
25 Interview: Rosemary Towler, 24 May 1999, tape ref. ATO/4.
26 L. Diack and D. Smith, 'Professional strategies of Medical Officers of Health in the post war period (1): "innovative traditionalism": the case of Dr Ian MacQueen, MOH for Aberdeen 1952–1974, a "bull-dog" with the "hide of a rhinoceros"', *Journal of Public Health Medicine* June 2002: 180–91.
27 Scottish Association of Mental Health *Annual Report 1960–1961*, Edinburgh, 1962, p. 19.
28 I.A.G. MacQueen, *Annual Report by the Medical Officer of Health for the Year 1962*, Aberdeen, 1963 p. 7.
29 Robert Smith, AULSC MS 3628.
30 ATO/10.
31 David Kemp, 'Aberdeen ready for the next battle', *Scotsman*, 26 June 1964, p. 7.
32 Interview: Dr A. Logie, 16 July 1999, tape ref. ATO/21.
33 Interview: Dr E. Russell, 23 February 1999, tape ref. ATO/2.
34 Interview: Dr M. McEntegart, 3 April 2000, tape ref. ATO/40.
35 *Sunday Times*, 7 June 1964, p. 7.
36 Grampian Television, press conference of 9 June.
37 'Beach bombshell,' *Press and Journal*, 19 June 1964, p. 1.
38 William Beattie and Wilson Russell, 'After 30 days, Aberdeen gets the great news', *Scottish Daily Express*, 18 June 1964, p. 1.
39 Magnus Magnusson, 'Aberdeen, Britain's gayest spot', *Scotsman*, 29 July 1964, p. 6.
40 SHHD, *Typhoid*, 1964, p 68.
41 SHHD, *Typhoid*, 1964, p 68.
42 Aberdeen Chamber of Commerce, Minute Book 11, p. 102.
43 Memo from Peter Humphreys-Davies dated 20 November 1964 to Mrs Hauff, PRO MAF 282/96.
44 Letter from Miss M.K. MacDonald to Mr Hogarth, both of the Scottish Office, dated 1 December 1964, PRO MH 148/357.
45 *Evening Express*, 17 December 1964, p. 1.
46 'Epidemiological notes. Typhoid in Aberdeen', *The Medical Officer*, 5 June 1964: 335.
47 Letter dated 12 June from Medical Officer of Health for Stirlingshire to Dr Ian MacQueen held by Northern Health Services Archive (NHSA).
48 I.A.G. MacQueen, 'Reflections on the Typhoid Report', *The Medical Officer*, 15 January 1965, 31–33; the committee is described in the following order by Dr MacQueen – Sir David Milne, Algernon Borthwick, James Howie, Gabrielle Pike and Dr Andrew Semple.
49 Society of Medical Officer of Health (Scottish Branch), Minutes of Meeting of Special Sub-Committee to Study Report on Aberdeen Typhoid Outbreak, 7 January 1965, Archives and Business Records Centre, University of Glasgow.
50 *Safety of Canned Food: Report of the Royal Society of Health on the Safety of Canned Foods*, 1965, London: Royal Society of Health, 1966, p. 144.
51 Ibid., p. 144.

52 L. Diack, 'Myths of a beleaguered city: Aberdeen and the typhoid outbreak explored through oral history', *Oral History* 29(1), spring 2001: 62–72.
53 I.A.G. MacQueen, *Report by the Medical Officer of Health for the Year 1964*, Aberdeen, 1965, p. 18.
54 *Health and Welfare* 23: 8 in NHSA, GRHB E1/7/9.
55 I.A.G. MacQueen, *Report of the Medical Officer of Health for Aberdeen for 1970*, p. 13, and 1972, p. 12.
56 L. Diack, T. Hugh Pennington, E. Russell and D.F. Smith, 'Departmental, professional and political agendas in the implementation of the recommendations of a food crisis enquiry: the Milne report and inspection of overseas meat plants', in D. F. Smith and J. Phillips (eds), *Food, Science, Policy and Regulation in the Twentieth Century: International and Comparative Perspectives*, London: Routledge, 2000, pp. 189–205.
57 T. Hugh Pennington, 'Recent experiences in food poisoning: science and policy, science and the media' in D. F. Smith and J. Phillips (eds) *Food Science, Policy and Regulation in the Twentieth Century. International and comparative perspectives*, London: Routledge, 2000, pp. 223–38.
58 J. Kitzinger and J. Reilly, 'The rise and fall of risk reporting: media coverage of human genetics research, "false memory syndrome" and "mad cow disease"', *The European Journal of Communication* 12(3), 1997, pp. 291–318.
59 The Pennington Group, *Report on the Circumstances Leading to the 1996 Outbreak of Infection with E. coli 0157 in Central Scotland*, Edinburgh: HMSO, 1997, preface.

Recommended further reading

L. Diack, 'Myths of a beleaguered city: Aberdeen and the typhoid outbreak explored through oral history', *Oral History* 29(1), spring 2001: 62–72.

L. Diack and D. Smith, 'Professional strategies of Medical Officers of Health in the post war period (1): "innovative traditionalism": the case of Dr Ian MacQueen, MOH for Aberdeen 1952–1974, a "bull-dog" with the "hide of a rhinoceros"', *Journal of Public Health Medicine*, June 2002: 180–91.

H. Hobson, P. Knightley and L. Russell, *The Pearl of Days: an Intimate Memoir of the Sunday Times*, London: Hamish Hamilton, 1972.

J. Kitzinger and J. Reilly, 'The rise and fall of risk reporting: media coverage of human genetics research, "false memory syndrome" and "mad cow disease", *The European Journal of Communication* 12(3), 1997: 319–50.

I.A.G. MacQueen, 'Reflections on the Typhoid Report', *The Medical Officer* 113, 15 January 1965: 31–3.

The Pennington Group, *Report on the Circumstances Leading to the 1996 Outbreak of Infection with E. coli 0157 in Central Scotland*, Edinburgh: HMSO, 1997.

T. H. Pennington, *When Food Kills: BSE, E. Coli and Disaster Science.* Oxford: Oxford University Press, 2003.

Scottish Home and Health Department, *Report of the Milne Committee of Inquiry into the Aberdeen Typhoid Outbreak of 1964*, London: HMSO, 1964.

D.F. Smith and H.L. Diack with T.H. Pennington and E.M. Russell, *Food Poisoning, Policy and Politics: Corned Beef and Typhoid in Britain in the 1960s*, London: Boydell Press, 2005.

D.F. Smith and J. Phillips (eds), *Food Science, Policy and Regulation in the Twentieth Century. International and Comparative Perspectives*, London: Routledge, 2000.

4 Uneasy prevention

The problematic modernisation of health education in France after 1975

Luc Berlivet

'We are working out social images, thus contributing to craft little by little a new culture of health. This is the way we will be able to contribute to the irreversible transformation of health behaviours.'

(Jean-Martin Cohen-Solal)[1]

This chapter explores the transformation of health education in France in the wake of the pioneer 'anti-smoking' legislation passed in June–July 1976. Although France's first ever health education campaign, which relied on the alleged informative power of the 'mass-media', focused solely on smoking, Simone Veil, Minister of Health of the right-wing government,[2] had a much greater ambition. These *'grandes campagnes nationales d'éducation pour la santé'* ('large-scale national health education campaigns') were seen as the perfect policy tool, actually the only one available for reducing the human and economic burden induced by a wide range of *'comportements à risques'* ('risky behaviour'), such as smoking, drinking in excess, unhealthy diet and lack of exercise, etc.

This rising interest in the uses of the 'mass-media' (the umbrella term used at the time for television, and to a lesser extent radio) as a means to influence reputed problematic social practices was certainly neither specific to France nor limited to the domain of public health. From road safety to the promotion of more effective energy conservation, through health education, the 1970s saw the development in Western industrialised countries of media campaigns aimed at persuading the public to modify a wide range of 'behaviour'. Since it was first implemented this new kind of public policy has aroused wide-ranging comments, both positive and critical, and despite the fact that for a time it epitomised modern government and attracted significant amounts of public money, analyses of this development by historians and social scientists are still scarce.[3] Most of the available literature on the topic comes from policy-makers or academics specialised in 'social marketing', and focuses on identifying what worked and what failed,[4] with little interest in explaining the emergence of this form of political action, or addressing the questions it raises on the evolution of modern states in the late twentieth century. This is surprising when one considers that health education, and later health promotion (a much broader approach to population welfare), are symbolic of the 'new public health' obsessed with the reduction of health risks that emerged in Western countries after the Second World War. Indeed, following the decline in infectious diseases this kind of preventive action quickly became the standard response to a growing number of 'risk factors' identified by epidemiologists for non-transmissible diseases.[5] By documenting the genesis and evolution of health education campaigns in France, this chapter aims to contribute to filling a significant gap in the historiography of modern public health in France.

In France, the rise of media campaigns as a common strategy in preventing disease rested with the Comité Français d'Éducation pour la Santé ('French Committee for Health Education').[6] From the autumn of 1976 to its transformation in 2002 into an Institute of Health Education and Prevention, this organisation was responsible for the preparation, planning, implementation and evaluation of campaigns that successively or concomitantly focused on: smoking; the risks of a sedentary lifestyle (1977);[7] improving the social integration of the disabled (1977); dental health (1978); '*l'abus d'alcool*' ('excessive drinking', 1984); the risk factors for cardiovascular diseases (1984); the hazards of illegal drugs (1986); AIDS (1987); domestic accidents (1990); 'the appropriate uses of pharmaceuticals' (1991);[8] advocating MMR vaccination (1993);[9] and hepatitis B vaccination (1995). The length and variety of the list testifies to the ambition and hopes invested in health education by successive French governments from the mid-1970s onwards, whatever their political orientation. Interestingly, their responsibility in organising high-profile media campaigns always overshadowed CFES's other activities. From the late 1970s onwards, senior staff had elaborated a general strategy in health education that stressed the necessity to extend campaigns by 'fieldwork actions' ('*des actions de terrain*'), including interventions in school, in the workplace, at holiday resorts and various other community settings. The understanding behind this view was that campaigns were necessary to throw some light on health issues in a dramatic way, while close interactions between trained health educators and the targeted population was the key to real, long-lasting behavioural changes. In other words, the 'problematisation' initiated by the broadcasting of the film and radio messages had to be reinforced and stabilised through face-to-face interactions.[10] In fact, analysing the difficulties experienced by CFES in training and maintaining a group of health education professionals, as well as financing these less visible activities, is essential to a real understanding of the fragility of health education in France.[11] However, in the limited space allowed by this chapter I will rather focus on the genealogy and evolution of the media campaigns, as this marks the very emergence of a new form of public health intervention.

The 1976 action on smoking was obviously not the first attempt to build on the alleged persuasive power of moving and speaking images: films had been shot and screened in different health education settings since the turn of the century,[12] and the French government had already sponsored a medical programme dedicated to advising the public in matters of health. Moreover, these exercises in health education followed pioneer 'propaganda' efforts in other domains, e.g. the interwar crusade against the 'depopulation' of France. What was new, however, was that the 1970s approach to health proceeded from a fascination (widely shared by 'modernisers' within the political and administrative elite) with the alleged persuasive power of audiovisual advertising. This implied that the Committee's staff would have to master every aspect of this communication format, if not to produce films and other materials entirely on their own, at least to interact effectively with communication experts and have the upper hand in the collaborative process. This task went far beyond the difficulties of engineering the campaigns as such (including the crafting of films and radio 'spots') to include the successful defusing of widespread criticism about the use of advertising methods in public health and other policy areas. Such attacks were certainly not specific to the French public sphere and came from both left- and right-wing critics. These criticisms were frequently contradictory, as alarm regarding the political dangers induced by attempts to regulate the 'lifestyle' of millions of citizens alternated with denunciations at the waste of public money on such a useless, ineffective enterprise. This latter theme developed into a public discourse on the limits of state power in modern developed countries: Murray Edelman's thesis on the rise of 'symbolic poli- cies' in response to governments' growing impotence proved influential in this respect.[13]

However, this chapter intends to point out that despite the multiple polit- ical issues involved in the development of health education, CFES's staff managed to gain some relative autonomy *vis-à-vis* successive governments. This autonomy stemmed from the ability of health education specialists to define themselves in political and administrative circles as experts in 'human behaviour' and the way to change it. Indeed, in the wake of the first national campaign these experts began to grapple with the complexity of human psychology and consequently developed an increasingly sophisticated strategy based on the mobilisation of symbols embedded in audiovisual support. This practical knowledge was unique in France at this time and allowed them to exercise a real command over the framing and implementa- tion of media campaigns, with the partial exception of AIDS prevention, as this issue was under stricter political control.[14] Interestingly, this apprentice- ship in the complexity of health communication went hand in hand with a concern to demonstrate the specific impact of campaigns in relation to the multiple reputed influences over social behaviour. A focus on the evaluation of interventions intensified, and the wording of questions included in CFES surveys on the reception of films and messages, grew in sophistication. This development operated on the apparent paradox whereby the promoters of an activity frequently castigated for its lack of effectiveness, and indeed virtually impossible to assess by modern public health standards, developed both a 'compulsion to evaluate' and a clear understanding of the limits of their search for evidence.[15] Nevertheless, as suspicion towards the usefulness of media campaigns is still widely shared in academia, it is perhaps worth reminding ourselves that difficulties in demonstrating the effectiveness of actions cannot be taken as demonstrations of their ineffectiveness.

The first part of this chapter analyses the inscription of tobacco smoking on the political agenda through the adoption of a law that set the tone of French policy for fifteen years, and paved the way for large-scale media campaigns. The centrality of large-scale communication implied a 'modernisation' of health education, and eventually the reorganisation and financial improvement of CFES. In the second part, I examine these transformations in detail, together with the planning and implementation of the first action against smoking. This important episode in the history of French public health policy provides a unique insight in the hyper-rational approach to human behaviour, and the means to reform it, which was elaborated by CFES in the mid-1970s. However, things did not go according to these rather grand plans, and the third part of the chapter will be devoted to a study of the transformation of what were called 'campaign strategies', from *c*. 1977–8. This *aggiornamento*, driven by strong unease regarding the pioneer experience in risk reduction, involved a systematic mobilisation of social science, both in the guise of academic publications and the kind of applied knowledge developed in market research.

The politicisation of smoking in mid-1970s France

Smoking entered the French biomedical scene in 1954, when an epidemiological investigation of the aetiology of lung cancer was set up to test the hypothesis of a possible relationship between smoking and cancer reported by British and US scientists in the previous years.[16] At the same time, newspapers, radio and then television had started airing concern about the danger of tobacco smoke. However, it took a further twenty years for this issue to become a 'political problem'. The politicisation of this issue did not stem from the mobilisation of public health specialists or voluntary organisations that had been instrumental in other countries, like the USA and the UK. Rather it took the form of a top-down agenda-setting process, and the name of Simone Veil, Minister of Health from 1974 to 1979, is still widely associated with tobacco control policies in France. However, she did not form this project on her own: it took a well established though quite singular oncologist, Maurice Tubiana, to alert her to the growing medical literature documenting the risks induced by tobacco smoke.

A radiologist and 'Professeur de physique médicale' (biophysics) in Paris, Tubiana had served since 1959 as head of the 'Radiations Department' at the Institut Gustave Roussy (IGR), the main French cancer clinic and most prestigious oncology research institute. In 1974, he became chairman of the 'Commission du cancer' of the Ministry of Health,[17] a position that made him one of the most prominent 'mandarins' in this field. While in the latter position he mostly worked along the same lines as his most respected predecessor and boss as head of the IGR, Pierre Denoix, Tubiana nevertheless departed from his approach on the smoking issue. Whereas Denoix considered smoking prevention to be a matter of medical counselling, in the clinics, his junior and somewhat impetuous colleague took advantage of his newly acquired position to promote a more political agenda. Not only did he decide to focus the first annual report of the Commission under his chairmanship on the dangers of smoking, but he also turned it into a pledge for government information on the risks induced by tobacco smoke. Maurice Tubiana's alertness on this issue, which was to establish him as a chief whistleblower amongst the French cancerologists for more than a decade, was based on his knowledge of and trust in the results of French and Anglo-American epidemiological investigations. In a medical community that was less prone than its British and US counterparts to trust statistics and act on them,[18] he was one of the few who defended the merits of this style of reasoning. In his memoirs, Tubiana credits Daniel Schwartz, the statistician in charge of the first French study on smoking and lung cancer, for showing him the potential of an epidemiology of non-communicable disease. The two young medical researchers became friends, and Tubiana never stopped defending medical statistics (both in the guise of clinical trials and epidemiology) against its critics.[19]

Important though it was, writing a report was not good enough for the impetuous Tubiana, who went on to convince policy-makers to engage in a crusade against smoking. He took advantage of a routine visit by Simone Veil to the IGR – and if the accounts of the meeting given by both sides and a journalist are anything to go by, the oncologist addressed the Minister rather directly: not only did he urge her to tackle the tobacco issue, but he also made plain to her that he thought a minister of health could not afford to give the wrong example and appear on TV smoking.[20] Simone Veil did not immediately take Tubiana's political advice, although she quit smoking quickly afterwards – apparently following the counsel given to her by Pierre Denoix during that same visit to the IGR.[21] It is still difficult to document precisely the rather fast process that saw the minister overcoming, in a few months, her anxiety regarding possible popular reactions, the mobilisation of vested economic interests, and political opposition towards any government initiative on smoking. Nevertheless, when interviewed, her main adviser on public health, and public relations specialist, stressed how they foresaw the opportunity to use an intervention against 'the abuse of tobacco' (I will come back to this interesting wording later) to reshape the political agenda and get her out of some serious difficulties.[22] Indeed, Simone Veil had been struggling since her first weeks in government to pass a law on the medical regulation of abortion, the first ever to set out a legal framework for 'voluntary interruptions of pregnancy' in France.[23] Although she enjoyed the full support of the President, Valéry Giscard d'Estaing, all along the legislative process, the Minister had to cope with fierce opposition from about two-thirds of the right-wing members of parliament, the very political support of the government, and the law would not have passed without the almost unanimous votes of the opposition. She had been morally wounded by the awful personal attacks she suffered during the heated parliamentary debate (including misogynistic and anti-Semitic insults shouted at a woman who had survived Auschwitz). Later, the film and pictures shot during the debate at the national assembly, which pictured Simone Veil hiding her face behind her hands to conceal her tears, became iconic of the controversial politics of abortion in mid-1970s France. Whereas her display of courage had won her many supporters within an increasingly liberal French society, she was also wary of being identified with this single issue, and saw smoking as an interesting topic that could help amend her public image.[24]

Unsurprisingly, Simone Veil and her entourage paid careful attention to the media coverage during the preparation, announcement and implementation of their *'plan anti-tabac'*. While few newspapers had announced (as early as late January and March 1975) that the Ministry of Health was drawing up such plans, they waited until 17 September 1975 to hold a press conference and announce that a bill aiming to regulate the uses of tobacco in public places and its advertising would be introduced before parliament that very autumn. It was simultaneously announced that this legal, 'repressive' approach to smoking was to be followed by a campaign of prevention. The Ministry of Health and its supporters in parliament were well aware of the need for a strong legitimisation of a state intervention that would go far beyond the routine fiscal policy of tobacco control, in a domain that had not attracted much interest since the pioneer but short-lived political mobilisations of the late nineteenth century.[25] Indeed, during the political debate, both in political arenas and in the media, a twofold justification for action was developed: the rising 'social cost of tobacco' was denounced as well as the risks of tobacco smoke for smokers, their children and foetuses (a sensitive argument less than a year after the heated discussion over abortion).[26] While the first argument drew on a kind of implicit utilitarian reasoning that deemed risk reduction (somewhat dubiously) a means of avoiding future medical expenses, the second thrust, in line with traditional principles of 'welfarism', referred to a state duty to protect and improve the citizens' well-being. As the question of protecting individuals, even against themselves, was consequently reopened, Simone Veil prudently declared that her project was alien to such authoritarianism.[27] Moreover, she always assured journalists and parliamentarians that her, somewhat humble, ambition was limited to stopping the increase in smoking and 'fight against excess of tobacco consumption': 'In the short term, the objective aimed at is essentially a stabilisation of the consumption, a result that seems better than the "serrated curves" [*'courbes en dents de scie'*] observed in some foreign countries, in the wake of spectacular, still much too intermittent actions'.[28] The text submitted to parliament (with the full political support of the Prime Minister and the President) aimed at undermining a variety of alleged social incitements to start, and then keep, smoking. Indeed, the arguments put forward to legitimise the possibility of a government ban on smoking in 'places dedicated to a collective use' ('*lieux affectés à un usage collectif*'),[29] opened by Article 16, mixed references to the dangers of 'passive smoking' with a kind of social contagion allegedly fuelled by the spectacle of smokers.

In 1970s France, like in many developed countries, advertising was definitely an important and controversial political theme. While lots of commentators, including a growing fraction of the political elite, were fascinated by what they saw as the manufacture of desire, many others, far beyond the radical left, attacked it as deceitful persuasion.[30] It is therefore no surprise that the law set out a principle of general prohibition, immediately balanced by an important exception. Advertisements were banned from television and radio (that is the media which have the biggest impact), and limited to the press, apart from 'publications intended for youth'.[31] Sponsoring of any sports events, apart from motor races, by the tobacco industry was also proscribed. Moreover, Article 8 intended to put an end to the display of glamour that had made the reputation of brands by specifying:

> adverts for tobacco and tobacco products [i.e. lighters, matches, etc.] cannot include any mention but the name of the product, its composition, the name and address of the manufacturer and, if need be, distributor; no graphic or photographic representation but the product, its packaging or the brand's logo ['*l'emblème de la marque*'].

In addition, it was decided that, within two years time, the average amounts in nicotine, tar and other 'substances produced during the combustion' should appear on any single pack of cigarettes (Article 9). An amendment introduced by a senator even made compulsory, within the same delay, the printing on cigarette and tobacco packs of a mention that does not translate easily: '*abus dangereux*'. Again, it was 'excess' (or 'overuse') solely that was deemed 'dangerous'.

A single article, 16, was meant to have the biggest impact on the ordinary life of the 42 per cent of French people under eighteen who admitted smoking at the time.[32] For all the risks of popular reactions from citizen-smokers, members of parliament from both the right and the left nevertheless backed enthusiastically the introduction of restrictions on smoking in public places. They did so to the point of amending the text in such a way that the decrees, provided for in Article 16, to implement the separation of buildings dedicated to a collective use between smokers and non-smokers, could not allow less than half the volume to the latter. The analysis of the three kinds of rationales put forward, both in parliament and in the press, to justify such a regulation provides a unique insight into the 'multiple realities' of smoking,[33] and especially passive smoking, as perceived by pioneers of tobacco control in mid-1970s France. Indeed, the need to avoid 'the toxic effects on non smokers' of 'passive inhalation'[34] was constantly reasserted, although only scarce data were available at the time: the results of the cohort studies that fuelled the controversy over the alleged rise in cancer risk induced by 'environmental tobacco smoke' were still to be published.[35] However, this scientific justification was constantly mixed with moral considerations.[36] At the same time, Simone Veil's supporters in the parliament were also deeply convinced that the spectacle of tobacco smokers, cigarette smokers in particular, had the power to induce a mimetic response, especially in teenagers (a population they depicted as all too eager to behave as adults), and described the ban on smoking in places dedicated to a collective use as a necessary move in their fight to stop the new generations from indulging in this harmful habit.[37] Nowhere was this belief in the socially contagious nature of smoking stronger than in the decree issued on the basis of the law itself.[38] Two series of proscription were included in this document: the first of them banned smoking from schools and leisure centres as a means to conceal the vision of smokers from young audiences, whereas even the prohibition of smoking in hospitals and health centres, included in the second kind of proscriptions, was partly based on the view that health professionals should not be allowed to set a subversive example, at the risk of undermining propaganda efforts.[39]

Surprisingly perhaps, when one remembers Simone Veil's worries and hesitations to act on Tubiana's advice, parliamentarians' reaction towards the governmental proposal for a new approach to public health policy proved remarkably positive. The text was unanimously adopted by both assemblies on 28 and 29 June 1976 at the end of a very brief procedure, by any French institutional standard. The linchpin to that huge political success lay in the shrewd persuasion strategy developed by the Minister, her staff and allies within various public arenas. Their constant efforts since September 1975 managed to convince the Ministry of Finance and representatives of the other vested interests that the proposed regulation on smoking would be almost harmless to the French economy.[40] In point of fact, the mid-1970s marked the beginning of a huge transformation of the 'issue network' surrounding tobacco in France,[41] due to an increasingly influential European law, necessary to the creation of the Common Market. National monopolies were gradually dismantled and the state-owned manufacturer Service d'Exploitation Industriel des Tabacs et Allumettes (SEITA), which still controlled 91.1 per cent of all the tobacco market in 1975,[42] was about to face fierce competition with US and British companies. In this context, the Minister of Health and her allies pretended that with the restrictions on advertising the foreign brands would never reach the level of notoriety achieved by such household names as 'Gauloise' and 'Gitane'.[43] In addition, the Ministry of Finance mandarins, who had SEITA under their control, seemed satisfied that the official limited goal of the policy was to stabilise the consumption of tobacco and that Simone Veil had ruled out, in advance, any real increase in prices (stable since 1972). This compromise between the two departments did not really threaten the excise revenue, and protected the government against the kind of problems generated by any sharp increase in the retail price index, as the index included the price of tobacco products.[44] At the same time, the 40,000 tobacco growers (whose number had plummeted from 107,000 in 1964) received reassurance that their exclusive contracts with SEITA would be renewed, including the clause guaranteeing the purchase price of their harvest.

An interesting paradox with this first French smoking policy is that, although it had been widely celebrated (the legislation was promptly renamed 'Veil law', after the Minister of Health), its implementation proved problematic, to the point that it eventually came to epitomise the difficulty of public health reform. In 1991, the then-Minister of Health, the socialist Claude Évin, drew precisely on these difficulties to legitimise the adoption of a tighter legal framework, including a complete ban on (direct and indirect) tobacco products advertising, and a more detailed regulation of smoking in public places. Meanwhile, Simone Veil had moved on from the 'repressive' dimension of her plan, an approach she explicitly considered to be a prerequisite to any prevention, and started to instigate 'modern' health education campaigns.

An exercise in hyper-rationalisation

When Simone Veil and her advisers first planned the development of media campaigns, there was already a tradition of state-sponsored health propaganda dating back to the establishment of an 'Office National d'Hygiène Sociale' (National Bureau of Social Hygiene) in 1924.[45] In 1972, Robert Boulain, the then Minister of Health, had also issued a statement to 'inform' the population of the risks associated with tobacco smoking. Simone Veil nevertheless took great care to break away from what she saw as an outdated approach. With the assistance of a handful of aides equally eager to take advantage of the possibilities opened by the 'modern' media (especially television), she built both on some foreign experiences in the domain, and the inspiration provided by the road safety campaigns organised by the French government since the early 1970s. The former came under their notice mainly through documentation circulated by the International Union for Health Education (based in Paris) and study trips to foreign countries.[46] In her capacity as Minister of Health, Simone Veil was on the interdepartmental committee in charge of the latter. What was needed though was an organisation that could draw on these experiences and handle large-scale communication campaigns.

According to Françoise Buhl (Veil's closest adviser) the Minister and her entourage first toyed with the idea of putting the departmental administration directly in charge of organising the anti-smoking campaign. However, the cumbersomeness of such a bureau did not fit very well with the model of highly reactive, lightweight, flexible organisations favoured by the liberal wing of the French right, to whom they all belonged, and commonly associated with the very idea of mass-media communication in the creed of the time. For that reason, they turned their attention towards the old-fashioned, and badly under-funded 'Comité Français d'Éducation pour la Santé', with the idea to turn it into a modern, well-staffed and highly effective quango. The organisation had been established in 1945 as the 'Comité Français d'Éducation Sanitaire'.[47] Between 1966 and 1972, after a long period when lack of funding and continuous institutional changes undermined its development, the Committee was renamed ('health education' was alleged to be more appealing than the old, bureaucratic 'sanitary education') and its structure eventually stabilised. A truly idiosyncratic organisation, it was technically a private non-profit body (escaping the rules of public service) although both its head and the chairperson of its board were appointed by the Minister. Moreover, the Committee's budget was virtually entirely resourced by the Department of Health, which therefore had its say on policy choices.[48] Until the mid-1970s, the propaganda media of health education were chiefly a magazine called *La Santé de l'homme* ('Human Health'), pamphlets, posters and lectures in schools (which sometime included the screening of brief 'educational' films). The diffusion and impact of such actions were not the major concern of CFES's staff (dominated by a handful of senior professors of medicine with an interest in public health). They rather concentrated on wording calls for moderation in drinking, and praising 'healthy living', in a rhetoric that was reminiscent of the great debate on 'degeneration' perils (in the specific way it had developed in France since the 1920s).[49]

Modernising health education meant breaking with this substance as much as the form: exhortations did not really fit with the kind of short, pithy audiovisual communication Veil and her collaborators had in mind. In order to implement this complete transformation, the Minister hired Michel Le Net, the energetic deputy director of the road safety agency, who had been in charge of pioneer media campaigns in this field since 1973.[50] A former adviser to the 'Secretaire d'État au logement' (the undersecretary in charge of housing policies) in 1971–2,[51] he was quite probably unique, in the sense that he had experience both in policy-making and in public communication. At first, the modernisation of the CFES initiated by Le Net did not go with any important increase in staff; the 'Délégué général à l'éducation pour la santé' rather relied on a handful of aides. Apart from a young medical doctor who had already started working on the uses of mass media in health education for the Committee, the others had neither previous connection with the quango, nor medical education. Le Net was much keener on hiring a statistician and economist from the department of research at the Ministry of Health; as I will show below, he considered quantitative methods to be crucial to the deciphering of human behaviour, as well as evaluating the true impact of public policies. The scaling up of prevention campaigns also implied a consequent increase in budget to allow for buying time slots on

Table 4.1 Evolution of the budget allowed to the CFES, 1974–88

Year	Budget (inflation-adjusted francs)	Percentage increase over the previous year
1974	2,522,000	–
1975	4,010,000	59%
1976	6,710,000	67%
1977	10,921,000	62%
1978	14,835,000	35%
1979	28,178,000	89%
1980	30,852,100	9%
1981	34,914,000	13%
1982	39,264,000	12%
1983	36,378,000	7%
1984	49,510,064	36%
1985	52,210,575	5%
1986	37,365,111	28%
1987	38,699,771	4%
1988	35,709,363	8%

Note:
Percentages have been rounded to the nearest number.

Source: These figures are extracted from É. Lévy, Deuxième rapport présenté au nom du
Conseil Économique et Social: l'éducation pour la santé (for the period from 1974–81)
and from L. Tondeur, 'Réflexion sur l'institutionnalisation de l'éducation pour la santé
en France, au travers du Comité Français d'Éducation pour la Santé', DEA, Mémoire
de Diplôme d'Etudes Approfondie en Sciences Politique [DEA thesis in political
science], Université Paris 1, 1994 (for the period from 1982–8).

radio and television, and producing a wide range of audiovisual material
(including films). Indeed, the funds allocated to the Committee jumped from
2.5 million Francs in 1974 to 28.2 million five years later (see Table 4.1).

Meanwhile, the new-model Committee had launched the first anti-
smoking campaign, based on the hyper-rationalist vision of human agency
developed by its new head. An '*Ingénieur des ponts et chaussées*' in his own
right, Le Net believed in an approach to public policy that was typical of the
French elite engineers. Characteristically, when interviewed he went as far as
to describe his 'scientific mind' as both the key to his success and what
turned critics against him:

The milieu of road safety, it's an engineers world [*un milieu d'ingénieurs*].
The Road Safety Delegate belonged to the '*Ingénieurs des ponts*', the

Director of Roads with the ministry belonged to the '*ponts*', there was a background of engineers, that is scientists, that is rational people. But medics did not think like that.[52]

As exposed in a preparatory document, the linchpin of a successful rational management of the campaign was to be a set of statistical indicators:

The objective of this management chart [*tableau de bord*] is to follow the evolution of knowledge, ideas and behaviour of the public as regards to smoking. It aims at displaying the shape of the mortality and morbidity curves that are linked to the use of tobacco products.[53]

In Le Net's rather plain view, the difference between *prosper hoc* and *post hoc* 'measures' would reveal the impact of the campaign. The first of the two surveys (alleged to present the baseline of public opinion on this matter) was implemented in September 1976 by pollsters hired by CFES; the campaign lasted from 1 October to 30 November; as early as January 1977, a 'post-test' (a replica of the previous survey completed with some tobacco sales statistics) came out, which was supposed to give a first hint of the action's impact.

An important press conference called by Simone Veil on 28 September launched the initiative. In two months time, nine different films, 20 seconds long, were broadcast forty-two times altogether on *Télévision Française 1*, and forty-five times on *Antenne 2*, the two French (state-owned) channels. At the same time, eighteen different oral messages (20 seconds long, on average) were aired 330 times overall on every radio (either publicly or privately owned). Most importantly, this pioneer action settled the *modus operandi* of French health education campaigns as based on broadcasting calls to prevention in the middle of commercial slots, instead of producing special, educative programs,[54] an approach that is still in use today. The communication elaborated since 1976, entirely framed on a format developed for advertising, intended consequently to build on the same kind of methods to reverse the positive representations of tobacco and alcoholic beverages patiently reinforced by generations of marketing experts. Tellingly, CFES staff never considered producing the audiovisual supports on their own; they hired advertising firms, thus initiating collaboration between two social worlds that proved crucial to the rise of health education and, more broadly, 'public communication' in France.[55] These expenses, added to the cost of advertisement slots, despite the bargains allowed by the 'Office de la Radio et de la Télévision Française' (ORTF, the public body in charge of both state-owned radio and television), the cost of the campaign increased to 2.9 million francs, out of the 6.7 million allocated to CFES in 1976.[56]

The 'educative' approach developed on television and radio was slightly different.[57] Films (some aiming at a general audience, others targeting a specific kind of smoker) drew on the evocative power of images to display a grim, repulsive version of tobacco, or to alert about specific aspects of smoking. In the former category was a 'spot' (CFES' staff had already picked up the parlance of French advertising professionals) displaying a cold, filthy and implicitly smelly ashtray full of butts; a second film went along the same line: non-smokers and ex-smokers were facing the camera and telling the various reasons they had to stay away from cigarettes, including the kind of offensive *sensory* onslaughts perpetrated by tobacco smoke (terrible odours at home, awful breath, smelly hair and clothes, etc.). Films belonging to the latter variety were more dramatic still. One of them displayed smoke clouds as a representation of smoking-induced air pollution. In another spot, a director had shot a child mimicking smokers with a fake cigarette, a remarkable evocation of the theory hammered all through the parliamentary discussion, the previous year, that the spectacle of smokers induced a mimetic response in impressionable youngsters. Even more striking, perhaps, was a film that intended to underline the dangers of smoking on the foetus. It showed a serene pregnant woman talking to a child, while both looked at the mother's swelling belly: 'You know, he/she [the French '*le*' theoretically encompasses both sexes] eats everything I eat, drinks everything I drink.' This prompted a question from the child: 'And when you smoke, does he/she smoke as well?' that, in turn, brought about plain anxiety on the mother's face. The oral messages produced for the campaign departed from this style of dramatisation: in accordance with representations of the time, radio was considered to be a medium that, contrary to television, allowed for more sophisticated communication. Although tobacco was still sometimes presented as the cause of disagreement (and an assault against the sensibility of fellow human beings, as in a spot that evoked smokers' 'smelly breath'), more conceptual issues were addressed. One of these messages, interestingly, quoted epidemiological data in order to inform about the shortening of life expectancy and the risks of life-threatening diseases induced by smoking. This was a clear appeal to the rationality of the audience.

CFES staff relied on a post-campaign survey to tell whether their strategy of persuasion had been successful. Although this investigation was based on nothing more than 450 face-to-face interviews (to make things worse, only 361 of them were fully exploited) the firm, specialised in market research, presented the interviewees (who had not been chosen by sampling but through the alternative 'quota' method) as 'representative of the French population aged fifteen and over'.[58] The results were rather mixed, with elements that were easy to emphasise as legitimising the new form of health education, while some other data tended to cast doubt on the effectiveness of the initiative. The 'memorisation' of spots was judged good by advertising standards (the investigators had no experience except in commercial communication): 11 per cent of the interviewees spontaneously mentioned the campaign when asked about the commercials they had recently seen, while 70 per cent recalled it after they were shown a list of promotions that included the anti-smoking films.[59] Still, by advertising standards, the understanding of the message behind the campaign, and the memorisation of the slogan: '*Sans tabac, prenons la vie à plein poumon!*' was rated 'good',[60] although the figures showed that only 34 per cent of the respondents had been able to verbalise it, either entirely or partially. The wide variety of films also played against their impact: only four out of the 361 interviewees that had seen at least one spot were able to describe four, or more, of the nine films. Much worse, when asked about the initiative, 55 per cent of the respondents judged it 'non-convincing', 57 per cent 'non-effective', and 86 per cent of the smokers (158 out of the 361) avowed they would not quit. At the same time, 49 per cent of the same interviewees declared they were 'very favourable to such an initiative', while a further 29 per cent were merely 'favourable'; 75 per cent described it as 'honest', 75 per cent 'serious' and 57 per cent 'objective'. Unsurprisingly, the Press and Information Division in the Ministry of Health put forward these last statistics in a document issued just after the end of the campaign.[61]

These contrasting preliminary results fuelled doubts about the so-called scientific approach advocated by Le Net, which had been raised by senior staff.[62] His hyper-rational representation of human agency was dubbed idealistic, while the various kinds of marketing experts hired by CFES had alerted them (in meetings and during their frequent conversations) about the difficulties they continually experienced in their efforts to grasp and change human behaviour. At the same time, the head of CFES was getting into trouble with Simone Veil, who found him much too rigid in his views, and not receptive enough to her ministerial desiderata. This double conflict led to the replacement of the engineer by Veil's public relations adviser, Françoise Buhl, who brought both a new style of management and a new approach to health communication.

What are the motivations behind risky behaviour? Towards a more sophisticated understanding of prevention

The late 1970s proved a critical period for the handful of French health education specialists challenged to 'professionalise' at great speed what was still a small, although highly visible, corner within a wide array of public health practices. Indeed, their doubts about the true impact of media campaigns (to which their fate was linked) developed in parallel with reservations on the morality and the political implications of their methods of prevention. This was never as visible as when Claude Vilain and Marc Danzon, who were Le Net's more senior collaborators, revolted against his authoritarianism. Both had been instrumental in the creation and growth of a Research and Studies Department, in charge of monitoring French attitudes towards tobacco as well as the evaluation of campaigns, and in the production of the audiovisual materials, in close collaboration with advertising professionals. They became even more central within the Committee after Françoise Buhl, who appreciated them and needed their fresh experience of mass media,[63] had taken over from Michel Le Net. Both Vilain and Danzon were equally eager to promote a kind of health education that would break away from the vision of prevention as 'normalisation' of human behaviour, which had informed public health discourse and practice in the past.[64] Leftist young professionals working for a right-of-centre government that needed their expertise, they were receptive to the counter-cultural movements of the time, critical of authoritarianism and wary of the so-called 'medicalisation' of society. The former, who graduated in statistics and held a masters (technically a 'Diplôme d'Études Supérieures') in economics, was deeply interested in the critical analysis of modern society in general, and Western medicine in particular. When interviewed he mentioned, unsolicited, reading the likes of Ivan Illich and Thomas Szasz with great interest, and discussing these views with friends and relatives.[65] In 1975, he had also taken a sabbatical year 'on the road' and travelled the world. Marc Danzon, one among the very few French physicians who became interested in mass-media communication, as early as 1972,[66] stressed the impact of the 'community health' approach on his views.[67] In 1980–1, they were joined by Jean Tavarès, a sociologist who had just completed a doctorate under the supervision of Pierre Bourdieu (at the 'École des Hautes Études en Sciences Sociales') and elaborated his own, though convergent, critical approach to prevention.[68]

Importantly, none of them ever disjoined, let alone opposed, the search for effectiveness in health education to the necessity to stop 'blaming the victim' and start taking individual experience into consideration.[69] On the contrary, they always believed that providing a serious scientific basis for prevention strategies would *ipso facto* 'purify' health education of any authoritarian-normative temptation, while respecting the subjectivity of the targeted audience was a *sine qua non* to any real improvement of campaign efficiency.[70] In other words, their critical stance on the evolution of Western civilisation did not stop them believing in a possible ideological neutrality of (true and good) science, nor in the possibility to reconcile scientific planning of human actions with consideration for individual experience. Françoise Buhl had every reason to endorse this programme in full. As head of CFES, she was unsurprisingly as keen as they were to improve the impact of health education; at the same time she also wanted to avoid giving rise to suspicion that her agenda was nothing but a manipulation of public opinion on behalf of the government. In this respect, she believed the stress on '*éducation pour la santé*' as a positive enterprise that aimed at strengthening individual control of one's health would help undermine such criticisms. Her intervention on a programme aired by Bavarian radio in 1980 made this view explicit: 'Under no circumstances should one scare the audience or make them feel guilty. On the contrary, we wish that anyone, conscious of the various risk factors he or she is confronted with, takes his or her health in charge'.[71]

This view, shared by Buhl and her closest collaborators (who were allowed some latitude in the preparation and implementation of action) paved the way to a true *aggiornamento* of CFES's doctrine: information was not good enough anymore. Accordingly, they turned to social sciences, social psychology in particular, both in the guise of academic research and applied social technologies of the kind developed by advertising professionals and marketing experts since the interwar period. The fix to any shortcomings were in a real, in-depth understanding of human behaviour, combined with a proper comprehension of the reception of images and oral messages by audiences.

A very crucial moment in this history was the discovery of 'Motivation Research', in late 1977. Although this new approach to marketing and advertising had been elaborated in the USA in the aftermath of the Second World War, it was not used in France before 1959, and did not become common practice before the mid-1970s.[72] A new attempt to build on psychology and social psychology to make advertisements more effective,[73] Motivation Research aimed at deciphering the emotional and symbolic background to purchases. In the aftermath of the pioneer smoking prevention campaign, under a backcloth of interrogations regarding the seeming irrationality of risky behaviour, Marc Danzon contacted Emeric Deutsch, who had been instrumental in the development of such investigations in France. Deutsch's career illustrated the numerous tight links between social scientists keen to 'apply' their knowledge and communication entrepreneurs at a time when this activity was becoming increasingly important in both economic and political life. The head of SOFRES Communication, the branch of the French pioneer and still dominant polling firm specialised in Motivation Research,[74] he also held an academic position and introduced social psychology to the curriculum at the Institut d'Études Politiques de Paris. Danzon and his aides asked him to investigate the reasons that led teenagers to start smoking. He set up a qualitative study based on in-depth interviews with children and teenagers aged eight to sixteen, and detailed his views on the problem in a comprehensive report.[75] According to Deutsch, the interviews with those of the teenagers who had already started to smoke revealed, in great detail, how they came to internalise pressure from their peers, which was strong enough to make them persevere in the practice despite their unanimous initial aversion to the acrid smoke and the harsh taste of cigarettes. The ultimate cause of smoking initiation was therefore the so-called 'social image of the cigarette', and especially the 'smoker myth' ('*mythe du fumeur*') that made teenagers want to emulate adults.[76] It is not overstating the importance of this report to say that Deutsch's analysis paved the way for the communication strategy on smoking developed by CFES until the present time. Since the campaign launched in 1978 to convince teenagers and young adults that 'stub a cigarette out' was a good way to 'win some freedom', the explicit goal of health education in this domain has constantly been to undermine the positive 'social image' of cigarettes, and (from the late 1980s onwards) to advertise the non-smoker as an active, fun-loving, independent-minded young person.[77]

However, Emeric Deutsch was not the only expert hired by the Committee to fix their communication, nor was smoking the only issue addressed by means of health education. Another important campaign, perhaps the most famous of all CFES's, provides interesting insights into their intensive use of social research. Launched in February 1984 with the aim of convincing French adults to avoid 'excessive drinking', the films and oral messages drew on in-depth preparatory research and a sophisticated model of drinking incitement. The background of Claude Vilain's main adviser on this occasion, Éliséo Véron, was remarkably analogous to Deutsch's: after a doctorate in sociology and many publications,[78] he had joined a marketing research firm as Scientific Director. The stakes were especially high: the initiative on alcoholism had been long delayed by the previous government for fear of reactions from organised interests and rural populations. CFES's staff were anxious to avoid being seen as blaming, or simply patronising drinkers, as they knew how sensitive the topic was. Excessive drinking was also the province of the Haut Comité d'Etude et d'Information sur l'Alcoolisme, although by the late 1970s they had lost most of the dynamism they had displayed from the mid 1950s to the early 1970s. The issue was therefore euphemistically reframed as 'excessive drinking' instead of alcoholism, and Véron was asked to set out a campaign strategy that would break away with the 'top-down' model of communication (as illustrated in the pioneer 1976 campaign when 'receptors' were subjected to 'information' diffused by a then unknown 'transmitting' body). With the assistance of a few aides, he engaged in a qualitative investigation into 'the typology of drinking opportuni-ties',[79] with a special interest in the social dynamic of drinking in three different 'spheres': at work, 'with friends and acquaintances', and in the family. In each case, they analysed the specific sociability to find out what kind of interaction led otherwise sensible adults to ingest much more alcohol than they had origi-nally planned, or even wanted to. They especially detailed the ritual of the 'round' ('*la tournée*' in French): interviewees were unambiguous on how committing this generalised exchange of drinking was. 'One cannot turn down a drink,' an interviewee said, without worrying about the reaction of the group one belongs to: the main apprehension was that this refusal might be wrongly interpreted as a snub, an affirmation of exteriority that would, in return, induce negative reactions from peers and, ultimately, marginalise the eccentric.[80] Consequently, Véron advocated the need to put forward to those willing to avoid drinking in excess a pragmatic way to escape the 'round' without fearing this could endanger their social positions. Following an intuition, he started to explore the common knowledge on excessive drinking expressed in popular sayings: three full pages of the report were filled with dictums and aphorisms relating to the dangers of alcohol.[81] The assumption was that such impersonal, widely diffused and often ironic views could not be confused with the tradi-tional medical (and pseudo-medical) advice on alcoholism that was so easily despised as patronising. The very products of the kind of sociability the inter-viewees were so eager to maintain, they differed in form if not content from these recommendations, and were seen as an impersonal 'voice of reason' the individuals could follow without feeling awkward *vis-à-vis* their friends, colleagues or relatives. Éliséo Véron summarised his point in his report:

> The dictum calls on popular wisdom. The one who enunciates it does not pose as a specific moral authority....The enunciator of a dictum is not therefore personally committed [in what he or she says] but increases his or her standing as he or she finds the right time to 'put it in'.[82]

The idea appealed very much to CFES and the copywriters hired for the occasion were asked to work along this line. They ended up with a series of eight films based on the same framework: individuals belonging to various social classes and age groups, and portrayed in different settings (at work, at the restaurant, at a party, etc.) started drinking together, until one of them made clear he or she did not want his or her glass to be filled again. He or she added words to body language by saying, in a funny way, as a matter of joke: '*Un verre ça va, trois verres: bonjour les dégâts!*'[83] All the films ended on the enunciation of a single slogan: 'For our health, let's opt for moderation!'

The campaign proved a great success, at least by social communication standards: according to a survey undertaken in 1984 on behalf of the Committee, 70 per cent of the interviewees spontaneously remembered and quoted the famous '*Un verre ça va...*', and were able to tell it referred to an initiative on excessive drinking.[84] An overview of the campaign dated 4 October 1984 proudly announced that 'The memorisation of and adherence to [the campaign] are the highest that have been recorded so far in the field of social communication, what is more on an especially difficult topic'.[85]

Moreover, 25 per cent of the interviewees who had watched the campaign on television or listened to it on the radio had discussed the films and the messages with their relatives or their friends: 'This last result' was perceived as 'especially interesting, as it is an indicator of the penetration of the action within the social fabric ['*le tissu social*']'.[86] Finally, this effort in preventing alcoholism was very often put forward by CFES, in their discussions with the more academic social scientists they wanted to enrol in their activities, as a model of health education that built on individual experience of risk instead of patronising the audience.

From the late 1970s onwards, senior staff at CFES had wished to establish close links with academically well-established social scientists and some public health scientists interested in the social dimensions of risky behaviour (especially the very few French researchers interested in social epidemiology). The reasons were twofold. First, they increasingly felt the need to follow up mass-media campaigns by 'fieldwork actions' ('*actions de terrain*'). Social knowledge about the various communities, as well as face-to-face communication processes, were two kinds of expertise alien to Motivation Research, and other varieties of marketing studies were seen as crucial in this respect. Second, and more symbolically, in these years of radical critics of the 'capitalist system', the few French social scientists interested in health, together with some public health scientists, had started setting out a discourse on the necessary reappropriation of health by individuals described as threatened by the 'medicalisation of society'.[87] As critical as they could be, individually, marketing and advertising experts, who were functionally associated with the expansion of this despised capitalist society, could not measure up to these academics. Yet, working closely with anti-authoritarian researchers was seen as a good way to protect them from widespread accusation. So widespread that in 1982 even a right-of-centre pioneer health economist could warn:

> Today, many are those who have realised that the forces of 'normalisation' and social control have taken new, and therefore more insidious, forms: the policeman and the judge have given way to the physician, the journalist, the teacher...and why not the health educator.[88]

CFES attempted to meet this challenge by building a strong and tight collaboration with various fields in health research. Their initial and crucial move took the form of a conference they organised on 21 and 22 March 1983. Sociologists, social psychologists, anthropologists, economists and psychologists interested in health, together with the few epidemiologists interested in the social determinants of disease, the very few public health researchers interested in health education and a group of 'social psychiatrists', had been previously approached by Tavarès, who had all the credentials to mix with academics. During the opening session, partly by conviction and partly to help scientists feel well disposed toward CFES's approach, senior staff members made several declarations of goodwill and displayed all the signs of their openness to criticism. In his opening presentation, Jean-Marie Cohen-Solal, who had succeeded Françoise Buhl as head of the Committee, directly addressed his academic guests:

> We do not consider your contribution [to health education research] as simply a means to potentialise our power of persuasion, or increase at any cost some kind of effectiveness....For your part, please consider our initiative as the query of an institution, if not in search for an epistemological rupture, at least in a situation of methodological doubt and serious self-questioning.[89]

Academics, in return, elaborated their views on health education and presented research they believed could serve to improve both mass-media campaigns and fieldwork follow-ups. Moreover, the conference allowed both parties to make contacts and start to know each other. The Committee intended to move forward in this nascent collaboration, and thus enrol the scientists, by funding some applied research on many aspects of risky behaviour through substantial grants. Unfortunately, in spring 1986, after a couple of years of reduction in public expenditure, the newly elected right-wing government decided on an even greater reduction in governmental budgets. As health education was not a priority anymore, CFES's budget plummeted (the situation did not improve before the beginning of the 1990s) and most of the senior staff, who had thought through and implemented the *aggiornamento*, including the plan for a collaboration with academic social and public health scientists, eventually left the Committee. The grant scheme intended to develop proper research in health education, a domain in which France was commonly castigated as backward, was never really put into practice. The grand plan for highly professional health education, co-ordinated by a well-respected CFES, fed by (finally) well-funded and active research in various social sciences, in an effort to help citizens 'reappropriate' their health, was in tatters.

The fiasco had critical consequences for the history of health education in France. On the one hand, a historic opportunity to develop some real research in 'fieldwork action' in support of mass-media campaigns, and train health educators in this practice, was lost, and has not yet occurred again. On the other hand, CFES had to rely solely on marketing and advertising experts in the planning of mass-media campaigns. This left their key activity open to criticisms: those unsympathetic to this kind of prevention would easily despise it as nothing but symbolic action.

Notes

1 'Intervention du Dr Jean-Martin Cohen-Solal, Délégué général du Comité Français d'Éducation pour la santé', *Actes de la XIIème conférence mondiale d'éducation pour la santé*, Dublin, 1985. p. 10. C. Rollet-Echalier, *La Politique à l'égard de la petite enfance sous la IIIe République*, Paris: PUF, 1990; R. Talmy, *Histoire du mouvement familial en France, 1896–1939*, Paris: Union Nationale des Caisses d'Allocations Familiales, 1962, 2 vols.

2 I translate the French 'ministre' as 'minister', although their status is usually more akin to those enjoyed by the British 'Secretaries of State'.

3 C. Ollivier-Yaniv (ed.), 'L'État communicant. Les formes de la communication gouvrenementale', special issue of *Quaderni. La revue de la communication* 33, 1997; L. Berlivet, 'Une Biopolitique de la santé. La fabrique des campagnes de prévention', in D. Fassin and D. Memmi (eds), *Le Gouvernement des corps*, Paris: Éditions de l'École des Hautes Études en Sciences Sociales, 2004, pp. 37–75. The dramatic AIDS epidemic also prompted research on public attempts to prevent contamination (see for example V. Berridge, *Aids in the UK. The Making of Policy, 1981–1994*, Oxford: Oxford University Press, 1996). Another interesting exception is Charles Webster's account of the difficulties of implementing health education and prevention in the NHS: *The Health Services since the War*, vol. 1: *Problems of Health care: the National Health Service before 1957*, London: HMSO, 1988, pp. 377–9.

4 For example: T.E. Backer, E. M. Rogers and P. Sapory, *Designing Health Communication Campaigns: What Works?* Newbury Park, CA: Sage, 1992.

5 On the rise of 'risk factor epidemiology' in the wake of pioneer British and US investigations of the relationship between smoking and lung cancer, and the questions it raised, see L. Berlivet '"Association or causation?" The debate on the scientific status of risk factor epidemiology, 1947–c.1965', in V. Berridge (ed.) *Making Health Policy*, Amsterdam: Rodopi, 2005. Interestingly, the AIDS epidemic did not overturn the pre-eminence of concerns about non-transmissible diseases that originated in the aftermath of the Second World War. First, the aetiology of AIDS was investigated through a broad range of scientific methods

including these very epidemiological techniques that had been developed in cancer and cardiovascular research, 'case-control studies' and 'cohort studies' (G.M. Oppenheimer, 'Causes, cases and cohorts: the role of epidemiology in the historical construction of AIDS', in E. Fee and D.M. Fox (eds), *AIDS: the Making of a Chronic Disease*, Berkley: University of California Press, 1992, pp. 49–83; J. Fujimura and D.Y. Chou, 'Dissent in science: styles of scientific practice and the controversy over the cause of AIDS', *Social Science and Medicine* 38, 1994: 1017–36; S. Epstein, *Impure Science. Aids, Activism and the Politics of Knowledge*, Berkeley: University of California Press, 1996, especially p. 405, note 100). Second, here again health education campaigns came to be seen as the necessary tools for persuading lovers to adopt 'safer-sex' practices and heroin addicts not to exchange syringes – in short, the only way to curb new contaminations.

6 Hereafter abbreviated to 'the Committee' or referred to by the acronym 'CFES'.

7 In brackets is the year of first airing of a media campaign on the topic. For more information on the recurrence of these topics and their comparative importance in the history of health education in France, see L. Berlivet, 'Une santé à risques. L'action publique de lutte contre l'alcoolisme et le tabagisme en France (1954–1999)', unpublished doctoral thesis, Univeristé Rennes I, 2000, Chapter 6.

8 This campaign was sponsored from the very start by CNAM-TS, the French compulsory health insurance scheme that covers salaried employees.

9 MMR stands for Measles-Mumps-Rubella ('Rougeole-Oreillons-Rubéole' in French).

10 M. Foucault, 'Le souci de la vérité', in *Dits et écrits. 1954–1988*, Paris: Gallimard, 1994, vol. IV: 1980–8, pp. 668–78 (initially published in *Le Magazine littéraire* in May 1984), and 'Entretien avec Michel Foucault', *Dits et écrits*, pp. 286–95 (initially published in *Masques* 13, spring 1982). The *modus operandi* of this '*problématisation*' has been analysed in Berlivet, 'Une biopolitique de la santé, pp. 37–75.

11 On the efforts of CFES to develop and organize what they called 'the network' of health education professionals, see Berlivet, 'Une santé à risques', chapters 5 and 7.

12 T. Lefebvre, 'Cinéma et discourse hygiéniste (1890–1930)', unpublished doctoral thesis, University of Paris III, 1996. Among the pioneers that started screening health education films in France was the Rockefeller Foundation; Louis-Ferdinand Destouches, who toured the French provinces lecturing on the perils of tuberculosis before reaching literary fame under the name of Céline: 'Interview avec Claude Bonnefoy', reprinted in *Cahiers Céline, vol. 2: Céline et l'actualité littéraire 1957–1961*, Paris: Gallimard, 1976, p. 214.

13 See M. Edelman's 'trilogy': *The Symbolic Uses of Politics*, Urbana: University of Illinois Press, 1964; *Politics as a Symbolic Action*, Chicago: Chicago University Press, 1971; and *Political Language: Words That Succeeded, Politics That Failed*, New York: Academic Press, 1977.

14 The development of these specific campaigns has been analysed by Geneviève Paicheler, *Prévention du sida et agenda politique. Les campagnes en direction du grand public (1987–1996)*, Paris: CNRS Éditions, 2002. This specific treatment signals the singularity of the politicisation of AIDS in France, compared to other public health issues; see. P. Favre (ed.), *Sida et Politique. Les premiers affrontements (1981–1987)*, Paris: L'Harmattan, 1992. Such a difference between the style of AIDS campaigns and actions aimed at reducing other health risks was (at least partially) due to the fact that, from 1989 to 1994, the CFES lost any responsibility for the former and a specific institution, the Agence Française de Lutte contre le Sida, was established for this purpose.

15 I trace the origin and the development of what I metaphorically call 'compulsion' in Berlivet, 'Une santé à risque', pp. 830–42. The airing of films and radio

spots over the entire French territory made impossible the organisation of any case-control studies, such as implemented in other domains (including health education interventions), as an extremely high proportion of the population had been exposed to the campaign. Indeed, only the tiny fraction of the population that had neither access to television nor radio programmes could have been used to assemble a 'control group', even back in the mid-1970s these individuals could hardly have been regarded as representative of the whole French population.

16 Between the many publications that came out of this case-control study, see for example: D. Schwartz and P. Denoix, 'L'enquête française sur l'étiologie du cancer broncho-pulmonaire: le rôle du tabac', *La Semaine des Hôpitaux de Paris* 33 1957: 424–37.

17 The 'Commission du cancer' was established in 1922 under the umbrella of the 'Conseil supérieur d'hygiène publique de France'. See P. Pinell, *Naissance d'un fléau. La lutte contre le cancer en France, 1890–1940*, Paris: A.-M. Métailié, 1992, pp. 160–5. See also M. Tubiana's memoirs: *La Lumière dans l'ombre. Le cancer hier et demain*, Paris: Odile Jacob, 1991.

18 See Berlivet, 'Une santé à risque', pp. 73–90; Robert Flament, one of the two physicians among the French pioneers of medical statistics led by Daniel Schwartz, in the 1950s, gave a vivid account of the contempt for the probabilistic way of thinking shown by his fellow interns: *Malades ou cobaye. Plaidoyer pour les essais thérapeutiques*, Paris: Albin Michel, 1994, pp. 24–5.

19 Tubiana, *La Lumière dans l'ombre*, p. 55. The Schwartzs and the Tubianas own neighbouring chalets in a French mountain resort and spend holidays together. Another exception to this widespread 'distrust in numbers' within the French medical elite was Pierre Denoix, a surgeon and cancerologist, who hired Daniel Schwartz to set up the aforementioned pioneer epidemiological investigation, and later secured him a position at the Institut National de la Santé et de la Recherche Médicale as well as funding for his statistical research unit. See Berlivet, 'Une santé à risque', Chapter 1.

20 Indeed, Maurice Tubiana, Simone Veil and her relatives all confirmed the meeting and the matter discussed (Berlivet, 'Une santé à risqué', pp. 347–8). An article that corroborates this version was published by the evening newspaper *La Croix* on 17 September 1975, that is to say months after the date of the meeting, under the headline: 'Mrs Veil launches the anti-tobacco campaign'.

21 Ibid. Interestingly, the account of the episode given by the journalist reads as a 'conversion narrative': 'Mme Simone Veil fumait. Comme beaucoup de Français et désormais, hélas, beaucoup de Françaises. Elle a discuté un jour avec le Professeur Denoix, directeur de l'Institut anti-cancer [sic] de Villejuif. Celui-ci l'a convaincue des dangers réels que représentent, pour le fumeur lui-même et pour les autres, contraints de respirer sa fumée, la consommation d'une trop grande quantité de tabac....Mme Veil a donc décidé d'arrêter de fumer et d'inviter les autres à en faire autant.' This way, Pierre Denoix's exercise in medical counselling on smoking (his own answer to the rise in lung cancers and respiratory diseases, as mentioned above) was to play a small, still symbolic, part in the political history of smoking. Françoise Buhl, Simone Veil's ministerial adviser on public health issues of the time, confirmed the chronology (interview, 23 January 1996).

22 Interview with Françoise Buhl. It would however be incongruous to bring her engagement in smoking down to a tactical consideration; on the contrary, this moment in French public health policy illustrates the traditional difficulties in analysing the complexities of decision-making processes.

23 Voted on 20 December 1974 by both assemblies after over a month of fierce debate, the law was promulgated on 17 January 1975 (initially for a limited five-

year period; a second act, voted in 1979, prorogued it). J.G. Padioleau, 'La lutte politique quotidienne: caractéristiques et régulation de l'agenda politique. L'exemple de l'interruption de grossesse', in *L'État au concret*, Paris: PUF, 1982, pp. 23–47.

24 Françoise Buhl also stressed how much Simone Veil (encouraged on this by her advisers) was eager to 'position herself more as Minister of prevention' (interview).

25 On the history of the 'Association Française contre l'abus du tabac', established in 1868, see D. Nourrisson, 'Tabagisme et anti-tabagisme en France au XIXème siècle', *Histoire, économie et société* 7, 1988: 491–547.

26 In her introductory speech before the Senate, Simone Veil declared: 'calculations building on well established information already allow to estimate this cost [of smoking] up to many billions of our Francs. To me, these data, alone, seems to justify our action' (*Journal officiel du Sénat; débats*, 12 juin 1976, p. 1889). At the same time, the member of the National Assembly in charge of reporting on the text was telling her colleagues that 'babies born from mothers who smoked' suffered a 'special frailty', due to the fact that 'their average weight [at birth] was lower than those of non-smokers (about 250 grams less and a smaller height, about 3cms less)'. M. Tisné, *Rapport au nom de la commission des affaires culturelles, familiales et sociales sur le projet de loi relatif à la lutte contre le tabagisme*, no. 2318, 25 mai 1976, *Journal officiel de l'Assemblée Nationale; documents parlementaires*, p. 25.

27 She was first quoted on this by a newspaper (*Le Figaro*, 16 September 1975) and developed her point in an interview to the influential newsmagazine *L'Express* (22 September 1975): 'Ce que je recherche, c'est que les Français, bien informés, prennent eux-mêmes leurs responsabilités vis-à-vis de leur santé. Ils pourront continuer de s'intoxiquer, mais en connaissance de cause.' This approach was to be reasserted by the Minister during the parliamentary debate; see the *Journal officiel de l'Assemblée Nationale; débats*, 12 June 1976, p. 4077

28 Ibid., pp. 4075–6. Unfortunately, Simone Veil did not disclose the identity of these 'foreign countries' mentioned as counter-model.

29 *Journal officiel; lois et décrets*, 10 July 1976, pp. 4148–9; Technically, the law delegated the regulation of smoking in public places, mainly buildings, to the government, although any administrative measure would have to be approved by the Conseil d'État.

30 Vance Packard's scathing attack on advertising (*The Hidden Persuaders*, New York: David McKay & Co, 1957) had been translated in French as soon as it was published, *La Persuasion clandestine*, Paris: Calmann-Levy, 1958. Indeed, negative reactions towards modern advertising in France dated back to the nascent rise of a consumer society modelled on the US way of life, in the 1950s: R.F. Kuisel, *Seducing the French. The Dilemma of Americanization*, Berkeley: University of California Press, 1993, pp. 88–9. The very belief in the power of advertising that underlay such fears was criticised by M. Schudson, *Advertising, The Uneasy Persuasion. Its Dubious Impact on American Society*, New York: Basic Books, 1984.

31 See Article 7. For a comprehensive analysis of the law, see F. Caballero, *Droit de la drogue*, Paris: Dalloz, 1989. Moreover, the second paragraph of Article 7 intended to prevent a switch in advertising medium by limiting the yearly surface authorised to advertisements for tobacco in the press to the mean of the surfaces really used for that purpose in 1974 and 1975. (A decree published in the *Journal officiel; lois et décrets,* on 21 March 1978, p. 1237, set up a commission in charge of monitoring the implementation of this paragraph, the: 'Commission d'observation des campagnes publicitaires'.)

32 This was the only statistic on smoking available to the Ministry at that time. The figure came out of a survey of 1,000 persons older than seventeen passed by

SOFRES (a polling firm) in December 1974. 21 per cent of the respondents declared they were smoking less than ten cigarettes per day; 15 per cent smoked between eleven and twenty cigarettes per day; while 5 per cent declared smoking more than twenty cigarettes per day.

33 'Multiple realities' refers to the phenomenological approach to society developed by the German-American sociologist A. Schütz: 'On multiple realities', in *Collected Papers, Volume I: the Problem of Social Reality*, ed. Maurice Natanson, The Hague: Martinus Nijhoff, 1962, pp. 207–59 (first published in 1945).

34 Tisné, Rapport au nom de la commission des affaires culturelles, p. 25.

35 On the role played by these epidemiological investigations on the controversies over the risks of passive smoking from the early 1980s onwards, see Berlivet, 'Une santé à risqué', Chapter 2.

36 The rhetoric of the report to the Commission in charge of health issues prepared by Monique Tisné (a Member of Parliament who strongly supported Simone Veil's approach to tobacco smoking all through the legislative process) was based on a mix of scientific statements and moral considerations. Her warning about the hazards of passive smoking only followed a paragraph stating the need for a regulation of smoking in order to reinstate a lost 'courtesy': as smokers did not refrain from smoking in public places any more, the government had become responsible for protecting non-smokers who, too often, did not dare 'manifest [their] trouble towards sometimes invading smoking habits'. *Rapport au nom de la commission des affaires culturelles, familiales et sociales*, p. 37. Interestingly, the French '*gêne*' (trouble) used by the member of parliament can refer both to a mere bother or a physical discomfort.

37 One will remember that this very representation of mimetic smoking underlined Maurice Tubinana's request to Simone Veil never to appear on TV with a cigarette. The rationale for such a prohibition had been already made explicit by a parliamentarian in his intervention before the National Assembly: '*exemplarity* is an important element of anti-smoking propaganda. Those who are called to teach should not only point at the consequences of cigarette smoking, but also ought to set an example, so the youngsters [*les jeunes*] would not be tempted.' Jean Fontaine, *Journal officiel de l'Assemblée Nationalel; débats*, 12 June 1976, p. 4081. The emphasis is mine.

38 Decree no. 77–1042, dated 12 September 1977, published in the *Journal officiel, lois et décrets*, 17 September 1977, p. 4609. For a juridical analysis of the text, see Caballero, *Droit de la drogue*, pp. 148–51.

39 Reporting on Simone Veil's plans, two years before, the most influential French newspapers had advised that: 'Because of the 'exemplar' role they can play, doctors, midwifes, nurses, teachers and educators should be especially targeted at by this [anti-smoking] campaign.', in 'L'action anti-tabac' est reconnue comme une grande cause nationale', *Le Monde*, 18 September 1975.

40 The Ministry of Finance was doubly interested in the proposed policy: first, because of its possible impact on tobacco consumption and, consequently, fiscal income; second, because at that time the business of tobacco was still under the control of a state monopoly, and with a strong state-owned manufacturer, SEITA, selling popular cigarette brands like 'Gauloise' and 'Gitane'.

41 M.D. Read, 'Policy networks and issue networks. The politics of smoking', in D. Marsh and R.A.W. Rhodes, *Policy Networks in British Government*, Oxford: Clarendon Press, 1992, pp. 124–47

42 J.G. Padioleau, 'La lutte contre le tabagisme: action politique et régulation de la vie quotidienne', in *L'État au concret*, Paris: PUF, 1982, p. 58.

43 The representatives of the foreign manufacturers did not miss the point; they attacked the disposition in the press (see 'Tabac le projet de Simone Veil' in *L'Express*, 24 May 1976), and lobbied the parliamentarians in a highly conspicuous

way, which was derided by another news magazine, *Le Nouvel Observateur*, 31 May 1976. The assumption was wrong, anyway, and SEITA's share of the tobacco market fell to 73.5 per cent in 1980; 58.9 per cent in 1985; 50.6 per cent in 1990; and 37.2 in 1997 (information provided by SEITA to the author).

44 The excise revenue had amounted to 5 billion and 945 million Francs in 1975; by then, taxes had risen up to 72 per cent of the price of cigarettes (Tisné, *Rapport*, p. 13). Evolutions of the retail price index were especially sensitive in postwar France, for it impacted on salary increases that were renegotiated every year by unions and employers' representatives.

45 Already, in 1917, the Rockefeller Foundation had integrated health propaganda (including films, as mentioned previously; an exhibition conveyed by car around the country; posters; and pamphlets) in the action plan of its 'Commission for the Prevention of Tuberculosis in France'. See L. Murard and P. Zylberman, 'Les fondations indestructibles: la santé publique en France et la Fondation Rockefeller', *Médecine/Sciences* 28, 2002: 625–32, and *idem*, 'La mission Rockefeller en France et la création du comité nationale de défense contre la tuberculose (1917–1923)', *Revue d'histoire moderne et contemporaine* 34, 1987: 257–81.

46 Here again, Françoise Buhl was instrumental. When interviewed, she remembered vividly her discovery of the documents on pioneer experiences issued by the International Union, as well as meetings with heads of the foreign institutions in charge of such campaigns. She was especially fascinated by her study trips in Scotland, Sweden and the USA, where she discovered the large-scale and meticulously planned actions set up by the American Heart Society.

47 An 'official' report on the institutional history of health education in France came out in 1982: É. Lévy, 'Deuxième rapport présenté au nom du Conseil Économique et Social: l'éducation pour la santé, séance de 22 et 23 juin 1982', *Journal officiel; avis et rapports du Conseil Économique et Social*, Thursday 7 October 1982.

48 Since the late 1980s, the Committee's accounting was also subjected to the rules of the public sector.

49 See L. Berlivet 'De l'éducation sanitaire à la promotion de la santé. La santé publique face aux accusations de moralisme', in A. Garrigou (ed.), *La Santé dans tous ses états*, Biarritz: Atlantica, pp. 243–70. It is therefore no surprise that commentators like Alfred Sauvy (a statistician, economist and demographer who had been instrumental in the stabilisation of the intellectual framework of the French '*populationiste*' movement) frequently offered to popularise their views in *La Santé de l'homme*. On Sauvy, see Paul-André Rosental, *L'Intelligence démographique. Sciences et politiques des populations en France (1930–1960)*, Paris: Éditions Odile Jacob, 2003.

50 The first in a long series of public communication campaigns was broadcast on television and radio in 1973 to popularise newly passed legislation that made seat-belts compulsory. See S. Decreton, 'Les trois temps de la communication de sécurité routière', *Quaderni. La revue de la communication* 33, 1997: 85–98.

51 Interview with Michel Le Net, 16 January 1996.

52 Ibid. Victim, perhaps, of this Manichean representation, Le Net constantly overestimates the role of medical and public health researchers on French health education policies. It was not until the 1990s that a few public health doctors started to train in health education.

53 *Tableau de bord anti-tabac*, 28 July 1976, p. 1; archives of the 'Service Études et Recherches', CFES. Four kinds of data were seen as necessary to a real following and control over action: 1) an 'indicator of knowledge and opinion' based on surveys passed before and after the campaign, and completed by an investigation in a maternity ward; 2) 'indicators of behaviour', based on the evolution in

tobacco sales and the demand for 'de-intoxication counselling'; 3) 'morbidity and mortality indicators' (still, only the latter was made available to CFES); 4) 'indicators of action', alleged to measure the 'persuasion effort' put into practice during the campaign, and based on the number of messages broadcast, the volume of edited pamphlet, etc.

54 This second possibility had been explored by the CFES before 1975, but considered unable to capture the attention of any large audience.

55 For more on the role of 'advertising gurus' and communication experts at different moments in the history of French health education, and in other fields of governmental communication, see: C. Ollivier-Yaniv (ed.), *L'État communicant. Les formes de la communication gouvrenementale*, Special issue of *Quaderni. La revue de la communication* 33, 1997; and M. Le Net, *La Communication publique*, Paris: La Documentation Française, 1993.

56 'Note documentaire no. 125 de la Division de la presse et de l'information du ministère de la santé, in *Premiers bilan d'éducation sanitaire sur le tabagisme*, undated, p. 2 (Documentation centre – CFES).

57 A tape edited for CFES in 1994 (entitled: '18 ans de campagnes') presented every single film produced for every health education in France since 1976. For more information on the implementation of the initiative (including the synopsis of radio-aired messages) see: *Dossier de presse: campagne d'information sur le tabagisme*, 28 September 1976 (Documentation centre – CFES).

58 Centre d'Études et d'Opinion (CEO), *Recall test de la campagne sur le tabagisme*, January 1977 (archives of the 'Service Études et recherches' – CFES). Four criteria only were used to fix these 'quotas' of interviewees, alleged to match the social structure of the French population: place and type of residency, age, and sex/gender.

59 Interviewees were only asked about films, without any mention of radio-aired messages.

60 Most slogans do not translate very well; this one meant literally: 'Without tobacco, let's take life at full lungs!' and ended every film as well as radio-broadcast message.

61 Premiers bilan d'éducation sanitaire sur le tabagisme.

62 Marc Danzon and Claude Vilain, who were Le Net's closest aides, both confirmed (when interviewed by the author, in February and June 1996) that their relations with him had started to deteriorate during the implementation of the campaign.

63 Interview with Françoise Buhl; Danzon was promoted 'Délégué général adjoint à l'éducation pour la santé' (this established him formally as Buhl's deputy), while Vilain became head of a 'Studies and Research Department' in fast expansion and of growing importance.

64 This vision of prevention as inculcation of individual responsibility towards an interdependent society, and normalisation of unhealthy behaviour, had been elaborated at great length (including enthusiastic reference to the doctrine of controversial French eugenicist Alexis Carrel) by a senior civil servant, Albert Legrand, in his report: *Sur l'éducation sanitaire et sociale*, Comité central d'enquête sur le coût et le rendement des services publics, 1972 (Documentation Centre – Ministry of Health). It was also the approach advocated by CFES before 1975, as attested in editorials published in *La santé de l'homme* (see for example Dr Aujoulat, '"Communications et changements", discours d'ouverture de la VIIème conférence mondiale sur l'éducation sanitaire et sociale, Buenos Aires, 7–12 septembre 1969', *La santé de l'homme* 165, November–December 1969: 7–11

65 I. Illich, *Medical Nemesis: The Expropriation of Health*, New York: Pantheon Book, 1975; translated in French as: *Némésis médicale*, Paris: Le Seuil, 1975. T. Szasz, *The Myth of Mental Illness*, New York: Harper & Row, 1961, and *The*

Theology of Medicine, Syracuse: Syracuse University Press, 1977; both books were translated in French: *Le Mythe de la maladie mentale*, Paris: Payot, 1975, and: *La Théologie de la médecine, fondements politiques et philosophiques de l'éthique médicale*, Paris: Payot, 1980.

66 He had already addressed this question in his medical thesis: Marc Danzon, 'Le médecin et l'éducation sanitaire moderne', thèse pour le doctorat en médecine, Université Paul Sabatier-Toulouse, 1972.

67 Interview with M. Danzon; 'community health' attracted some attention in late 1970s France, under the influence of the Canadian reforms prompted by the 'Lalonde report' that came out in 1974.

68 In 1985, when Marc Danzon left CFES for a senior position at the World Health Organization, Claude Vilain was promoted 'Délégué général adjoint à l'éducation pour la santé', and Jean Tavarès took over as head of the 'Studies and Research Department'.

69 This criticism of health education was set out by Robert Crawford at the time; see: 'You are dangerous to your health: the ideology of victim blaming', *International Journal of Health Services* 7(4), 1977: 663–80. Although I cannot trace precisely the impact of Crawford's view on CFES staff, it has to be mentioned that public health professionals had started discussing such criticism in many Western, industrialised countries.

70 For more detailed explanations on the rationale behind this 'scientific idealism', see Berlivet, 'De l'éducation sanitaire à la promotion de la santé'.

71 Françoise Buhl, 'Intervention de Mme Buhl à la semaine internationale d'information sur l'éducation pour la santé par la radio et la télévision', Munich, 17–21 November 1980 (CFES archives – File 'Éducation pour la santé').

72 Gérard Lagneau, *Sociologie de la publicité*, Paris: PUF, 1983, p. 68. Pierre Martineau's book: *Motivation et publicité, un guide de la stratégie publicitaire*, Paris: Hommes et Techniques, 1959, was the first attempt to import Motivation Research in France. For an account of the early years of the advertising profession in France, see: Marie-Emmanuelle Chessel, *La Publicité: naissance d'une profession 1900–1940*, Paris: CNRS Éditions, 1998.

73 The mobilisation of social sciences in advertising started in the 1920s; see: E.E. Leach, 'Mastering the crowd: collective behaviour and mass society in American social thought, 1917–1939', *American Studies* 27, 1986: 99–114, and M.A. McMahon, 'An American courtship: psychologists and advertising theory in the progressive era', *American Studies* 13, 1972: 5–18.

74 The Société Française d'Études par Sondages (SOFRES) was set up in 1963 under the supervision of a statistician named Jacques Antoine, following in the path of Jean Stoetzel, the French pioneer in public opinion research whose Institut Français d'Opinion Public (IFOP) was established as early as 1938. Loic Blondiaux, *Le Fabrique de l'opinion*, Paris: Seuil, 1998, pp. 522–3.

75 SOFRES-Communication, *Les Jeunes et le tabac. Étude psycho-sociologique*, Février 1978 (Archives of the 'Service Études et recherches' – CFES). The study was based on forty-four 'non-directive' interviews, although only forty-four of them were really used.

76 Ibid. See especially pp. 37 and 91–2.

77 The slogan of the 1978 campaign read: '*Une cigarette écrasée, c'est un peu de liberté gagnée!*' For a thorough analysis of the increasing sophistication of the social psychological model of communication behind the successive campaigns, see Berlivet, 'Une santé à risque', pp. 717–53, and 'Une biopolitique de la santé'.

78 Including a quite famous book on the media coverage of a nuclear incident in Three Mile Island (USA): E. Véron, *Construire l'événement*, Paris: Minuit, 1981.

79 SORGEM, *Stratégies de communication pour la prévention de l'excès de consommation de boissons alcoolisées*, 7 October 1983, p. 31 (Achives of the 'Service

Études et recherches' – CFES). Here again, the research was based on non-directive interviews.
80 Ibid., p. 19ff.
81 Ibid.
82 Ibid., p. 14
83 This pseudo-saying (it was set out for the occasion by a famous copywriter
    named Daniel Robert) is almost impossible to translate. It contrasts 'A [single]
    glass' presented as 'all right', with 'three glasses: what a mess'. The semiotic
    impact of the very colloquial French idiom *'bonjour les dégâts'* is very strong, as
    it allows for various layers of interpretation by referring both to 'a mess' and
    some 'harm' (*'dégâts'*). Originally, the copywriter had proposed an even more
    colloquial pseudo-dictum: *'Un verre c'est bon, trois verres c'est con!'* but CFES's
    senior staff worried about the reactions to a governmental funded communica-
    tion campaign that used rude words and unashamedly claimed that 'a drink is
    good'.
84 SOFRES Médical, *Sondage d'impact sur la campagne alcool*, May–June 1984
    (Archives of the 'Service Études et Recherches' – CFES). The proportion rose to
    80 per cent of both the executives and blue-collar workers interviewed, and 89
    per cent of the interviewees between 15 and 17.
85 *Un verre ça va, trois verres...bonjour les résultats!* (*sic*), 4 October 1984, in
    Dossier alcool, Year 1984 (CFES – Archives)
86 Action nationale 'Un verre ça va...trois verres bonjour les dégâts', Évaluation à
    court terme, 7 August 1984.
87 See the contributions of the most eminent social scientists in the field, social
    epidemiologists and psychiatrists of the time published (without any editor's
    name) in: *Recherches en sciences humaines et éducation pour la santé*, Paris:
    CFES, 1985.
88 Lévy, Deuxième rapport présenté au nom du Conseil Économique et Social.
    L'éducation pour la santé, p. 904.
89 J.M. Cohen-Solal, 'Allocation d'ouverture', *Recherches en sciences humaines et
    éducation pour la santé*, p. 10. Later he added: 'Nous mettons cartes sur table et
    sommes prêts à aller avec vous au bout de la réflexion, y compris de vos réflex-
    ions critiques. La critique n'est pas forcément hostile. Que votre diagnostic soit
    sans complaisance. De notre côté nous n'hésiterons pas à interpeller votre tour
    d'ivoire théorique.'

Recommended further reading

L. Berlivet, 'Une biopolitique de la santé. La fabrique des campagnes de prévention',
    in D. Fassin and D. Memmi (eds), *Le Gouvernement des corps*, Paris: Éditions de
    l'École des Hautes Études en Sciences Sociales, 2004, pp. 37–75.
T. Lefebvre, 'Cinéma et discourse hygiéniste (1890–1930)', unpublished doctoral
    thesis, University of Paris III, 1996.
C. Ollivier-Yaniv (ed.), 'L'État communicant. Les formes de la communication
    gouvrenementale', special issue of *Quaderni. La revue de la communication* 33,
    1997.
J.G. Padioleau, 'La lutte contre le tabagisme: action politique et régulation de la vie
    quotidienne', in *L'État au concret*, Paris: PUF, 1982, pp. 49–77 (initially published
    in the *Revue Française de science politique* 27, 1977).
E. Toon, 'Teaching American children about health', in J. Golden, R. Meckel and
    H.M. Prescott (eds), *American Children and Youth in Sickness and Health*, West-
    port, CT: Greenwood Press, 2004.

Part III

Industrial models, public health and health services

5 Managerialism *avant la lettre*?

The debate on accounting in the NHS Hospitals in the 1950s

Tony Cutler

This paper seeks to examine a relatively neglected area, the early history of attempts to apply management techniques to the British National Health Service (NHS) and the role of research both in structuring proposals for changes in management practice and in assessing the impact of such changes. In particular it focuses on debates on accounting methods in NHS hospitals in the first decade of the Service. The issues raised by this debate are signifi-cant because, as will be argued below, this period has frequently been perceived as 'pre-managerial'. In social scientific accounts, the emergence of a salient role for management in the public sector has been seen as a feature of the last quarter of the century. Such accounts are, in part, reasonable. Commentators on contemporary public sector management are right to point to the sustained and systematic character of the application of manage-ment techniques in public sector services over the last twenty-five years[1]. However, it will be argued that the debate on accounting in NHS hospitals represents variants of a public sector managerialist project '*avant la lettre*'. As such it has potential lessons for the evaluation of the more recent system-atic attempts to apply managerial techniques in public sector services.

The paper is divided into four sections: the first examines how current theories of new public management (NPM) have implicitly periodised the history of public sector management into a phase of 'public administration' that is followed by a period in which NPM comes into operation. The second section argues, in contrast to this periodisation, that the attempt to change internal accounting practices in NHS hospitals in the 1950s can be seen as an instance of managerialism '*avant la lettre*'. The third section considers the limits of the impact of that project and the final section discusses the reasons for these limits and what lessons the debates on accounting in NHS hospitals may have for current discussions of NPM.

The NHS in the 1940s and 1950s: a case of 'public administration'?

A key concept in current debates on the application of managerial tech-niques to public sector services is 'new public management' (NPM). NPM refers to a set of techniques, practices and organisational structures that have been applied in public sector services in a systematic way, broadly over the last quarter of a century. Since the approach is seen as 'new' this implies a contrast with a different set of practices that operated 'before' NPM. This 'before' phase is characterised by Dunleavy and Hood[2] in the title of their article 'From old public administration to new public management'.

NPM is conceptualised as the successor to 'public administration'. This in turn raises the issue of the central distinctions between these approaches to the organisation of public services. In discussing the shift from 'public administration' to 'NPM' Dunleavy and Hood[3] point to the importance of accounting practices; thus they see the move to NPM as involving 'reworking budgets to be transparent in accounting terms with costs attributed to outputs not inputs, and outputs measured by quantitative performance indicators'. In NPM the focus is on the costs of the products of public sector services or 'outputs'. In turn these can be linked to 'quantitative performance indicators' that serve as the measures of such 'outputs', which requires the use of what Hood[4] has termed 'explicit standards and measures of performance'.

This approach to management control has implications for organisational structures and practices since, as control is via evaluation of performance in relation to standards or objectives, it must be possible to locate responsibility for such performance. Thus, in characterising NPM Hood[5] argues that 'accountability requires clear assignment of responsibility'.[6]

NPM is discussed as effectively a polar opposite to 'public administration'. In public administration, where costs of public sector services are discussed, this is seen as referring to 'inputs'. This, means, for example, that costs will be presented in terms of expenditure on labour of various kinds (e.g. medical, nursing) or certain types of provisions (e.g. drugs). What, it is suggested, is likely to be absent is measures of the cost of outputs or what is 'produced' by such inputs.

In turn, this suggests that accountability and control are procedural. Thus, for example, presentation of expenditure in terms of what resources are spent on is consistent with parliamentary accountability. Hence, in the context of NHS organisation in the 1950s, requiring Hospital Management Committees (HMCs), Regional Hospital Boards (RHBs) and Boards of Governors (BGs) (of teaching hospitals) to present expenditure in this form allowed for a check that expenditure was being undertaken for purposes regarded as 'appropriate' by parliament. However, such approaches could be seen as inimical to *managerial* concepts of accountability. Thus, if only inputs are costed then such data might be of limited use for internal management purposes because the information collected does not refer to 'outputs' or standards of performance.

Finally, if managerial accountability is absent or downplayed then the correlative requirement for clear lines of managerial (as against procedural) accountability are absent. Thus activities that generate costs (e.g. clinical activity) could be initiated by organisational actors (notably doctors) who are neither managerially responsible for such costs nor accountable to other actors (hospital administrators) for them.

Thus contemporary NPM theory contains an implicit periodisation. Prior to the emergence of NPM public services were 'administered'. This meant that, while costs of inputs may have been known, there was no link to services produced. This was part of a general lack of managerial accountability. Professionals and administrators were not required to justify service expenditure in relation to performance targets. Such links were only attempted with the advent of NPM. In the next section the aim will be to raise various critical questions relating to this periodisation by examining the debate on accounting practices in NHS hospitals in the first decade of the Service.

The critique of 'public administration'? The debate on NHS hospital accounting in the 1950s

Departmental costing enters the policy agenda

To situate the debate on accounting practices in the NHS in the 1950s it is necessary at this point to give a chronological overview of key developments. The presentation of hospital accounts under the NHS were, initially, governed by Statutory Regulation No. 1414, which was laid before parliament in June 1948 and came into operation on the 'Appointed Day' (5 July 1948).[7] A crucial feature of the Regulation was that expenditure was shown in relation to different types of input. Thus the most significant (current) expenditure area, 'hospital maintenance', was broken down into eight subcategories including salaries and wages; provisions; and drugs, dressings, medical and surgical appliances and equipment.[8] This approach was termed 'subjective' because costs were expressed under given 'subject' headings.

The regulations were effectively based on practices that had originated in voluntary sector hospital accounting. These involved both presenting expenditure under 'subject' headings and giving an overall cost measure in terms, particularly, of average cost per in-patient week. The rationale for this practice was to show the actual/potential donor how expenditure was divided and what it cost to provide an in-patient bed.[9] While the attraction of contributions was not a factor for the NHS, external accountability was. Thus the regulations were designed to govern the way estimates and expenditure out-turns were presented by RHBs and BGs to the Minister. This, however, left the question as to whether the subjective approach would also be the basis for *internal* hospital accounting. On this latter issue the regulations were not specific. They merely stipulated that 'Each Board of Governors and Hospital Management Committee shall prepare annual cost accounts in such a form as the Minister may require.'[10]

As the argument later in the section will show there was a significant body of expert opinion in hospital accounting that was critical of the subjective approach. Such expert opinion favoured presenting cost and output data for separate hospital departments. This 'departmental' approach to hospital accounting moved on to the policy terrain through the auspices of the Central Health Services Council (CHSC). In June 1949 the CHSC had established a Hospital Administration Committee.[11] In December 1949 this committee presented an Interim Report which included the proposal that 'complete unit costing of a number of hospitals should be put in hand'.[12] While the term 'departmental costing' was not used, the reference to 'unit' costing suggests that a departmental approach was implied since advocates of a departmental approach favoured relating costs to specific 'units' of output.

This proposal involved a research project and the Committee stated that 'the obvious bodies to carry out this experiment are the King's Fund and the Nuffield [Provincial Hospitals] Trust'.[13] It is not clear from the Interim Report (or in the papers in the relevant Public Record Office file) why the two organisations were the 'obvious bodies'. However, there are a number of reasons why they may have been selected. In the case of the Nuffield Provincial Hospitals Trust (NPHT) research on departmental approaches to hospital accounting had been instituted at the Radcliffe Infirmary in 1937 and a paper (not in the CHSC files) had been sent to the CHSC in 1949.[14] In the case of the King's Fund (KF) a decision was made in 1939 to appoint a 'consultant on hospital finance'.[15] This was designed, in part, to be a role where the consultant would advise hospital management on their accounting practices.[16] The person appointed was Captain J.E. Stone, then Secretary to the Birmingham Hospital Centre, who had been Chief Accountant at St Thomas's hospital.[17] Stone was the author of a standard work, *Hospital Organisation and Management*,[18] and was a strong advocate of a departmental approach.[19]

The Hospital Administration Committee's proposal that the Minister of Health invite the KF and NPHT to undertake the accounting research was endorsed by the CHSC,[20] and the Minister issued an invitation to the two bodies to undertake the work in May 1950.[21] As an interim measure, a committee of treasurers of RHBs was set up to recommend an appropriate form for 'a relatively simple system of cost analysis'[22] and these recommendations were embodied in the first NHS *Hospital Costing Returns*, which were first published, for fiscal year 1950–1, in 1952. The approach taken in these returns, which retained a broadly subjective framework, will be discussed in detail below.

The process of developing a departmental approach was moved forward with the publication of the KF report in September and the NPHT report in October 1952. Both reports were circulated to RHBs, the Association of Hospital Management Committees and the Teaching Hospitals Association for comment in November 1952,[23] and responses had been received by June 1953.[24] Following these responses three policy options were considered: further research on hospital costing could be undertaken; a decision by the Ministry that departmental costing should be introduced for particular departments could be made; or a working party could be set up to develop proposals for a modified internal hospital accounting regime.[25]

To put these options in context it is necessary to point to a key feature of the responses from hospital authorities. While there was sympathy with the objectives of the departmental approach, only one response (Newcastle RHB) wanted it to replace the subjective form of costing. The reasons for this scepticism will be discussed in more detail later in the paper but in part this response reflected resource concerns. The NHS in the 1950s was subject to stringent expenditure controls[26] and departmental approaches would both require more sophisticated collection of financial and operational data, which would increase administrative costs.[27]

What this meant was that departmental approaches were seen as, at least in the short to medium term, to operate as 'supplementary'[28] to subjective approaches. This was why further research was an option. However, this raised difficulties, amongst which was the problem that experimental work would be pursued in particular hospitals, but this would raise difficulties for non-participant hospitals if it was decided to move to implement a general departmental scheme.[29]

There were also problems with the Ministry determining which services should be costed on a departmental basis. As is explained below, while both the KF and NPHT endorsed a departmental approach, they differed on key details of how this should be implemented. Furthermore there was no consensus amongst hospital authorities, in their responses to the reports, on such issues of detail.[30] This suggested that imposing a departmental approach would put the Ministry in a difficult position.[31] Thus the working party was adopted *faute de mieux*. Given the reservations expressed by the hospital authorities in their responses any departmental accounting scheme was to be supplementary to subjective costing and was to be designed to impose 'the minimum additional burden on hospital authorities'.[32]

The decision to appoint a working party was announced in September[33] and the membership announced in November 1953.[34] The membership included Stone as the representative of the KF and McLachlan, the accountant to the NPHT.[35] The other ten members were drawn from the Ministry and the financial (e.g. treasurer or finance officer) or non-financial (e.g. secretary) administrative staff of RHBs, HMCs and BGs. The Working Party submitted its report in June 1955.[36] The findings of the Working Party and research evaluating the impact of the internal hospital accounting scheme implemented on the basis of its proposals are discussed in detail below. However, at this point it is necessary to examine the issues at the centre of the debate on NHS accounting in the 1950s and how they relate to the NPM/public administration distinction discussed above.

'Subjective' costing

As was pointed out earlier a committee of RHB treasurers had been asked to devise an interim scheme for hospital costing. Table 5.1 shows, in an abbreviated form, how they considered that internal cost accounting data should be presented. Rather than giving a full list of cost headings, major cost items are included and selected more minor cost categories are shown to give some idea of the relative (estimated) cost of different items. The illustrative data is given for certain London teaching hospitals, and the aim of the discussion is to locate this form of cost presentation in the debates on cost control in hospitals during this period.

Table 5.1 Average cost per week of maintaining a patient, selected London teaching hospitals, NHS costing returns, 1950–1

		Barts	*London*	*Royal Free*	*Guy's*	*Middle-sex*
1	Available staffed beds	542	826	854	635	712
2	Occupancy rate	91	92	87	88	92
3	Out-patient attendances	338,909	585,715	508,351	386,524	359,748
4	Provisions	£3.47	£2.19	£3.26	£3.65	£2.85
5	Patient's clothing	£0.05	£0.05	£0.02	£0.03	£0.01
6	Drugs, dressings	£3.33	£2.96	£2.88	£3.47	£2.94
7	Bedding	£0.20	£0.25	£0.27	£0.21	£0.21
8	Cleaning	£0.20	£0.20	£0.21	£0.31	£0.22
9	Total running costs	£7.55	£5.93	£7.00	£7.56	£7.00
10	Medical salary	£10.04	£5.80	£5.57	£9.72	£6.68
11	Nursing salary	£6.62	£4.35	£5.56	£5.79	£5.10
12	Other staff wages	£11.18	£10.92	£10.02	£9.93	£10.22
13	Staff uniforms	£0.55	£0.18	£0.26	£0.26	£0.35
14	Fuel, light, power, water	£1.52	£1.35	£1.60	£1.22	£1.27
15	Maintenance	£1.45	£0.64	£0.51	£1.58	£0.38
16	Total standing charges	£34.37	£24.68	£25.04	£29.15	£25.86
17	Direct credits	£3.13	£2.09	£2.07	£1.92	£2.63
18	Net standing charges	£31.24	£22.59	£22.97	£27.23	£23.23
19	Extraordinary expenditure	–	£0.97	£0.71	£0.66	£0.72
20	Total inclusive net cost	£38.80	£29.50	£30.69	£36.63	£31.52
21	Adjusted for out-patient attendances	£28.20	£20.71	£22.35	£26.47	£24.27
22	Adjusted for occupancy	£26.19	£19.31	£20.25	£23.70	£22.71

Source: Adapted from Ministry of Health, Hospital Costing Returns.

A striking feature of the table is the attention given to individual items of expenditure. This feature is de-emphasised in the adapted version presented in Table 5.1. In the full costing returns there were cost data for eight separate items under the broad heading of 'running charges' (five of which are shown in Table 5.1), and cost data for a further twelve items given under the general heading 'standing charges' (of which eight are shown in Table 5.1).

This was intrinsic to the 'subjective' approach to the presentation of cost data and would seem to correspond to a 'public administration' approach. As was indicated above, concepts of NPM characterised it as focusing on costs of 'outputs' whereas 'public administration' approaches cost 'inputs'. However, arguably this oversimplifies the picture. The above account suggests a substantial indifference to the use of cost data by hospital management as a means to improve hospital performance. However, a closer examination of the RHB treasurers' work shows that there was a clear intent that accounting data in the costing returns should be used to judge hospital efficiency.

The costing returns: a (cautious) managerial reform?

The argument outlined above has suggested that the presentation of hospital cost data as embodied in the Hospital Costing Returns exhibited an indifference to the use of cost data for internal management purposes. However, there are aspects of the returns which suggest that the potential use of such data for management control *was* seen as significant.

A characteristic feature of NPM approaches has been the attempt to draw conclusions on performance standards by comparing units providing what at least are seen to be similar services. For example, the Department of Health published its first 'star ratings' of NHS acute trusts against twenty-one performance indicators in September 2001. Trusts in the highest ranking category (three stars) were seen as embodying standards of practice to which less well 'performing' trusts should aspire and the Chief Executives of such trusts were to be invited to 'provide direct advice' on national policies.[37]

Such a concern with comparative performance can be seen in the Costing Returns. Data presented were explicitly comparative since they showed costs in either individual hospitals, groups of hospitals under HMCs or (as in Table 5.1) BGs. There is also what might be seen as an 'overall' cost performance indicator since data is presented on the 'average cost of maintaining a patient per week'. The returns sought to present data on hospitals classified by type[38] that were designed to allow for comparison of units of a similar character.

These figures were presented in 'net' terms by deducting 'direct credits' such as payments for accommodation by staff (see row 17). There were also attempts to refine this indicator by presenting it in three variant forms. Row 20 gives a 'total' inclusive net cost figure. However, this encompasses costs incurred for in-patient and out-patient activity. The Report of the RHB treasurers had pointed out that 'the differing incidence of out-patient expenditure distorts comparative hospital costs to such a degree that some provision should be made for this factor'.[39]

There was also an attempt to produce data in a standardised form; thus an adjustment for the occupancy rate was made (Table 5.1, row 22). This reflected the fact that certain costs (e.g. maintenance of the fabric of a hospital building) will not vary with occupancy levels and hence could be contributory to a higher unit cost. In addition the broad classification of costs was designed to distinguish costs 'which tend to vary directly with the number of patients'[40] classified as 'running costs' (cf. rows 4–9, Table 5.1), and those 'which tend to remain unaltered by normal variations in occupancy'[41] classed as 'standing charges' (rows 10–16, Table 5.1).

Thus, while the Costing Returns worked within 'the limitations of the present costing scheme',[42] they _were_ regarded as serving an internal management function. Thus it was claimed that 'comparisons between the average costs of comparable hospitals and investigation into the reasons therefore should...lead to improvements in methods of administration and to economies'.[43] Equally the managerial rationale could be seen as reflected in the form of cost presentation. The grouping of hospitals by type could be viewed as facilitating comparisons as would the adjustment for variations in out-patient attendances. The further adjustment for occupancy levels could be seen as a means of distinguishing factors within and outside internal management control. For example, by their nature, many isolation hospitals would be likely to operate with low occupancy rates that would increase (unadjusted) costs per patient week.

Such comparative data was not unproblematic. For example, hospitals classed as 'mainly general' were defined as 'more than 50 per cent general' (i.e. with cases falling under the categories of medical, surgical, gynaecological and obstetric cases).[44] Such hospitals also would have 'a specific allocation of beds for the chronic sick'.[45] This meant that hospitals with a considerable variation in the percentage of beds for the chronic sick would be classed under the same hospital type and this would have implications for costs. Equally 'wholly general' hospitals could contain a considerable variation of, for example 'medical' and 'surgical' cases, and there were no data allowing for any differentiation of medical and surgical specialties let alone differentiation of case-mix within specialties. Nevertheless the Costing Returns can be seen as a cautious instalment of a managerial reform project. However, if this was a cautious version of a managerial reform project there was also a more radical variant that sought to jettison the 'subjective' approach altogether.

Clearly the ground for managerial reforms? The critique of 'subjective' cost data

As was indicated earlier, the KF and NPHT reports embodied a departmental approach to internal hospital accounting. This involved a critique of the subjective approach and it is now necessary to examine the basis of this critique.

The Costing Returns embodied an overall cost indicator, that of maintaining an in-patient per week. For the critics of the 'subjective' method, however, this overall indicator was problematic. Central to this critique was the conception that hospitals were complex institutions involving a plurality of activities. What followed was that cost data and cost units ought to be differentiated according to the nature of the activity involved. Thus, for example, the 'product' of a hospital boiler house was steam; of a cleaning function, a volume of space cleaned; of a radiology department, varieties of diagnostic X-rays. For the critics it made no sense to divide costs generated by these diverse activities into a single unit, the 'in-patient week'. Thus the KF report[46] argued that there were 'so many variations between hospitals' (e.g. in range of services provided or age and layout of buildings) that 'an all-in unit of cost cannot be accepted as a reliable unit of cost'[47].

The corollary of the use of the *single* divisor (e.g. the in-patient week) meant that the *individual* 'subjective' headings (provisions, heating, radiology, medical salaries, etc.) were not connected to any *specific* activity measures. Thus taking the example of an X-ray department, the KF report pointed out that the costs of the department were included under distinct subject headings such as 'salaries and wages' and 'medical and surgical appliances and equipment' (the latter covering plates and film).[48] This meant that 'stated thus the cost of the X-Ray department…is incapable of being considered in relation to any activity';[49] in a similar vein the NPHT report argued that subjective approaches involved the problem that 'there is nothing to show what service the hospital is giving'.[50]

The logic of this critique was the rejection of the 'subjective' approach. Such cost data were seen as inconsistent with organisational divisions within hospitals. For example, whereas doctors and nurses worked in specific wards, or at least could have their working time allocated to such wards, the cost of their working time, under 'subjective' headings, was grouped under, respectively, medical and nursing salaries. What was needed was the preparation of internal accounts on a departmental basis. This would establish the basis for managerial accountability. The NPHT report[51] argued that 'for costing to have its full value each departmental head should be made aware of those items which are within his or her control'; and the KF report[52] argued that a departmental costing system would mean that 'increases and decreases in expenditure are automatically revealed and brought to the notice of the officers responsible'.

The two organisations produced different reports that embodied distinct methods of departmental accounting. In the case of the NPHT report a 'prime' or 'direct' cost approach was used. What this meant was that the costs of each department were traced (as far as was possible) in terms of 'direct' costs. This can be illustrated by taking the example of medical in-patient department costs.[53] Direct costs for this department consisted of salaries and wages of medical staff, of nursing staff and the cost of materials.[54] Within 'materials' provisions were excluded because they were charged to another 'department', catering.[55] Equally, although the ideal was direct use of labour by the department some estimation was required to allocate the labour time and hence cost of housemen or student nurses.

In contrast, the KF report initially broke departments into three categories: patient departments, specialist services and general services.[56] In terms of broad classifications the NPHT divided departments into two categories, 'medical', which subsumed the KF 'specialist services' such as laboratories,[57] and 'non-medical services', which broadly corresponded to the KF 'general services' such as the boiler house.[58] However, the central difference between the two documents was that the KF report advocated charging general service expenditure to the patient and specialist departments. Thus the aim was to provide a *total* cost for these departments.

The reason for the difference in approach related to views taken on allocation of such general service expenditure in the two reports. In some cases such costs could be directly traced. For example, where laundry was supplied to a particular ward it would be possible to charge this to the ward. However, in other instances such direct charging was not an option. For example, maintenance work on the external fabric of a building or on the entrance had to be allocated via a formula. In the KF case, for example, this

Table 5.2 Sample of departmental cost statement: medical wards

Expenditure heading	Unit cost	Cost
Consultant salary	£1,078.113	£0.09
Registrar/senior house officer salary	£578.77	£0.05
Housemen salary	£380.16	£0.03
Nursing salary	£5,910.76	£0.50
Ward maid salary	£499.99	£0.04
Dressings	£360.12	£0.03
Instruments/medical appliances	£171.85	£0.01
Hardware/crockery	£105.38	£0.01
Printing/stationery	£105.02	£0.01
Furniture	£180.75	£0.02
Cleaning, bedding, maintenance materials	£52.06	
Total	£9,423.00	£0.80

Notes:
Period: 1 October 1951 to 31 December 1951:
group A: hospital A
Unit of cost: in-patient days
Beds available: 143
Percentage occupancy: 89.64
Available in-patient days: 13,156
Actual in-patient days: 11,794
Patients admitted: 541
Average length of stay: 21.80

Source: Nuffield Provincial Hospitals Trust, *Report of an Experiment in Hospital Costing*, London: Oxford University Press, 1952, p. 58.

was based on the share of hospital space taken up by the department.[59] The NPHT report was uneasy about the use of such formulae for allocation of overheads. The report argued that attempts to show total costs for medical and specialist service departments 'had ... to be based on a succession of arbitrary allocations';[60] and reliance on 'direct costs' was 'sufficient to provide all that is needed for the financial administration of hospital management committees and boards of governors'.[61]

A clearer idea of how costing was designed to aid hospital management can be seen if this work is considered in more detail. To do this the NPHT report will be examined. It was substantially longer than that of the KF and allowed for more detail in the presentation of the illustrative material. Tables 5.2 and 5.3 show two of the NPHT 'samples of departmental cost statements' for a medical ward and a laundry. An examination of both will illustrate what was seen as the advantage of departmental costing. In both cases costs are presented alongside measures of activity: in-patient days for the medical ward; and pieces washed for the laundry. In this sense there is a distinction with 'subjective' cost accounting in that activities are connected to costs. Equally expenditure is connected to a given organisational function, the medical wards and the laundry. Total costs are divided by 'units' to give the unit cost figure. For example, in the case of the medical ward, total expenditure over the period covered (£9,423) is divided by the 'unit of cost' 11,794 (actual) in-patient days to yield a cost per in-patient day of 80 pence. The 'problem' of the single divisor is avoided because 'units of cost' are differentiated according to what is seen as appropriate to the department; in-patient days in the case of the medical ward; cost per '100 pieces' in the case of the laundry. Consequently the unit cost information could be regarded as

Table 5.3 Sample of departmental cost statement: laundry

Expenditure heading	Cost	Unit cost
Superintendent salary	£76.13	£0.10
Other salary	£381.39	£0.49
Hardware, crockery, cleaning, furniture, furnishings	£73.46	£0.10
Work done by other hospitals	£81.62	£0.10
Total	£612.60	£0.79

Notes:
Period: 1 October 1951 to 31 December 1951: group D: hospital F
Unit of cost: 100 pieces
Pieces washed: 78,257
Weekly pieces washed: own laundry 5,417; other hospital 603
Pieces washed: white coats 1,625; aprons 9,156; dresses 1,575; overalls 156; theatre gowns 3,696; blankets 281; counterpanes 740; pillow slips 6,970; sheets 8,266; draw sheets 5,412; hand towels 2,841; bath towels 1,408; roller towels 564; other 35,567

Source: Nuffield Provincial Hospitals Trust, *Report of an Experiment in Hospital Costing*, London: Oxford University Press, 1952, p. 60.

adapted to the needs of 'departmental management'. Further the combination of cost and activity data could be viewed as providing a 'pointer' to management, e.g. in the case of the medical ward changes in unit costs could be linked to occupancy rates and average length of stay.

Thus it is possible, in this period, to discern a managerialist project with cautious and radical variants. However, this project operated within certain limits and these are examined in the next section.

Managerialism *avant la lettre*: the limits of the project

The limits of the managerialist project can be considered under two headings: those related to the range of costs and activities covered by the internal hospital accounting regime recommended by the 1955 Working Party; and the conceptual limitations of the recommended framework when set in the context of the objectives of 'departmental costing'.

The principal revised internal accounting scheme adopted by the Working Party was termed the 'main costing scheme' and was subject to a size limitation. In acute and 'mainly acute' hospitals this was to apply where annual hospital expenditure exceeded £150,000 per annum,[62] although it was hoped to progressively shift this limit to £100,000.[63] In other types of hospitals that met this expenditure condition the application of the main scheme was to be at the discretion of RHBs, in the case of non-teaching hospitals and the Ministry, and in consultation with the Teaching Hospitals Association, in the case of teaching hospitals.[64] Hospitals that did not meet this expenditure 'hurdle' were to continue to use the interim scheme drawn up by the RHB treasurers.[65] These recommendations were accepted by the Minister of Health who announced, in March 1956, that departmental costing, in its supplementary role, would come into operation in April 1957.[66]

The effect of this limitation, whose rationale will be discussed in the next section, was to severely limit the share of hospital expenditure covered by the main scheme. An attempt to estimate the impact of this restriction was made by Montacute. He was released by his RHB (South Western) to undertake an evaluation of the departmental costing scheme introduced in line with the recommendations of the Working Party.[67] The work was undertaken while he had held a research fellowship at Manchester University and the field research was funded by the NPHT.[68] The research involved a questionnaire sent to 214 finance officers in hospitals using the main scheme. He received responses from 144 officers (a 67.3 per cent response rate) and he supplemented the information from this source by making sixty-four visits to RHBs, HMCs and BGs.[69]

His study sought, *inter alia*, to investigate the percentage of overall hospital maintenance (current) expenditure in England and Wales covered by hospitals using the main scheme. He estimated that such hospitals accounted for 28.5 per cent of expenditure in non-teaching hospitals and 56.7 per cent of expenditure in teaching hospitals.[70] Overall 32.3 per cent of expenditure in hospitals in England and Wales was covered by main-scheme hospitals.[71]

Thus main-scheme hospitals accounted for only one-third of total hospital expenditure in England and Wales. However, Montacute's findings also suggest that this figure overestimated the impact of the main scheme. Internal hospital costs can be divided into three types: 'hotel' functions, medical service departments, and costs directly linked to clinical treatment. As the term suggests, 'hotel' costs refer to hospital functions that are broadly similar to activities needed to sustain a hotel 'guest' such as catering, cleaning, laundry and heating. Medical service departments refer to specialist departments whose activities are ancillary to and driven by clinical decisions. Examples of the latter are X-rays, radiotherapy and physiology departments. Finally there are the costs of direct clinical treatment, particularly medical and nursing salaries.

Montacute anticipated that the use of the scheme for financial control purposes would vary significantly between the different types of activities, and his findings confirmed this expectation. He argued 'the 'hotel' side of the hospital service lends itself to costing more readily than the 'treatment' side'.[72] One of the questions he asked was whether 'special investigations' of individual departments within the hospitals concerned had been undertaken as a result of cost data collected. Of the 144 respondents seventeen indicated that no such special investigations had taken place.[73] The remaining 127 'hotel' functions, including catering, cleaning and laundry, averaged 1.0 investigations per authority; in contrast in-patient and out-patient departments averaged 0.3 investigations per authority.[74] Thus 'clinical' departments were subject to cost-driven 'special investigations' at only one-third of the level applied to 'hotel' activities.

Critics of the subjective approach wanted its replacement. The KF and NPHT issued a joint statement following the completion of their reports which proposed 'that the existing accounting based on subjective analysis of expenditure be discontinued'.[75] In this respect the restriction of departmental accounting to a supplementary role involved a compromise for the critics of the subjective approach. Nevertheless Stone was not dissatisfied with the outcome of the Working Party report, which he argued represented 'a big advance in hospital accounting looked at from the management angle'.[76] Stone's enthusiasm was arguably related to the fact that the proposed structure for hospital internal accounts did include a number of attempts to introduce departmental costing along the lines suggested by the KF and NPHT reports. Thus it was proposed that laundry costs be divided by weighted units of items laundered, and that catering expenditure be expressed in terms of cost per person fed per week.[77]

However, a fundamental limitation related to the medical (in-patient and out-patient) departments. In the case of in-patient costs, for example, the 'units' selected were in-patient weeks or cases. Such measures had two related problems. In the case of the 'in-patient week' there was no measure of a medical output since the 'output' stipulated made no reference to the type of treatment provided. In turn this led to the related problem of how meaningful comparisons between medical departments would be since, for example, higher costs per in-patient week could reflect differences in the mix of cases dealt with.

A crude way of tackling the comparability issue would be to limit comparisons to wards engaged in broadly similar medical activity. However, even this was problematic because, under the main scheme, patient departments involved *combining* wards to form departments.[78] Equally it is important to stress that this absence of a medical output for the patient departments was already a problem in the work of critics of the subjective approach. Thus, as was illustrated in Table 5.2 (above), the 'unit of cost' used for medical wards in the NPHT report was 'in-patient days'. If, however, the revised system of internal hospital accounts was subject to these limitations this raises the question of the basis for these limits and the possible lessons for the current NPM project. These issues are addressed in the final section.

Managerialism *avant la lettre*: determinants of the limits of the project

The reasons for the limits of the managerialist project to radically reform internal hospital accounting in the NHS in the 1950s can be related to two broad issues: the constraints imposed by a regime of economy; and the impact of clinical autonomy on the anticipated role of departmental costing.

The effects of economy were complex and some aspects were prejudicial to the managerialist project. In the previous section it was pointed out that an important limitation on the scope of the main costing scheme was that it was only to apply to larger hospitals. This limitation reflected concerns regarding the cost of a more sophisticated internal accounting system. The remit given to the Working Party enjoined members, with respect to the recommended accounting practices, to have 'full regard to the present needs to limit the cost of introducing and operating such a system to the minimum'.[79] The restriction of the main scheme to larger hospitals related to the view that only in hospitals with a relatively large budget would the costs of introducing the new practices be justified.

As was indicated in the previous section, the impact of the size restriction on the main scheme meant that two-thirds of expenditure in hospitals in England and Wales was not covered by the main scheme. The logical corollary was that this occurred because the majority of hospitals were small. In turn this reflected the fact that the hospital stock in the late 1950s was inherited from the pre-NHS period.

Given the timescales involved in capital programmes this was, to a considerable extent, inevitable. However, it also related to the impact of economy. Within the overall restraint on NHS spending, *capital* programmes were more severely restricted than current spending. Precise comparisons with the pre NHS period were difficult but Abel-Smith and Titmuss in their key study on the cost of the NHS, published in 1956, estimated that capital expenditure on hospitals in England and Wales in 1952–3 was, in real terms, around one-third of the level prevailing at the end of the interwar period.[80] In this respect the regime of economy had a paradoxical effect. Economy encouraged the search for greater control over costs but the severity of restrictions on capital expenditure meant that an inheritance of hospitals that were disproportionately small made up most of the capital stock of the NHS; in England and Wales in 1952 of 2,559 hospitals, only 220 had 500 or more beds and over 1,500 had under 100 beds.[81] Consequently most of this stock was unsuitable for the more sophisticated modes of financial control envisaged in departmental accounting. Economy concerns could thus have contributed to the limits of departmental costing via the size restriction on the main scheme in the context of an inherited capital stock dominated by small hospitals. However, there was another source for the limits of this project and this was its implications for clinical autonomy.

The dominant view amongst RHBs, HMCs and BGs that the subjective approach should not be discontinued has been discussed above in relation to responses to the KF and NPHT reports. However, the documentary source for these responses[82] gives only a summary account of their views. A more complete account can be found in evidence given by hospital authorities to the Guillebaud Committee, which had been appointed, in 1953, to investigate the costs of the NHS. In this evidence frequent reference was made to the effects of clinical autonomy on the operation of hospital accounting regimes. Thus representatives of North West Metropolitan RHB argued

> in the case of certain unit costs – e.g. in the operating theatre – it was difficult to understand what executive action could be taken once the information had been obtained. It was well known for example that some surgeons were slower than others and would remain so even when unit costs revealed their slowness'.[83]

Similar reservations were expressed by other RHBs; thus the East Anglia Board representatives thought that the 'value' of cost accounting techniques was 'unknown in medical departments'.[84]

There was similar scepticism in the Treasury where it was argued, with respect to evidence of variations in hospital costs, 'will doctors [in a high-cost hospital] be told they must spend less time with their patients? Are we anywhere near getting round to a position in which such a thing could be said and who would say it?'[85]

The 'who would say it' question was a telling one and the issue was not confronted in the KF and NPHT reports where it was not entirely clear who was to act on the cost information provided on 'departments' such as wards or out-patient clinics. Furthermore, while service departments such as radiology could examine how they undertook the work required of them, clinical autonomy meant that the *requests* for such services were outside the departmental purview. This was admitted in the NPHT report where it was stated

> it is useful to know that a pathological investigation is done in an efficient way but it would be equally useful to know whether the number of investigations is above or below the average having regard to the types of patients treated.[86]

However, the report was very cautious with respects to attempts to apply such a norm, observing that 'it is hoped that with the co-operation of specialists in every field it might be possible to arrive at formulae which would give broad indicators of the right usage of many services which a hospital gives'.[87]

A similar indication of caution was the absence of examples of the use of accounting data to change practice in areas under direct clinical control. Thus, for example, in a section of the NPHT report giving examples of 'the value of cost accounting in hospital administration'[88] the positive examples of the use of cost data are drawn from the laundry, catering, stores and administration of salaries and wages.[89]

The exploration of the reasons for the limits on the project to reform internal hospital accounting practices during the 1950s raises the question of what lessons might be drawn from this experience. It will be suggested that this experience can be 'read' in distinctive ways. One 'reading' effectively returns us to the NPM/public administration distinction discussed above. The limits could be seen as imposed by the situating of a managerialist project in a 'pre-managerialist' era. For example, the lack of will to implement such changes could be regarded as indicated in the underresourcing of the programme.

In a similar vein deference to clinical autonomy could be seen as reflecting a 'pre-managerial' mind set in which responsibility for initiating expenditure was divorced from management accountability for the outputs of such expenditure. Furthermore the 1950s experience could be contrasted with, for example, the Management Budgeting initiative of the 1980s. The latter stemmed from the Griffiths Report of 1983 that was crucial to the introduction of the general manager role in the NHS. With respect to accounting practices, the report argued NHS units should develop 'management budgets which involve clinicians and relate work-load and service objectives to financial and manpower allocations'.[90] This text appears to be situated in the era of public sector managerialism with the corollary that clinical practice would no longer be 'off limits' as in the more attenuated venture of departmental costing in the 1950s.

Such a reading of the 1950s experience also has a prescriptive implication. The limits discussed above stemmed from an insufficient commitment to support effective management practices. This reading is then consistent with Pollitt and Bouckaert's[91] observation that 'a good deal of the rhetoric associated with public management reform contrasts the new (= good) with the old (= bad)'. Departmental costing failed because it was stifled by 'bad' 'old' public administration.

However, as Pollitt and Bouckaert observed with respect to public management reform more generally, such approaches are 'misleadingly neat and over-simple'.[92] The first problem is that the 'new' is portrayed as a success yet such a position is difficult to sustain with respect to projects designed to 'involve' clinicians in managing budgets in hospitals. The Management Budgeting initiative itself was short lived and, in a review of the scheme, the then-Director of Financial Management of the NHS argued that it had 'not generally been seen as making any worthwhile contribution to the planning and costing of patient care'.[93] The scheme was relaunched with the Resource Management (RM) initiative and this was designed to be more palatable to doctors by using a rationale that distanced the project from narrower financial considerations.[94] However, the evaluation of this 'softer' variant of clinical budgeting, commissioned by the Department of Health, argued that 'in general service providers did not feel that RM had yet produced significant benefits'.[95]

Of course, these more recent 'failures' could be related to a further failure to sufficiently embrace the 'good' and the 'new'. However, it is perhaps worth concluding by suggesting that, in turn, this argument is problematic. To do this it is necessary to return to the debates of the 1950s. In part the reform project in hospital accounting could be seen as stemming from the model of 'standard' costing in industrial applications of management accounting. For example, the report by the Anglo-American Productivity Council, published in 1952, discussed a variant of management accounting, 'standard product costing', where industrial engineering techniques were used to set appropriate technical standards in terms of requirements of materials and labour. In turn these are translated into cost terms via 'appropriate prices' for materials and labour, and allocation of overhead expense,[96] and cost targets are set.

However, even amongst advocates of departmental costing in hospitals there was scepticism with respect to such views. In the KF report it was argued 'standard costs, as we understand them imply a "blueprint" precision which is obviously impossible of attainment in the treatment of patients which indeed could only be attained on the emergence of the "standard patient"'.[97]

Arguably, these concerns remain relevant to the application of accounting techniques to clinical practice. The most forceful version of such an approach would be if a 'standard cost' approach could be used. However, this, in turn, would presuppose that 'standard' forms of treatment could be identified. Such issues have a distinctly contemporary ring since they relate, for example, to current debates on 'evidence-based medicine' (EBM). While linking costs to clinical interventions pose major problems in their own right the project, at least in its strongest form, requires the possibility of standardising medical practice on the analogy with identifying 'best' practice in an industrial setting. Yet even advocates of EBM have expressed doubts on the viability of such a conception of medicine. Thus Naylor, the head of a publicly funded institute concerned with diffusing evidence as the basis for medical practice, has argued that 'the present application of the evaluative sciences will affirm rather than obviate the need for the art of medicine.'[98]

An important theme of this collection is the relationship between research, and the formation and implementation of health policy. In the context of the NPM/public administration distinction, approaches to health service administration in the 'pre-managerial' era have been portrayed as not 'evidence based'. This is consistent with the argument discussed by Pollitt and Bouckaert[99] that NPM represents a major advance over 'pre-managerial' practices. The analysis in this paper suggests a different view. It is clear that considerable effort went into research on hospital accounting practices in the 1950s; in turn this raised debates that in many respects prefigure current controversies in public sector management. Managerialism *tout court* appears be engaged with questions that were anticipated in 'managerialism *avant la lettre*'.

Notes

1 C. Pollitt and G. Bouckaert, *Public Management Reform: a Comparative Analysis*, Oxford: Oxford University Press, 2000, pp. 88–90.
2 P. Dunleavy and C. Hood, 'From old public administration to new public management', *Public Money and Management* 14, 1994: 9–16.
3 Ibid., p. 9.
4 C. Hood, 'A public management for all seasons', *Public Administration* 69, 1991: 3–19.
5 Ibid., p. 4
6 Ibid.; see also T. Cutler and B. Waine, *Managing the Welfare State: Text and Sourcebook*, Oxford: Berg, 1997, p. 4.
7 *Statutory Rules and Orders 1948, Volume II*, London, HMSO, 1948, p. 743.
8 Ibid., p. 736.
9 F. Prochaska, *Philanthropy and the Hospitals of London: the King's Fund 1897–1990*, Oxford: Oxford University Press, 1992, p. 71.
10 *Statutory Rules and Orders 1948*, p. 741.
11 Public Record Office, Central Health Services Council: Minutes of a Meeting, 21st June 1949, CHSC (49), 2nd meeting, MH 133/32.
12 Public Record Office, Central Health Services Council: Interim Report by the Hospital Administration Committee, CHSC (49), December, MH 133/32.
13 Ibid.
14 Nuffield Provincial Hospitals Trust, *Report of an Experiment in Hospital Costing*, London: Oxford University Press, 1952, p. 10.
15 King Edward's Hospital Fund for London: Appointment of a Consultant on Hospital Finance, March 1939, King's Fund Archive (London Metropolitan Archive) A/KE/694/1–88.
16 Ibid.
17 Prochaska, *Philanthropy*, p. 143.

18 J. Stone, *Hospital Management and Organisation*, 1st edn, London: Faber & Gwynne, 1927.
19 Prochaska, *Philanthropy*, p. 143.
20 Public Record Office, Central Health Services Council: Minutes of a meeting, 13th December 1949, CHSC (49), 4th meeting, December, MH 133/32.
21 King Edward's Hospital Fund for London, *Report on Costing Investigations*, London: King Edward's Hospital Fund for London, 1952, para 2.
22 Ministry of Health, *Hospital Costing Returns for the Year Ended 31st March 1951*, London: HMSO, 1952, 1.
23 Public Record Office, Teaching Hospitals Association: Report on Hospital Costing, June 1953, MH 137/54.
24 Public Record Office, Chatterton to Marre, 9 June 1953, MH 137/54.
25 Ibid.
26 C. Webster, *The Health Services since the War: ii. Government and Health Care: the British National Health Service 1958–1979*, London: the Stationery Office, 1996, p. 5.
27 Public Record Office, Chatterton to Marre, 9 June 1953, MH 137/54.
28 Ibid.
29 Ibid.
30 Ibid.
31 Ibid.
32 Ibid.
33 Public Record Office, Hospital Costing, September 1953, MH 137/54.
34 Public Record Office Hospital Costing, Ministry of Health Appoints Working Party, November 1953, MH 137/54.
35 Ibid.
36 Public Record Office, Chatterton to Marre, 25 June 1955, MH 137/55.
37 Department of Health, *NHS Performance Ratings: Acute Trusts*, London: Department of Health, 2001.
38 Ministry of Health, Hospital Costing Returns, p. 5.
39 Public Record Office, Interim Report of the Costing Sub-committee Appointed by the Committee of Regional Boards, February 1950, MH 137/13.
40 Ministry of Health, Hospital Costing Returns, p. 2.
41 Ibid.
42 Ibid., p. 4.
43 Ibid.
44 Ibid., p. 5.
45 Ibid.
46 King Edward's Hospital Fund for London, *Report on Costing Investigations*, para. 94.
47 Ibid.
48 Ibid., para. 91.
49 Ibid.
50 Nuffield Provincial Hospitals Trust, *Report of an Experiment*, p. 24.
51 Ibid., p. 17.
52 King Edward's Hospital Fund for London, *Report on Costing Investigations*, para. 120.
53 Nuffield Provincial Hospitals Trust, *Report of an Experiment*, p. 110.
54 Ibid., pp 110–11.
55 Ibid., p. 123.
56 King Edward's Hospital Fund for London, *Report on Costing*, para. 38.
57 Nuffield Provincial Hospitals Trust, *Report of an Experiment*, p. 114.
58 Ibid., p. 119.
59 King Edward's Hospital Fund for London, *Report on Costing Investigations*, para. 156.

60 Nuffield Provincial Hospitals Trust, *Report of an Experiment*, p. 29.
61 Ibid., p. 58.
62 Ministry of Health, *Report of the Working Party on Hospital Costing*, London: HMSO, 1955, para. 11.
63 Ibid.
64 Ibid.
65 Ibid., para. 19.
66 Public Record Office, National Health Service: Hospital Costing, HM (56) 24, 27 March 1956, MH 137/55.
67 C. Montacute, *Costing and Efficiency in Hospitals: a Critical Survey of Costing as an Aid to the Management of Hospitals*, London: Oxford University Press, 1962, pp xi and xiv.
68 Ibid., p. xi.
69 Ibid., p. xiv.
70 Ibid., p. 71.
71 Ibid.
72 Ibid., p. 82.
73 Ibid., p. 100.
74 Ibid.
75 King Edward's Hospital Fund for London, *Report on Costing Investigations*, Appendix 1.
76 Public Record Office, Stone to Chatterton, 13 June 1955, MH 137/54.
77 Ministry of Health, *Report of the Working Party*, Appendix A.
78 Ibid., para. 13.
79 Ibid., para. 6.
80 B. Abel-Smith and R. Titmuss, *The Cost of the National Health Service in England and Wales*, Cambridge: Cambridge University Press, 1956, 1, p. 138.
81 Acton Society Trust *Hospitals and the State, Part I Groups, Regions and Committees, Hospital Management Committees*, London: Acton Society Trust, 1957, pp. 30–1.
82 Public Record Office, Teaching Hospitals Association: Report on Hospital Costing, June 1953, MH 137/54.
83 Public Record Office North West Metropolitan Regional Hospital Board, Oral Evidence to the Guillebaud Committee, GC (53), 6th Meeting, 29 and 30 September 1953, MH 137/227.
84 Public Record Office, East Anglia Regional Hospital Board, Oral Evidence to the Guillebaud Committee, GC (53), 6th Meeting, 29 and 30 September 1953, MH 137/227.
85 Public Record Office, Hospital Costing (Workman to Chatterton), 4 January 1956, T 227/802.
86 Nuffield Provincial Hospitals Trust, *Report of an Experiment*, p. 50.
87 Ibid.
88 Ibid., pp. 44–5.
89 Ibid., p. 45.
90 R. Griffiths, *NHS Management Inquiry*, London: Department of Health and Social Security, 1983.
91 Pollitt and Bouckaert, *Public Management Reform*, p. 58.
92 Ibid.
93 T. Packwood, J. Keen and M. Buxton, *Hospitals in Transition: the Resource Management Experiment*, Milton Keynes: Open University Press, 1991, p. 14.
94 Ibid., p. 16.
95 Ibid., p. 150.
96 Anglo-American Productivity Council, *Management Accounting*, London: Anglo-American Productivity Council, 1950, p. 41.

97 King Edward's Hospital Fund for London, *Report on Costing Investigations*, para. 118.
98 C. Naylor 'Grey zones of clinical practice: some limits to evidence-based medicine', *Lancet* 345, 1 April 1995: 840–2.
99 Pollitt and Bouckaert, *Public Management Reform*, p. 58.

Recommended further reading

T. Cutler, 'The cost of the National Health Service: problem definition and policy response 1942–1960', unpublished Ph.D. thesis, London School of Hygiene and Tropical Medicine, 2000.

P. Dunleavy and C. Hood, 'From old public administration to new public management', *Public Money and Management* 14(3), 1994: 9–16.

King Edward's Hospital Fund for London (King's Fund) *Report on Costing Investigations*, London: King Edward's Hospital Fund for London, 1952.

Nuffield Provincial Hospitals Trust (NPHT) *Report of an Experiment in Hospital Costing*, London: Oxford University Press, 1952.

J. Stone, *Hospital Management and Organisation*, 1st edn, London: Faber & Gwynne, 1927.

6   From evidence to market

Alfred Spinks's 1953 survey of new fields for pharmacological research, and the origins of ICI's cardiovascular programme

Viviane Quirke

Introduction

In 1953 Alfred Spinks, an organic chemist who had joined ICI's Dyestuffs Division in 1942, drew up a survey of new fields for pharmacological research at ICI.[1] For this task, he began by seeking guidance from the company's Medical Department on the requirements for new drugs in medical practice.[2] ICI were relative newcomers in the pharmaceutical field, and needed such information to gain an understanding of the market. The guidance Spinks obtained included epidemiological data and prescription statistics. In addition, Spinks searched through US and British pharmacological journals for potential research topics, and assessed their profitability and likelihood of success. He based his assessment not only on death rates, but also on the chronicity of conditions such as rheumatic diseases, and on the research activities of competitors in the UK and USA.

This essay describes how the evidence gathered, interpreted and presented by Spinks helped to shape ICI's research strategy. Among the topics identified in Spinks's survey, cardiovascular function became ICI's most important programme, leading, after the appointment of the pharmacologist J.W. (now Sir James) Black in 1958, to the development of a new class of drugs, the beta-blockers. In this essay, I will focus on the period leading up to Black's arrival, which is generally absent from accounts of the discovery of the beta-blockers, and which provides fresh insights on the move from infectious to chronic diseases that characterised the postwar period. This move is often depicted as a change from medical intervention to lifestyle public health.[3] However, this essay suggests that it was underpinned by pharmaceutical innovation, and that scientists such as Alfred Spinks, and companies such as ICI, played an active part in its realisation.

From infectious to chronic diseases

The shift in emphasis from infectious to chronic diseases in postwar medical research has been widely acknowledged.[4] However, little is known about its rationale and mechanism of this shift.[5] The archives of the pharmaceutical industry, and, when these are inaccessible, company histories, offer a hitherto little used resource. They suggest that, in the 1950s and 1960s, several British pharmaceutical companies set up research programmes to develop drugs against chronic diseases, identified as a major cause of morbidity and mortality in the postwar period.[6] However ICI, perhaps precisely *because* they were relative newcomers in the pharmaceutical field, had one of the earliest, and most clearly articulated, programmes of research to tackle chronic diseases, referred to as 'diseases of organic dysfunction'.

In her book on the history of ICI, Carol Kennedy has suggested that the main reason for ICI's success in pharmaceuticals was commercial. ICI's expertise in synthetic organic chemistry was unrivalled in the UK, and had enabled them to corner the market for antimalarials in the Empire and, later, the British Commonwealth. However, with the gradual shrinking and increasingly competitive nature of this market in the postwar period, they were faced with a need for a 'change of direction'.[7] Quoting Garnet Davey, a former research director of the Pharmaceuticals Division, Kennedy has written: 'It was clear that we would have to go into what I would call the diseases of dysfunction, the ones that affected western civilisation: heart diseases, arthritis, hypertension.'[8]

The ICI archives reveal a more problematic story than popular – and *a posteriori* – accounts. They suggest that the rationale for tackling chronic diseases was complex. It was linked to ICI's late entry into pharmaceuticals, to the scientific and technical expertise inherited from Dyestuffs, to the management culture that evolved within its Pharmaceutical Division, and to a favourable context. After the introduction of the sulphonamides in the 1930s, the launch of the antibiotic era in wartime, and the childhood immunisation campaigns of the postwar period, the victory over infectious diseases appeared imminent.[9] Furthermore, the National Health Service (1948), and the new Patents Act (1949), created a potentially profitable framework for medical and pharmaceutical research into chronic diseases. This opened up a window of opportunity that was exploited by ICI, like many other British pharmaceutical companies. However, unlike many of their competitors, ICI were late entrants into pharmaceutical research, and this led them to seek new niches, and new approaches for drug development. Before moving on to a detailed study of Spinks's survey of fields for pharmacological research, I therefore begin with a short history of IC Pharmaceuticals.

IC Pharmaceuticals

From Dyestuffs to Pharmaceuticals

Following the discovery by Gerhard Domagk in the laboratories of the German firm Bayer of the antibacterial activity of the red azo dye Prontosil,[10] Ernest Fourneau's team at the Pasteur Institute in Paris had discovered that the active part of the molecule was sulphanilamide, which was not covered by patents.[11] This led to the decision to set up a Medicinal Chemicals Section within the

Dyestuffs Division of ICI at Blackley, north of Manchester, in 1936.[12] The decision was made under the 'prodding' of C.F. Cronshaw (Research Director of Dyestuffs, later Division Chairman, and in 1943 Main Board Director), as well as under pressure from the company's academic advisers. These included Warrington Yorke (Professor of Tropical Medicine at Liverpool University), Robert Robinson (Professor of Organic Chemistry at Oxford University) and Carl Browning (Professor of Bacteriology at Glasgow University).[13] The new section at first comprised six Ph.D. chemists led by Sam Ellingworth, the only one of the group to have had previous medicinal experience. Its brief was not only to manufacture well-established drugs for other companies to sell, which Dyestuffs had done on occasion even before 1936,[14] but also to develop new drugs by adopting a 'research approach'.[15] For this, the section was given £15,000 p.a. for five years, and if by the end of that period nothing of interest had been discovered, it was to be disbanded.[16] To begin with, the chemists remained dependent for biological evaluation upon researchers working in the laboratories of various university medical schools, under the co-ordination of a panel of biological and chemical consultants. However, by 1937, the company had started recruiting biologists to work in a multidisciplinary team, and much of their research was concerned with the study of sulphonamide drugs. This led in 1940 to the synthesis by Dr F.L. Rose, an azo dye chemist who had joined ICI in 1932, and was transferred to the Medicinal Chemicals Section in 1936, of Sulphamezathine.[17] Less toxic than M&B 693 (Sulphapyridine), which is famous for having saved Winston Churchill's life when he was suffering from pneumonia during the war, Sulphamezathine was to rival May & Baker's compound and become widely adopted by the medical profession.

The Second World War and developing links with the state

In 1939, the onset of war led the British government to set up agency agreements with a number of companies, by which it paid for the cost of plant devoted to war production.[18] In this fashion, ICI came to play an important part in several major wartime research programmes, most notably the Tube Alloys (atom bomb) programme.[19] ICI also became involved in pharmaceutical projects that were crucial to the war effort, in particular the development of synthetic antimalarials and penicillin.[20] This involvement not only strengthened the position of pharmaceuticals within the group, but it also created new ties between the company and the state.

ICI, like other British firms, were asked to 'crack the German patents',[21] and to devise manufacturing processes for the drugs that were still (as the antisyphilitic drug Salvarsan had been in the First World War) only made in Germany. Among these were the antimalarials Pamaquin and Mepacrine, for which ICI was requested by the Allied military medical authorities to find a replacement.[22] Despite the secrecy surrounding the chemical structure of Mepacrine, Rose's colleague, Frank Curd, succeeded in working it out, and finding a production method for it in 1939. ICI's early efforts in the field proved invaluable when, in 1941, the route to the East Indian quinine plantations was severed by the Japanese invasion, and the company was able to begin large-scale production of the synthetic drug at the Grangemouth works.[23] By 1942, rising profits from antimalarials led the company's main board to establish a selling company, IC (Pharmaceuticals) Ltd, and in the same year enter the field of veterinary medicine.[24]

The year 1942 was significant for ICI in other respects. When, following the Japanese invasion, a vast UK–US antimalarial research programme was initiated under the co-ordination of the two national Medical Research Councils, ICI became heavily involved. The aim of this programme was to develop a new drug that would be easy to synthesise, and would act as a prophylactic (i.e. in the early stages of the protozoal infection, before the malaria parasite invades the bloodstream), unlike many of the compounds then in use. Rose, who was promoted to Section Leader in 1942, was assisted in this search by Curd, now his deputy. The parasitologist Garnet Davey was recruited in 1942 with the object of devising a biological screen, and despite his reluctance to work in industry appears to have agreed to join the company as a means of contributing to the war effort.[25] In addition, the team included Alfred Spinks, who had also been recruited in 1942, and who, although a chemist, was put to work on the pharmacodynamics (i.e. absorption, distribution, metabolism and excretion) of sulphonamide and antimalarial compounds. At first, ICI's management objected to the vast amount of time spent on these studies, which Rose had initiated in his work on the sulphonamides. However, Rose's promotion, and Spinks' personality and skill, ensured that the study of chemical structure–drug absorption relations became a matter of research policy within the Section.[26] The combined efforts of the team led, in 1945, to the development of Paludrine, which was used extensively in the Malaysian campaign, and long afterwards remained one of the most widely used antimalarials, alongside the US drug Chloroquine.[27]

In 1942, ICI also joined in the collaborative scheme to manufacture penicillin, at first by surface culture, and then by deep fermentation, a process highly favoured by the company's consultant, Robert Robinson. This scheme brought together British pharmaceutical companies, which had formed an association called the Therapeutic Research Corporation (TRC), university workers represented by the Medical Research Council (MRC), and the Ministry of Supply, as well as US companies, researchers and government agencies.[28] ICI joined the TRC in November 1942, after setting up a penicillin plant at Trafford Park, Manchester, which became an agency factory.[29] In 1943, the scheme to manufacture penicillin was followed by another, to uncover the chemical structure of penicillin with a view to its synthesis, and then again, because of their considerable synthetic and manufacturing capacity, ICI became key partners in the collaboration.[30]

With twenty-five agency factories, ICI were the British government's largest wartime industrial agent. The scientific and technical expertise acquired, and the contacts developed during the war, proved crucial to the postwar development of IC Pharmaceuticals. Whilst antibiotics and fermentation technologies were outside ICI's main area of expertise, but nevertheless remained as a legacy of the company's wartime activities,[31] the experience of synthesising, testing and manufacturing antimalarials, and the profits made from their sale, were to have a considerable impact on the company's postwar R&D.[32] An offshoot of the antimalarial work was the antiseptic Hibitane, which involved the 'same sort of chemistry', and long remained one of ICI's top-selling drugs.[33] In addition, clinical observations of the hypotensive side-effects of some antimalarials were to provide ICI's chemists with chemical leads in the development of antihypertensive agents.[34]

But perhaps an even more important outcome of the war was the links built up between ICI and government agencies, especially the MRC. An indication of the good relations developed between ICI and the Council was the appointment of its Secretary, Sir Edward Mellanby, as company consultant after his retirement in 1949.[35] Following the creation of the National Health Service, ICI also cultivated good relations with the Ministry of Health (MH), and recognised the importance of maintaining the goodwill of its ministers.[36] These links led ICI to become much sought-after partners in a number of nation-wide collaborative schemes. During the war, ICI had provided anaesthetists with a specially purified trichloroethylene, Trilene, and afterwards continued research on anaesthetics.[37] In 1953, as a result of explosions that were related to the increasingly popular use of electrical devices in surgery, the MH, having consulted with the MRC, recommended that a search be carried out for a non-volatile anaesthetic. In 1955, ICI, like other British companies, were therefore invited by the MRC to join in a co-operative scheme to develop such an anaesthetic.[38] However, by then ICI, having anticipated the Ministry's recommendations, were already making good progress with halothane (Fluothane). The compound had been synthesised in 1953 by Charles Suckling, a chemist who had been recruited in 1942 to work in the Mond Division on fluorine gases for the Tube Alloys Project.[39] Because of ICI's head-start, the collaborative scheme became a one-to-one partnership between the MRC and ICI whose drug, which required specially designed apparatus, became widely adopted by the community of anaesthetists, and brought profits as well as prestige to the company.[40]

Reflecting the growing importance of pharmaceuticals within the company, in 1944 the ICI Board set up a separate Pharmaceutical Division. However, Dyestuffs Division continued to be strongly represented on the Pharmaceutical Board, and in control of the research laboratories and manufacturing plant until 1955.[41]

Making the move to Alderley Park

The move towards a wholly independent Pharmaceuticals Division was, therefore, very gradual, and the company's strategy in pharmaceutical R&D was, understandably for a relative newcomer onto the pharmaceutical market, cautious. ICI 'hedged their bets', and developed a three-pronged approach that involved:

- Manufacturing and/or marketing competitors' products to gain experience in a variety of fields.
- Building on their strengths: mainly synthetic organic chemicals (sulphonamides developed as hypoglycaemic agents, synthetic analogues of cortisone, etc....).
- Developing new products and, in order to do so, new approaches to drug development (more efficient screening methods, and a pharmacological research programme to assist with ICI's capability in synthetic organic chemistry).

By the time of the move to Alderley Park in 1957, the third approach had gained in importance, and Spinks played a key role in this transformation. However, he acted within the framework of ICI's management structure, which evolved in response to internal changes, such as the expansion and decentralisation of research within the Divisions,[42] and also in response to external, scientific and medical developments.

Following the recent successes of the chemotherapeutic approach to the treatment of infectious diseases,[43] in 1947 a Chemotherapeutic Research Committee, chaired by Dr C.M. Scott, and with Sam Ellingworth as Secretary, was added to the Management and the Sales and Services Committees of the Pharmaceutical Division.[44] The remit of the Chemotherapeutic Research Committee (henceforth 'The Committee') was: 1) to advise the Delegate Board of IC Pharmaceuticals concerning all chemotherapeutic research, including both its chemical and biological aspects, and research in pharmacy; 2) to be responsible for annual research reports; 3) to advise with respect to the appointment of and relations with consultants; 4) to meet at three-monthly intervals; and 5) to submit minutes to the Delegate Board.

The research programme for 1948 was laid out at the first meeting of the Committee. New projects included:

1 amoebiasis;
2 haelminthology;
3 acid-fast bacilli;
4 antibacterials (general);
5 virus infections;
6 tissue growth;
7 anticonvulsants;
8 speculative work on remaining projects:
9 malaria, trypanosomiasis, spirochaetosis, leichmaniasis, analgesics, spasmolytics and respiratory stimulants, mycology, pest control, process development.[45]

The term 'speculative' was used at ICI to signify a theoretical approach to drug development, based on scientific hypotheses, in contrast with more routine chemical investigations.[46] By the time of its second meeting, the

Committee had identified hypertension as an important topic of investigation, requiring such a 'novel approach'.[47] At another meeting in 1951, it was put forward as a new research target, together with local analgesics and anaesthetics, antispasmodics, and anticoagulants.[48] In 1953, although the American example had shown minor improvements to existing products to be profitable, the Committee stated that a flow of new products was required for the company to prosper.[49]

Thus, in the context of setting new therapeutic targets, and of developing novel approaches in order to ensure the flow of new products, plans began to be made to build pharmaceutical laboratories. By March 1953, definite plans were laid out for a new research centre at Alderley Park, in Cheshire, defined as a 'centre for speculative chemotherapeutic research'.[50] Its estimated cost was £1,250,000. Although there were no clear directives as to the proper amount to be spent on research, so far research expenditure at IC Pharmaceuticals had represented roughly 10 per cent of its turnover, a figure similar, it was remarked, to that 'applied to IG Farben (pre war) and USA pharmaceutical firms [postwar]'. Expected turnover in 1957–60 was expected to reach £5,000,000 p.a.; therefore it seemed likely that £500,000 p.a. would be spent on research.[51]

The USA, therefore, provided a working model for IC Pharmaceuticals.[52] The creation in 1949 of a central research laboratory in the grounds of the Frythe, near Welwyn, was symptomatic of the growing importance of the American model in R&D. The Frythe laboratory fulfilled the wish, expressed even before the Second World War, that ICI should be endowed with laboratories where scientists might engage in fundamental research 'freed from the urgencies and distractions of applied research',[53] and was inspired by the Du Pont Experimental Station at Wilmington.[54] This wish would also – to some extent – be fulfilled with the creation of Alderley Park, where, from the start, cardiovascular function was to be a major focus of study, as part of a wider programme to tackle chronic diseases.

ICI's cardiovascular research programme

The origins of the programme

Contrary to popular accounts, such as Kennedy's history of ICI, it appears that, although of all chronic afflictions hypertension was recognised as most serious, and worthy of the company's attention as early as 1948,[55] a broad programme to study diseases of 'organic dysfunction' was not set up until 1954.[56] Furthermore, it had to compete for resources with protozoal and bacterial diseases until 1958, if not later. A major impetus was given to the programme after it had been realised in 1958 that ICI was falling behind in terms of sales of antimalarials.[57] ICI's share of British export business in antimalarials had decreased from 98 per cent in 1949, to about 50 per cent in 1957, when it represented roughly £500,000, of which Paludrine made up £280,000. In addition, it was anticipated (rather optimistically) that the mass eradication campaigns planned by the World Health Organization would eventually lead to a cessation of demand for these drugs. Nevertheless, infectious diseases in general, and malaria in particular, continued to be of major concern to the company well into the 1960s, when problems of drug resistance provided it with fresh challenges.[58] Thus, ICI's cardiovascular programme could be said to have grown out of, rather than simply replaced, the company's anti-infective programme, in three ways: 1) increasing clinical usage of anti-infectives since the Second World War led to observations of the hypotensive side-effects of some antimalarials; 2) these provided chemical leads for research into antihypertensive compounds; 3) by reinvesting profits from anti-infective drugs new research programmes, such as that on hypertension, could be set up.

With a view to establishing a Pharmacological Section, and in preparation for the move to the new pharmaceutical laboratories, in 1950 Spinks was sent to Oxford University, to acquire the necessary knowledge in the biological sciences. He was chosen because he had distinguished himself in his work on the pharmacodynamics of sulphonamide and antimalarial drugs, at a time when very little formal teaching in pharmacology existed, and because this work had helped to put the company's approach to drug development on a more 'rational' basis.[59] Furthermore, he clearly showed promise as a future research manager. However, his return to university did not happen without a certain amount of board-level opposition, which had to be overcome by Spinks's supporters, most notably the research director of the Dyestuffs Division Mr Clifford Paine, the research manager of the Pharmaceuticals Division Dr W.A. Sexton, and Frank Rose.[60] Their lobbying succeeded, and Spinks enlisted on a two-year undergraduate course in physiology, beginning in 1950. During his vacation time, he worked in Henry Blaschko's laboratory in the Pharmacology Department, headed by Professor J.H. Burn.[61] He obtained a first-class degree in June 1953.

On his return to Blackley, a Pharmacological Section was set up in August 1952, but this had as yet no special apparatus, and the two laboratory assistants were untrained in pharmacological techniques. The topic selected for study was, therefore, diuresis, which was capable of commanding sales of £100,000 p.a., and according to Spinks 'seemed to fulfil most closely the three requirements of simplicity of apparatus, simplicity of techniques, and availability of compounds'.[62] Then, in March 1953, he drew up a survey of new fields for pharmacological research, which he presented to the Chemotherapeutic Research Committee. He began 'in characteristic fashion', for this was not the first time that he had prepared a survey,[63] by 'addressing a formal letter to the Medical Director seeking guidance on the current needs for new drugs in clinical practice'.[64] However, this time it was more than a literature survey. The evidence Spinks presented was quantitative, including epidemiological data, and statistics on drug prescriptions, which although notoriously difficult to obtain in the UK,[65] probably were obtained from the MH by the company's Medical Department. The evidence also included a survey of research topics in the USA and UK, which Spinks may have compiled himself from the US *Journal of Pharmacology and Experimental*

Table 6.1 Death from various causes, England and Wales, 1949 (as percentage of total deaths)

Main heading	Subheading	Percentage
Infective and parasitic diseases	All	6.1
	TB	3.9
General	All	1.3
	'Rheumatism'	0.35
	Diabetes mellitus	0.7
Blood etc.	All	0.8
CNS	All	12.8
	Cerebral haemorrhage	6.7
	Cerebral thrombosis	4.6
Circulatory system	All	34.6
	Arteriosclerosis	2.7
	Heart, valvular	2.7
	Heart, myocardial degeneration	18.1
	Heart, coronary disease	8.4
Respiratory system	All	11.4
	Bronchitis	6.0
	Pneumonia	4.1
Digestive system	All	3.4
	Ulcer	0.95
	Appendicitis	0.3
Cancer	All	16.4
Urinary and genital system	All	3.65
	Nephritis	2.2
Skin and bones	All	0.2
Congenital malformation	All	0.95
Senility		2.55
Violence		3.65
Other		2.2

Source: CPR 3: A. Spinks, 'Survey of new fields for pharmacological research', 24 March 1953.

Therapeutics, and the *British Journal of Pharmacology and Chemotherapy* (a journal started a few years earlier by Burn).[66]

What qualitative evidence, or tacit knowledge, Spinks brought back from Oxford is unclear. However, Burn's biographical memoir suggests that Spinks came in contact with experimental methods and results concerning the action of sympathomimetic amines (drugs that mimic stimulation of the sympathetic nervous system) on the heart and other tissues, as this was one of Burn's chief areas of interest at the time of Spinks's stay in Oxford.[67] In Blashko's lab, he may also have become acquainted with the work on dopa decarboxylase, which laid the foundations for the development of the anti-hypertensive agent L-methyldopa.[68] Although Spinks's future work on

Table 6.2 Survey of a sample of 17,301 prescriptions on form EC10 for September 1949

| Drug class | Drug | Prescriptions | |
		Subtotal	Total
Hypnotics and sedatives	Barbiturates	1,636 ⎱	2,643
	Bromides	1,007 ⎰	
Stomachics			1,678
Tonics			1,553
Mild analgesics and antipyretics	Aspirin	330	1,528
	Codeine, etc.	565	
	Others	633	
Cough mixtures	Expectorant	402	1,382
	Sedative	174	
	Combined	806	
Vitamins	A&D	175	739
	B1	177	
	B complex	126	
	C	66	
	E	27	
	Multiple	168	
Penicillin			681
Bronchodilators, analeptics, antispasmodics	Adrenaline	29	637
	Ephedrine	152	
	Aminophylline	69	
	Compound	160	
	Atropine	227	
Iron			623
Laxatives			587
Sulphonamides			498
Cardiac drugs	Glucosides	250	481
	Nitrites	231	
Hormones	Insulin	68	477
	Oestrogens	234	
	Liver	50	
	Others	125	
Misc. (see Table 6.3)			412
Antihistaminics			302

(Continued on next page)

Table 6.2 (continued)

Drug class	Drug	Prescriptions	
		Subtotal	Total
Urinary preparations			264
Amphetamine			218
Strong analgesics	Morphine	57 ⎫	
	Diamorphine	37 ⎬	156
	Pethidine, physeptone, etc.	62 ⎭	

Source: CPR 3: A. Spinks, 'Survey of new fields for pharmacological research', 24 March 1953.

antihypertensive agents was almost certainly influenced by the research carried out in Burn's department in 1950–3, the epidemiological data gathered by ICI's Medical Department occupied a prominent place in his survey, for more clearly than any other evidence, it located the greatest need for drugs.

Spinks's survey

The first table listed the causes of death in England and Wales in 1949. It showed that the highest percentage of deaths was attributed to diseases of the circulatory system, which broken down into subheadings highlighted myocardial degeneration as the principal cause of death.

However, Spinks stressed that, in choosing fields of study, considerations other than death rates had to be taken into account. These included the *chronicity* of the conditions, which hinted at a potential mass market for drugs:

> Thus, no one doubts the great importance of the rheumatic diseases as a field for research in spite of the trifling death rate attributable to them. Some cardiovascular affections also wholly or partly cripple the sufferer for many years; and others, like hypertension, are ultimately so dangerous that palliative treatment over a number of years might be justified in spite of a lack of serious crippling symptoms. Other diseases, apart from the rheumatic group, figure less prominently in Table 6.1 than their incidence and importance would suggest; notable examples are the ulcer group, and diabetes mellitus....The study of senescence is to be kept in mind as a possible major field of research; but initially it might better be approached by way of a more specific topic: cardiovascular research is an obvious possibility.[69]

The second table consisted of a survey of 17,301 prescription forms for September 1949. Whereas hypnotics and sedatives headed the list, cardiac drugs, by contrast, came nearer to the bottom. Table 6.3 completed Table 6.2, by providing details of the 'misc.' category, that of 'rarely prescribed drugs', which included antimalarials.

Table 6.3 Rarely prescribed drugs (misc. in *Table 6.2*)

Calcium
Anthelmintics
Mersalyl (thought to be administered from doctors' own stores)
Cold vaccines
Vaccines
Antimalarials etc.

Source: CPR 3: A. Spinks, 'Survey of new fields for pharmacological research',
    24 March 1953.

Table 6.4 gave the distribution of current pharmacological and related research effort in the USA, and indicated that cardiovascular research was at the top of the American biomedical agenda, with the largest part of the research carried out by government research establishments, followed by universities and, finally, by industry. However, Spinks commented that in the USA 'the weight of influence is from industry to universities', whereas in the UK 'the influence is often in reverse direction'. Amongst the topics studied in the American cardiovascular field, 61 per cent were concerned with hypertension, and most of these consisted in the study of veratrum analogues and antiadrenaline agents.

Table 6.6 showed that, by contrast, British pharmacological research was dominated by the study of sympathomimetics, a legacy of the research tradition created by Henry Hallett Dale. Spinks commented: 'British pharmacology still clings to the field initiated, some think exhausted, by Sir Henry Dale'.[70] By contrast, only a small proportion of research laboratories carried out cardiovascular research (mainly ganglionic block and veratrum analogues). This suggested to Spinks that, if ICI were to enter the field of cardiovascular research, they would be among the first to follow the trend shown by the US data, and would find relatively little competition in the UK.[71]

Spinks confirmed the Committee's earlier findings that hypotensive agents were 'the largest potential fields',[72] with a market for a successful drug capable of reaching £100,000 p.a. by 1956.[73] He then proceeded to identify research priorities according to 1) probable profitability, and 2) likelihood of success:

1 profitability: cardiovascular topics, senescence, oral contraception, growth, gastric secretion, diabetes;
2 likely success: cardiovascular, gastric secretion, growth, oral contraception, diabetes, senescence.

Among cardiovascular topics:

1 profitability: hypertension, myocardial degeneration, atherosclerosis, coronary dilators, arrhythmias;
2 likely success: arrhythmias, coronary dilators, hypertension, atherosclerosis, myocardial degeneration.[74]

Table 6.4 Distribution of current pharmacological (and related) research effort in the USA

Subject		% of total effort		
		Government	University	Industry
Cardiovascular research (subdivisions in Table 6.5)	23.7	2.0	17.4	4.3
Sympathomimetics (amphetamine 2.6)	6.9		5.8	1.1
Anticonvulsants	6.9		3.7	3.2
Antirheumatics (adrenal cortex and related topics)	6.7		2.0	4.7
Hypnotics	5.8		4.9	0.9
Analgesics	5.5	2.6	2.3	0.6
Curarising agents	4.6		3.2	1.4
Anaesthetics	4.6	0.9	3.7	
Antibacterials	4.3		2.6	1.7
Diuretics	3.8		2.9	0.9
Acetylcholine	3.8		3.8	
Gastric secretion	0.9			0.9
Antihistamines	0.6			
Other misc.	3.9			

Note: As calculated from numbers of authors publishing papers on stated topics in vols 103, 105 and 106 of the *Journal of Pharmacology and Experimental Therapeutics*.

Source: CPR 3: A. Spinks, 'Survey of new fields for pharmacological research', 24 March 1953.

In this very systematic way, Spinks reasoned that cardiovascular topics were both potentially the most profitable, and the most likely to lead to a successful outcome. Amongst cardiovascular topics, although hypertension would be the most profitable, it would also be one of the more difficult to tackle. Nevertheless, if the American example was anything to go by, he thought that hypertension was worthy of the company's attention:

> The incidence of hypertension in the US is about 25 per cent according to a recent Mayo Clinic Symposium. It is possible that continued palliative treatment will come into general use even in the absence of dangerous or alarming symptoms. If this possibility were ever realized (none of the drugs thus far encourages optimism) the project would dwarf any conceivable anti-infective market.[75]

Spinks then went on to set the research agenda for a hypertension project, which became the agenda for the whole of the cardiovascular programme at ICI:

Table 6.5 Distribution of research on cardiovascular topics in the USA

Topic		% effort	
Hypertension		61	
Cardiac stimulants		15	
Arrhythmias		10	
Coronary dilators		2.5	
Others		11.5	
	Veratrum	20.5	
HT	Antiadrenaline agents	19.5	61
	Ganglionic block	13.5	
	Vasodilators	7.5	

Source: CPR 3: A. Spinks, 'Survey of new fields for pharmacological research',
     24 March 1953.

I should therefore support entry only on the following terms:

1   fullest possible use should be made of our chemical advantage: a) by establishing screens that allow a high rate of compound turnover; b) by establishing general screens that indicate all predictable modes of action;
2   competitive experimental drugs should be rapidly made and assessed even at the expense of a fair proportion of our effort;
3   we should endeavour to obtain close clinical contacts and review our interest in the field frequently in the light of clinical progress and the status of competitive drugs;
4   an early commercial entry would be useful although not essential.[76]

The evidence Spinks provided was, of itself, convincing. It was tangible, quantitative evidence, presented at a time when the company was turning to statistics in an effort to improve the efficiency of its screening and experimental methods.[77] It was also supported by Spinks's clear reasoning and powers of persuasion, which played an important role in the management's acceptance of his ideas.[78] In the following section, I show how the company subsequently translated this evidence into R&D strategy.

Implementing Spinks's survey

This survey put the company's research programme on diseases of organic dysfunction, which, after several years in limbo, began in earnest in 1954, on a more secure footing.[79] Only from then on, can one properly talk of a research programme into chronic diseases, and at ICI this was to be, essentially, a *pharmacological* programme, in which hypertension was to provide a focal point.

Table 6.6 Distribution of current pharmacological (and related) research effort in Britain

Subject		% total effort		
		Government	University	Industry
Sympathomimetics (adrenaline etc.)	13.9		13.9	
Curarising agents	8.1	0.8	6.1	1.2
Parasympathomimetics (acetyl-choline etc.)	7.8		7.8	
Antibacterials (except TB)	6.6		3.9	2.7
Tumour inhibitors	6.2		1.5	4.7
Trypanocides	5.8	1.2	3.1	1.5
Histamine and antihistaminics	5.2	1.5	3.7	
Cardiovascular research	5.2	0.8	2.1	2.3
ganglionic block	3.1	0.8		
veratrum	1.2		1.2	2.3
Choline esterases etc.	4.3		4.3	
Analgesics	4.3		3.1	1.2
Spasmolytics	3.5		2.3	1.2
Antitubercular drugs	3.1		1.9	1.2
Antiviral agents	3.1			3.1
Antimalarials	1.9			1.9
Antirheumatics	1.5		1.5	
Other misc.	19.8			

Note: As calculated from numbers of authors publishing papers on related topics in vols 6 and 7 of *British Journal of Pharmacology and Chemotherapy*.

Source: CPR 3: A. Spinks, 'Survey of new fields for pharmacological research', 24 March 1953.

The impact of Spinks's survey can be seen in the joint annual research plans of the Research Department (Medicinals Division) and Biological Departments, with the addition of a pharmacological section to the list given above (on p. 151):

17 Pharmacology:

a   diuretics
b   anticoagulants
c   local anaesthetics
d   hypotensive agents
e   pancreatic function
f   gastric secretion
g   inflammatory conditions[80]

When Spinks had presented his survey, he had felt the need to justify the inclusion of so many topics for research. He did this in a way reflecting the climate of optimism that reigned in the early 1950s concerning the victory over infectious diseases, but also the uncertainties about the outcomes of the research programme:

> The chief reason for including so many [topics for research] is the necessity of gaining know-how in a number of fields. There is little doubt that within the next 20 years (given stable conditions) there will be a decline in the importance of infective diseases. Many diseases will disappear. The structural and functional diseases will remain. We should be prepared eventually to transfer some of our interests to them, and to that end it is desirable that we should start work on a number of novel projects even if initially we try only to test their feasibility.[81]

Despite such uncertainties, Spinks succeeded in convincing the management of pharmaceutical research at ICI. In 1955, effort on pharmacological topics was increased by the formation of a new unit, led by J.M. Thorp, who began the study of atherosclerosis.[82] Spinks himself, working with the chemist Dr E.H.P. Young, took the lion's share of the programme, working on hypertension, as well as diuretics, anticoagulants, local anaesthetics and sedatives.[83] An embryonic cardiovascular programme had therefore begun to take shape, even before the move to Alderley Park. Spinks's work on hypertension led to the development of the ganglion-blocker pempidine (marketed under the name of Tenormal).[84] Although pempidine presented advantages over other antihypertensive agents, in that it could be taken orally, ganglion-blockers had unpleasant side effects, and were soon superseded by better drugs. However, Spinks's contribution to ICI's cardiovascular programme survived in many ways, not least in the company's continuing commitment to a broad-based pharmacological approach to drug development, and in a clear research agenda (see above, p. 159). Perhaps it was in recognition of this contribution that, in 1976, the beta-blocker atenolol was marketed under the name of 'Tenormin'.

Alderley Park opened in 1957, and at the same time the Pharmaceutical Division broke away from Dyestuffs, coming directly under the Main Board of ICI from that date.[85] Spinks played a prominent part in the design and occupation of the laboratories, and in the appointment of new researchers, including Drs Brian Newbould and James Black, who according to Spinks's biographers 'sought and found support for his work on beta-receptors'.[86] Subsequently, Spinks rose up through the company, becoming in 1961 Manager of the first Biochemistry Department, which included a natural products group that had been transferred from the Frythe laboratories.[87] He was made Research Director, replacing Sexton in 1966, then Deputy Chairman, and in 1970 succeeded Rose on the ICI Main Board, responsible for the R&D of the entire organisation. In the 1970s he played an important part as adviser to government on scientific and industrial policy.[88] In his report on biotechnology, which was instrumental in establishing the UK biotech industry in the 1980s,[89] he showed the same qualities of clarity of exposition and persuasiveness displayed earlier, in his 1953 survey, which had helped to establish ICI's cardiovascular programme. Of him, the chairman of Dunlop, on whose board Spinks was invited to serve in 1979, has said that he was 'an eminently wise, shrewd and experienced businessman who could read a balance sheet as easily as a DNA helix'.[90]

Spinks's survey had consisted in quantitative evidence about the market for drugs. This evidence, combined with his powers of persuasion, had helped to shape the company's research strategy, and prepared the ground for James Black's arrival at Alderley Park in 1958. There are indications that, after completing their ganglion-blocker project, ICI had been preparing to alter their course and look at centrally, instead of peripherally, acting agents.[91] However, Black's work represented a radical departure from the approach until then adopted by most pharmaceutical companies to the problem of heart disease. The radical nature of the beta-blockers as a pharmaceutical innovation was, ultimately, to change the market for cardiovascular drugs.[92] Therefore, this essay ends with a brief history of the beta-blockers.

James Black, and the development of the beta-blockers at ICI

If little has been written about the period leading up to the development of the beta-blockers at ICI, by contrast the history of the beta-blockers themselves is much better known.[93] Garnet Davey, who had recently become manager of the Biological Research Department, invited Black to come and work at Alderley Park on coronary artery disease.[94] With Spinks working on hypertension, and Thorp on atherosclerosis, a proper cardiovascular research programme was now in existence, and this was reflected in the title of the research reports, on 'Anaemia, allergy, rheumatism, and cardiovascular diseases', edited by A.F. Crowther.[95] Davey appears to have cushioned Black against potential opposition to his original approach to angina pectoris,[96] by which he 'turned the problem on its head', suggesting that rather than *increasing* the supply of oxygen *to* the heart, one should try to *decrease* the demand of oxygen *from* the heart.[97] Raymond Ahlquist's theory of alpha and beta-receptors, which had largely been ignored by the pharmacological community at that time, provided him with a means of achieving this objective.[98] Thus protected, and benefiting from the collaboration of ICI's organic chemists John Stephenson and, subsequently, A.F. Crowther, R. Howe and L.H. Smith, Black was able to test his ideas unhindered, at least in the early stages, before commercial imperatives were brought to bear upon the project.[99] Within only two years of his arrival, Black had developed the first clinically effective beta-blocker, pronethalol (Alderlin), whose name was derived from Alderley Park. It underwent small-scale trials in 1961, and was launched in 1963. By then, Spinks had been promoted to Manager of the Biochemistry Department, and the hypertension project, which had become Black's responsibility, was soon eclipsed by the beta-blocker project.[100] After carcinogenic studies had shown that Alderlin caused thymic tumours in mice, it was withdrawn from the market, and was replaced by another compound, propanolol (Inderal). Inderal had been synthesised earlier as part of the vast chemical effort to obtain wide patent coverage of the field, and had been tested in one of the pharmacological screens in 1962. It was marketed in 1965.[101] Following extensive trials, which began in 1964 and gathered pace throughout the 1960s, Inderal became the preferred treatment for angina pectoris and cardiac arrhythmias. Later, it also was used in the treatment of hypertension, after it had been found in the clinic that it reduced blood pressure.[102]

In 1964, having acquired a considerable reputation for his work on the beta-blockers, and eager to try out his ideas in another field of research, Black left ICI for the British subsidiary of the American company SmithKline & French, where he developed the H2-antagonist cimetidine (Tagamet), for the treatment of gastric ulcers.[103] After Black's departure, ICI continued to do research on beta-blockers, partly, as competitive activity increased, in order to maintain their foothold in the field, and partly so as to introduce better drugs onto the market. Inderal had been found to provoke bronchoconstriction, and therefore was contraindicated in asthmatic patients. In 1970, ICI launched practolol (Eraldin), which acted selectively on the heart, but in 1975 had to be withdrawn because it was suspected of causing blindness in certain patients.[104] By then, it was felt that the market was saturated with beta-blockers, and atenolol (Tenormin), unlike its predecessors, was marketed primarily as an antihypertensive drug, with the statement: 'one tablet, once a day, simplicity in hypertension'.[105] In 1987, that is to say over ten years after its launch, Tenormin and its related products generated sales worldwide of about £500 million, out of a total of £1,000 million.[106] However, these figures need to be offset against innovation costs, which between 1975 and 1985 amounted to £600 million invested in R&D, to evaluate 100,000 new compounds, only forty-seven of which reached the development stage and three reached the market.[107]

Thus, Black's original approach helped ICI to gain an 'early commercial entry', whilst the skill of Crowther's team of chemists enabled the company to obtain extensive patent coverage. This established ICI as prime movers and enabled them to keep abreast of competitors in the beta-blocker field.[108] In addition, as Spinks had recommended in his research agenda for hypertension (see above, on pp. 156–160), ICI developed close contacts with clinicians, by which their drugs were to gain wide acceptance within the medical community.[109] Other than Brian Prichard, whose work with the beta-blockers as antihypertensive agents came to be seen as having great significance in the clinical development of beta-blockade, the company's earliest collaborators included Prof. A.C. Dornhorst, St George's Hospital, London; Prof. M.L. Rosenheim, University College Hospital, London; Dr

R.M. Fulton, Stockport Hospitals Group, who was assisted by Dr K.G. Green of ICI's Medical Department; and Dr J.P.P. Stock, N. Staffs Hospitals Group.[110]

In the 1960s and 1970s, the numbers of investigators expanded considerably, in universities as well as in hospitals. Laboratory data on the pharmacodynamics of the beta-blockers provided guidance to clinicians on the dosage and therapeutic regime to adopt, and feedback from the trials and clinical performance of the beta-blockers informed ICI's research strategy, leading to further, and sometimes better, drugs. Together, laboratory data and clinical feedback became part of a growing body of evidence upon which modern health research and practice in the cardiovascular field have, since then, largely been based.[111] To borrow an expression used by Black in an interview, the beta-blockers came to represent one leg of a 'three-legged stool', which included diet and exercise, as well as drugs.[112]

More perhaps than any other treatment for heart disease, the beta-blockers have contributed to a change in disease perception, that is to say of the level of severity at which treatment could be instituted, and to a radical change in meaning (for instance, of what hypertension actually is).[113] Therefore the beta-blockers, which emerged from an appraisal by ICI of the potentials of the market for drugs, have contributed to changing the market itself by creating new categories of disease, and by creating new needs. A measure of these needs is the proportion of the world's best-selling drugs which the beta-blockers and similar drugs have come to represent. By 1987, 36 per cent of the total value of the world's top-twenty selling medicines was accounted for by H2- and beta-blockers, and nearly three-quarters of these were invented and developed in the UK.[114]

Conclusion

That these developments occurred in Britain requires an explanation. In the 1950s, several pharmaceutical companies abroad had beta-blocker projects, which took off after ICI's drugs had reached the market. If they were behind ICI, it was either because they had failed to connect their beta-blockers with cardiovascular diseases (for example the American companies Eli Lilly and Mead Johnson), or, in the case of the Swedish company AB Hässle, because they were late in patenting their drugs.[115] It has been argued that ICI benefited from the close contacts they built with the British community of cardiologists, who were keen to test and adopt their drugs, first their ganglion-blockers, and then their beta-blockers.[116] However, this argument does not take into account the fact that hypertension, which provided ICI with a point of entry into cardiovascular research, and more widely into chronic diseases, was an important topic for a number of other British pharmaceutical companies in the 1950s. These companies could also, presumably, have taken advantage of contacts with British cardiologists.

An explanation must therefore take into account Black, ICI and the national context in which the pharmaceutical side of its business developed in the 1950s. Black's contribution has been widely acknowledged, not least by the award of the Nobel Prize for Physiology or Medicine in 1988.[117] However, the role of ICI, and of the British context in which he developed the beta-blockers, has not been so widely discussed. This essay has shown that ICI, whose synthetic chemical capability was unrivalled in the UK, also had one of the earliest and best-articulated cardiovascular programmes, within a broader programme of research into chronic diseases. This ensured a 'good fit' between ICI's scientific, technical and commercial objectives, which, once realised in the beta-blockers, conferred upon them a considerable advantage as prime movers in the field.

ICI owed this programme in large measure to Alfred Spinks, his command of different types of evidence, and his ability to convince. However, like Black, Spinks was only one of a number of outstanding scientists the company was able to attract. A study of the early history of the Pharmaceutical Division suggests a variety of reasons for this. ICI had entertained excellent relations with their academic consultants even before the war,[118] and this gave the company access to a wide pool of talented chemists. ICI, the British government's largest industrial agent during the Second World War, were able to recruit top-quality scientists, some of whom, like the biologist Garnet Davey, might not have considered joining if it had not been for the war effort. Others, like Spinks, may otherwise not have been allowed to cross from chemistry to biology, and carry out innovative research at the boundary between the two disciplines. ICI's new research centre, which was the result of the company's growing commitment to pharmaceuticals since the war, attracted the pharmacologist James Black, who 'from time to time...had heard about this fairytale place ICI were building at Alderley Park'.[119] Between 1942, the date of Frank Rose's promotion to head of the embryonic Pharmaceuticals Division, and 1958, the date of Black's arrival at Alderley Park, a distinctive management culture had developed within ICI's hierarchical structure.[120] It was one in which research directors could, if they saw fit, protect their researchers against potential opposition from their superiors. This allowed ICI scientists the financial backing, as well as the freedom, to make their mark, not only on the company's R&D, but also on its research policy in the 1950s. Spinks's 1953 survey of new fields for pharmacological research, and Black's subsequent work on the beta-blockers, amply demonstrate this.

ICI's late, but successful, entry into pharmaceuticals led them to explore new niches, and new approaches, for drug development. This was done in the context of the shift in emphasis from infectious to chronic diseases that characterised postwar medical and pharmaceutical research. At ICI, this shift was the result of a drop in sales of antimalarials, and of a climate of optimism about the victory over infectious diseases. Furthermore, it was associated with a company-wide effort to rationalise its R&D, in which quantitative evidence and statistical methods played a key role. It also reflected the nationwide effort to rationalise therapeutics and health policy, in which medical statistics and randomised clinical trials had a crucial part.[121]

In *Inventer la biomédecine*, Jean-Paul Gaudillière has observed that this development was distinctive of Britain, where unlike in France the NHS provided a favourable context for a statistical approach to debates about public health, in particular about the risks associated with chronic diseases.[122] Although it is beyond the scope of this essay to explore fully such a comparison,[123] the history of ICI's cardiovascular programme is indicative of the close ties between companies and government, developed within the scientific–military–industrial complex during the Second World War, and sustained within the biomedical complex afterwards, which linked universities, hospitals, companies and government. However, Spinks's survey of new fields for pharmacological research, and its subsequent impact on ICI's research strategy, show that rather than passive observers of trends unfolding before them, industrial scientists were active participants, and pharmaceutical companies were major players in the move from infectious to chronic diseases. By making themselves indispensable to the formulation and implementation of national health policies, a situation of mutual interdependence was created between these companies and the state, which has profound implications for public health today, and therefore needs to be better understood. I hope that this essay will have provided some elements towards such an understanding.

Notes

1 A.W Johnson, F.L. Rose and C.W. Suckling, 'Alfred Spinks, 1917–1982', *Biographical Memoirs of Fellows of the Royal Society* 30, 1984: 567–94 (588).
2 Ibid., p. 584. Little is known, unfortunately, about this, and other companies' Medical Departments.
3 V. Berridge, 'Science and policy: the case of postwar British smoking policy', in S. Lock, L.A. Reynolds and E.M. Tansey (eds), *Ashes to Ashes: the History of Smoking and Health*, Amsterdam: Rodopi, 1998, pp. 143–63. See also Berridge and Loughlin, in their introduction to this volume.
4 Ibid. See also J.V. Pickstone, 'Production, community, and consumption', in R. Cooter and J.V. Pickstone (eds), *Medicine in the Twentieth Century*, Amsterdam: Harwood Academic, 2000, pp. 1–19, and J. Goodman, 'Pharmaceutical industry' in the same volume, pp. 141–54.
5 For a sceptical view of the benefits of medical science to public health, see T. McKeown, *The Role of Medicine: Dream, Mirage, or Nemesis?* Oxford: Blackwell, 1979. For a different view, see J. Le Fanu, *The Rise and Fall of Modern Medicine*, London: Abacus, 2001.
6 For example: R. Davenport-Hines and J. Slinn, *Glaxo: a History to 1962*, Cambridge: Cambridge University Press, 1992; E. Jones, *The Business of Medicine*, London: Profile Books, 2000; G. Tweedale, *At the Sign of the Plough: 275 Years of Allen & Hanbury's and the British Pharmaceutical Industry, 1715–1990*, London: Murray, 1990; J. Slinn, *May & Baker, 1834–1984*, Cambridge: Hobsons, 1984; G. Macdonald, *One Hundred Years Wellcome, 1880–1980: in Pursuit of Excellence*, London: the Wellcome Foundation, 1980.

7 C. Kennedy, *ICI: the Company That Changed Our Lives*, London: Paul Chapman Publishing, 1986, p. 129.

8 Ibid., p. 130.

9 See Le Fanu, *The Rise and Fall of Modern Medicine*, pp. xv–xvi, 192.

10 J. Lesch, 'Chemistry and biomedicine in an industrial setting: the invention of the sulfa drugs', in S.H. Mauskopf (ed.), *Chemical Science in the Modern World*, Philadelphia: University of Pennsylvania Press, 1993, pp. 158–215.

11 D. Bovet, *Une Chimie qui guérit: histoire de la découverte des sulfamides*, Paris: Payot, 1988.

12 See W.J. Reader, *Imperial Chemical Industries: a History*, vol. 2, London: Oxford University Press, 1975. Also W.A. Sexton, 'The research laboratories of the Pharmaceutical Division of ICI', *Chemistry and Industry*, 3 March 1962: 372–7 (372).

13 Kennedy, ICI, pp. 120–1.

14 C.W. Suckling and B.W. Langley, 'Francis Leslie Rose, 1909–1988', *Biographical Memoirs of Fellows of the Royal Society* 36, 1990: 491–524 (498).

15 Sexton, 'The research laboratories of the Pharmaceutical Division of ICI', p. 372.

16 K. Holland, 'IC Pharmaceuticals', *Pharmaceutical Journal*, 12 September 1985: 286–8 (286). See also Suckling and Langley, 'Francis Leslie Rose', p. 498.

17 Ibid.

18 Reader, *Imperial Chemical Industries*, pp. 249–313. See also Kennedy, ICI, p. 78.

19 Ibid., Ch. 6: 'ICI's atom bomb'.

20 Much more is known about the history of penicillin than about synthetic anti-malarials. Unfortunately, the work on synthetic antimalarials at ICI was done in such secrecy that no records were made of the meetings of the Consultative Committee directing the research. See Kennedy, ICI, p. 124.

21 Ibid.

22 Johnson *et al.*, 'Alfred Spinks', p. 578.

23 Suckling and Langley, 'Francis Leslie Rose', p. 503.

24 Holland, 'IC Pharmaceuticals', p. 286. Also Kennedy, ICI, p. 129.

25 Ibid., p. 125.

26 Johnson *et al.*, 'Alfred Spinks', pp. 571–2.

27 Suckling and Langley, 'Francis Leslie Rose', pp. 503–5.

28 On the British side, see J. Liebenau, 'The British success with penicillin', *Social Studies of Science* 17 1987: 69–86. On the joint British–US effort, see G.L. Hobby, *Penicillin: Meeting the Challenge*, Yale: Yale University Press, 1985.

29 Kennedy, ICI, pp. 127–9. See also J.G. Cook, 'Penicillin at Trafford Park', *ICI Magazine*, November 1947.

30 The outcome of this programme was the publication of a volume edited by H.T. Clarke, entitled *The Chemistry of Penicillin*, Princeton: Princeton University Press, 1949.

31 'Fermentation Products Department', Pharmaceutical Division, ICI Ltd, January 1972.

32 Reader has argued that the agency system helped to avoid profiteering, and that this policy was highly acceptable to ICI, who in the war saw the opportunity to fulfil their patriotic duty. In Reader, *Imperial Chemical Industries*, pp. 254–7. However, the huge success of ICI's products seem to have provided the basis for the postwar expansion of IC Pharmaceuticals, which Reader says very little about. See Kennedy, ICI, Ch. 8.

33 Ibid., p. 126. Also Suckling and Langley, 'Francis Leslie Rose', p. 512.

34 J.A. Woodbridge, 'Social aspects of pharmaceutical innovation: heart disease', Ph.D. thesis, University of Aston, Birmingham, 1981, p. 26.

35 ICI (AstraZeneca) CPR 3: minutes of meetings on 13 June and 23 October 1949.

36 CPR 1: 'Minutes of meetings of the Group B Pharmaceuticals Conference, 1948–54'.

37 Holland, 'IC Pharmaceuticals', p. 286.

38 For more on this scheme, see See V. Quirke, 'Experiments in collaboration: the changing relationship between scientists and pharmaceutical companies in Britain and France, 1935–1965', D.Phil. thesis, Oxford University, 1999, pp. 260–6.

39 See F.R. Bradbury, M.C. McCarthy and C.W. Suckling, 'Patterns of Innovation: part II – the anaesthetic halothane', *Chemistry and Industry*, 5 February 1972: 105–10. Also Kennedy, ICI, pp. 130–5.

40 In 1957, of the new products introduced by ICI, Fluothane had the highest expected turnover. CPR 2: development memo for Oct. 1957. Fluothane created profits that helped to establish the Pharmaceutical Division. Interview with Bernard Langley and Norman Ellmore, Wilmslow, 15 October 2002.

41 Reader, *Imperial Chemical Industries*, p. 459. See also Kennedy, ICI, p. 129.

42 Reader, *Imperial Chemical Industries*, Ch. 25: 'ICI at mid-century'.

43 For a contemporary account, see for instance M.L. Goldsmith, *The Road to Penicillin: a History of Chemotherapy*, London: Lindsay Drummond, 1946. For a more recent analysis, see M. Weatherall, *In Search of a Cure: a History of Pharmaceutical Discovery*, Oxford: Oxford University Press, 1990, Chs. 8, 9 and 10.

44 CPR 3.

45 See CPR 3: minutes of 1st meeting of the Chemotherapeutic Research Committee, 19 January 1948.

46 Ibid. A member of the Committee, Dr J. Madinaveitia, for example, drew its attention to the 'importance of biochemical work as a basis for new ideas and new lines of synthetic work'.

47 Ibid., minutes of the 2nd meeting of the Chemotherapeutic Committee, 31 March 1948.

48 Ibid., minutes of meeting, 19 July 1951.

49 Ibid., minutes of meeting, 31 March 1953.

50 Ibid., special meeting, 16 March 1953.

51 Ibid.

52 Ibid., minutes of meeting, 18 December 1951; also memo by D.G. Davey on his visit to the USA, 5–23 April 1954.

53 Reader, *Imperial Chemical Industries*, p. 448. He quotes from M.T. Sampson and R.M. Winter, 'The Butterwick Research Laboratories', 12 April 1949, ICIBR (Research Director).

54 Reader, *Imperial Chemical Industries*, p. 92. ICI had a longstanding agreement with Du Pont. Ibid., pp. 38–9.

55 CPR 3: 31 March 1948.

56 CPR 8: Research Directors' Conference on diseases of organic dysfunction, 1 December 1954. See also CPR 33: ICI Ltd Pharmaceutical Division, Research Department, Biological Group (Diseases of Organic Dysfunction), 1954–5.

57 CPR 2: minutes of a special meeting on antimalarials, 31 January 1958.

58 Ibid., development memo, May 1960.

59 Johnson *et al.*, 'Alfred Spinks', p. 582.

60 Ibid., p. 583.

61 See G.V.R. Born and P. Banks, 'Hugh Blaschko, 1900–93', *Biographical Memoirs of Fellows of the Royal Society* 42, 1996: 41–60. Also E. Bülbring and J.M. Walker, 'Joshua Harold Burn, 1892–1981', *Biographical Memoirs of Fellows of the Royal Society* 30, 1984: 43–89.

62 CPR 3: A. Spinks, 'Survey of new fields for pharmacological research', 24 March 1953.

63 On his arrival at Blackley in 1942, he had been asked to make a literature survey on the subject of analgesics, and 'characteristically he produced a masterly document', in Johnson *et al.*, 'Alfred Spinks', p. 571.

64 Ibid., p. 584.

65 CPR 2: development memos for January and March 1959. By then, ICI were considering joining the Taylor, Harkins and Lea Interdatis scheme or subscribing

to the Prescription Survey provided by Nielsen in order to obtain such information. However it was noted that 'The BMA were procrastinating about the Interdatis scheme.'

66 Bülbring and Walker, 'Joshua Harold Burn', p. 56.

67 Ibid., pp. 72–6. Burn and Spinks published a joint paper, 'Thyroid activity and amine oxidase in the liver', in *British Journal of Pharmacology* 7, 1952: 93. Note that J.H. Burn and H.H. Dale had been close collaborators early in their careers.

68 Born and Banks, 'Hugh Blashko', pp. 54–7.

69 CPR 3: Spinks, 'Survey of new fields'.

70 Ibid.

71 Spinks seems to have been unaware at this stage of other British companies' growing interest in hypertension, which led to the simultaneous discovery by May & Baker and ICI of pempidine. See Slinn, *May & Baker*, p. 159.

72 CPR 3: Spinks, 'Survey of new fields'.

73 CPR 8: Research Directors' Conference on distribution of research effort, 6 June 1956.

74 CPR 3: Spinks, 'Survey of new fields'.

75 Ibid.

76 Ibid.

77 See CPR 31: Research Department Period Report, Biological Group (Statistical Research Section), July–December 1954. The section was under the direction of O.L. Davies, who contributed to a series of ICI books on statistical methods, *Statistical Methods in Research and Production,* and sat on the panel of the journals *Applied Statistics* and *Journal of the Royal Statistical Society*. The use of statistical data in industry was in Britain, to some extent, the legacy of the quantitative approach to problem solving developed during the war in Operations Research. See Claude S. George, *The History of Management Thought*, Englewood Cliffs: Prentice Hall, 1968, Ch. 11.

78 Johnson *et al.*, 'Alfred Spinks', p. 572. Spinks's 'persuasiveness with authority' had already enabled him to acquire new instruments, despite stringent wartime import controls.

79 CPR 8: 1 December 1954.

80 CPR 11: Joint plan for 1954.

81 CPR 3: Spinks, 'Survey of new fields'.

82 CPR 35: Research Report of the Biological Group (Pharmacological Section) for July-Dec. 1955.

83 CPR 33: Research Department, Biological Group (Diseases of Organic Dysfunction) report, October–December 1954.

84 Johnson *et al.*, 'Alfred Spinks', p. 584.

85 Sexton, 'The research laboratories of the Pharmaceuticals Division of ICI', pp. 373–4; Holland, 'IC Pharmaceuticals', p. 286.

86 Johnson *et al.*, 'Alfred Spinks', p. 585.

87 Ibid.

88 Ibid., p. 588. [Spinks Report] *Biotechnology: Report of a Joint Working Party of the Advisory Council for Applied Research and Development and Advisory Board for the Research Councils and the Royal Society*, London: HMSO, 1980.

89 S. Wright, *Molecular Politics: Developing American and British Regulatory Policy for Genetic Engineering, 1972–1982*, Chicago: Chicago University Press, 1994, pp. 409–10. See also Slinn, 'The bioscience industry', unpublished, 2001.

90 Johnson *et al.*, 'Alfred Spinks', p. 589.

91 R. Vos, *Drugs Looking for Diseases: Innovative Drug Research and the Development of the Beta-blockers and the Calcium Antagonists*, Dordrecht: Kluwer, 1991, pp. 81–2.

92 V. Quirke, 'Putting theory into practice: James Black, receptor theory, and the development of beta-blockers at ICI, c. 1958–78', *Medical History* (forthcoming, 2006).

93 For examples A.M. Barrett, 'Design of β-blocking drugs', in E. Ariëns (ed.), *Drug Design*, vol. 3, New York: Academic Press, 1972, pp. 205–28; R.G. Shanks, 'The discovery of beta adrenoceptor blocking drugs', in M.J. Parham and J. Bruinvels (eds), *Discoveries in Pharmacology*, vol. 2, Amsterdam: Elsevier, 1984, pp. 38–72; Vos, *Drugs Looking for Diseases*; J.A. Woodbridge, 'Social aspects of pharmaceutical innovation'.

94 Kennedy, ICI, pp. 136–7.

95 CPR 50, 50/3: Research Department Period Report 'Anaemia, allergy, rheumatism and cardio-vascular diseases', 22 January 1959.

96 Woodbridge, 'Social aspects of pharmaceutical innovation', p. 152.

97 V.P. Gerskowitch, R.A.D. Hull and N.P. Shankley, 'The "pharmacological toolmaker's" rational approach to drug design: an appreciation of Sir James Black', *Trends in Pharmacological Sciences* 9, 1988: 435–7 (435).

98 Vos, *Drugs Looking for Diseases*, p. 77.

99 See Woodbridge, 'Social aspects of pharmaceutical innovation', pp. 182, 189, 268.

100 Vos, *Drugs Looking for Diseases*, p. 84.

101 Ibid., p. 91. Also Kennedy, ICI, p. 138. For the work on propanolol, Black was assisted by Dr R.G. Shanks. See Shanks, 'The discovery of beta adrenoceptor blocking drugs', in Parnham and Bruinvels, *Discoveries in Pharmacology*, p. 55.

102 Shanks, 'The discovery of beta adrenoceptor blocking drugs', p. 66. Woodbridge, 'Social aspects of pharmaceutical innovation', p. 196. In 1969, ICI obtained clearance from the Committee on the Safety of Medicines to market Inderal for hypertension. Ibid., p. 212.

103 Ibid., p. 189.

104 For this, ICI introduced a compensatory scheme. Ibid., p. 235. Also Holland, 'IC Pharmaceuticals', p. 287.

105 Woodbridge, 'Social aspects of pharmaceutical innovation', p. 259.

106 Holland, 'IC Pharmaceuticals', pp. 286–8.

107 Ibid., p. 287

108 Barrett, 'Design of β-blocking drugs', p. 217.

109 Vos, *Drugs Looking for Diseases*, pp. 90–1; Shanks, 'The discovery of beta adrenoceptor blocking drugs', pp. 57–8.

110 Woodbridge, 'Social aspects of pharmaceutical innovation', p. 170.

111 See for example the entries for propanolol and atenolol in J.A. Henry (ed.), *New Guide to Medicines & Drugs*, London: Dorling Kindersley, 2001, pp. 201, 386. Note that indications for these drugs include the treatment of anxiety and migraine. See also L. Opie, *Drugs for the Heart*, 5th edn, Philadelphia: W.B. Sanders, 2001. Opie was a close collaborator of ICI in the mid-1970s, when he was director of the MRC Ischaemic Heart Disease Research Unit, Department of Medicine, University of Cape Town. In CPRB 99.

112 Quoted in Woodbridge, 'Social aspects of pharmaceutical innovation', p. 267.

113 Ibid., p. 36.

114 Holland, 'IC Pharmaceuticals', p. 287.

115 Vos, *Drugs Looking for Diseases*, pp. 104–10.

116 Ibid., pp. 90, 120.

117 See Gerskowitch *et al.*

118 These have been described by G.K. Roberts in 'Dealing with issues at the academic-industrial interface in inter-war Britain: University College London and Imperial Chemical Industries', *Science and Public Policy*, 24, 1997: 29–35.

119 Kennedy, ICI, p. 136.

120 See the organisation chart in Reader, *Imperial Chemical Industries*, Fig. 17, pp. 444–5.

121 See Berridge, 'Science and policy', in Lock *et al.*, *Ashes to Ashes*, pp. 146–8. On the rise of medical statistics in Britain, see E. Magnello, 'The introduction of mathematical statistics into medical research: the roles of Karl Pearson, Major Greenwood, and Austin Bradford Hill', in E. Magnello and A. Hardy (eds), *The Road to Medical Statistics*, Amsterdam: Rodopi, 2002, pp. 95–123.

122 J.-P. Gaudillière, *Inventer la biomédecine: la france, l'amérique et la production des savoirs du vivant (1945–1965)*, Paris: La Découverte, 2002, Ch. 6, esp. pp. 243–5. For a comparison between European pharmaceutical industries, see also S. Chauveau, 'Entreprises et marchés du médicament en Europe occidentale des années 1880 à la fin des années 1960', *Histoire Economique et Sociale* 1, 1998: 49–81.

123 For more on this, see V. Quirke, 'French biomedicine in the mirror of America', essay review of Gaudillière's *Inventer la biomédecine*, in *Studies in History and Philosophy of Science* 35, 2004: 765–76.

Recommended further reading

A.M. Barrett, 'Design of β-blocking drugs', in E. Ariëns (ed.), *Drug Design*, vol. 3, New York: Academic Press, 1972, pp. 205–28.

A.W. Johnson, F.L. Rose and C.W. Suckling, 'Alfred Spinks, 1917–1982', *Biographical Memoirs of Fellows of the Royal Society* 30, 1984, pp. 567–94.

C. Kennedy, *ICI: the Company That Changed Our Lives*, London: Hutchinson, 1986.

W.J. Reader, *Imperial Chemical Industries: a History*, vol. 2, London: Oxford University Press, 1979.

R.G. Shanks, 'The discovery of beta adrenoceptor blocking drugs', in M.J. Parnham and J. Bruinvels (eds), *Discoveries in Pharmacology*, vol. 2, Amsterdam: Elsevier, 1984, pp. 38–72.

R. Vos, *Drugs Looking for Diseases: Innovative Drug Research and the Development of the Beta-blockers and the Calcium Antagonists*, Dordrecht: Kluwer, 1991.

7 The 'invisible industrialist' and public health

The rise and fall of 'safer smoking' in the 1970s

Virginia Berridge and Penny Starns

Hostility to the tobacco industry is axiomatic in contemporary public health. In 2003 on the ASH (Action on Smoking and Health) website, we read that:

> Tobacco is unique: the only product that kills when used normally – 120,000 deaths per year in the UK. ASH is leading the fight to control the tobacco epidemic and to confront the lies and dirty tricks of the tobacco industry.[1]

TV documentaries such as the *Tobacco Wars* or *The Secrets of Big Tobacco* tell of the forty-year struggle to hold US tobacco companies to account for the damage cigarettes have caused. Journalist histories *The Smoke Ring* and *Dirty Business – Big Tobacco at the Bar of Justice* recount a thrilling story of corporate greed and duplicity, of big business that cared little for the health of its customers.[2,3] The popular UK television series *Yes Minister* had a classic episode exposing the close relationship between government ministers and the industry, which brought a humorous spin to the relationship, based on real-life events.[4]

But there is also a different history of industry, government and public health interests that has been less visible or discussed. This chapter approaches that history through the story of the rise and fall of 'safer smoking' in the 1960s and 1970s, and through a case study of the activities of the Wills tobacco company at that time. This is a UK-specific story; the US story has predominated and is often taken to be a universal model.[5] It is also an account of a complex balancing act within policy between risk reduction and elimination of risk, in which both science and public health were involved. It shows that the traditional view of smoking policy – of a governments in thrall to 'big tobacco' with public health battling against the industry's malign influence – is less than the full historical picture. Industry, government and public health forged alliances that the issue of 'safer smoking' epitomised. This chapter aims to bring that forgotten part of the policy history into view. It also draws on recent work on the role of the 'invisible industrialist' in the history of scientific research. This chapter shows how industry, science and government also developed relationships in the public health field.[6]

The British government and the tobacco industry had a long history of co-operation. Tobacco was a key import and its duty a major source of government revenue. During the Second World War the industry was brought under strict government control and the Board of Trade appointed a Tobacco Controller, Sir Alexander Maxwell, who before the war had been a leading leaf merchant.[7] He was advised by two bodies representing the two sides of the industry – the Tobacco Manufacturers Advisory Committee (TAC) and the Tobacco Distributors Advisory Committee (TDAC), the former of which took the lead. Leaf was imported for the Board of Trade by Imperial Tobacco, the main national tobacco company, and distributed through leaf pools organised by the TAC. Tobacco was an industry like any other, its interests closely allied with government. It was the TAC wartime set-up that was in place when the first research showing the relationship between smoking and lung cancer was published in 1950. It was Maxwell of the TAC who sent a secret offer to Harold Himsworth, secretary of the Medical Research Council (MRC), offering £250,000 for the purposes of research.[8] After discussion within the government about the propriety of the MRC accepting money from an industrial body, it was agreed that the difficulty could be resolved if the gift was made to HM Government, who would then allocate it. The gift was to be made, so John Boyd Carpenter at the Treasury wrote to the Marquess of Salisbury, Lord President, for research into smoking and lung cancer, and 'presumably of the means of removing the elements in the tobacco which may have this effect'.[9] This offer was in line with the previous co-operative relationships that had marked government relationships with the industry.

Public health and safer smoking: the 1962 Royal College of Physicians' report and the industry response

The aim of what came to be called 'safer smoking' lay behind this initial offer. This strategy was clearly of importance to the industry, which hoped that tobacco could be modified to remove whatever was implicated in the rise in lung cancer deaths. It is forgotten that this was a parallel objective for public health interests who were concerned about smoking. The first report on smoking of the Royal College of Physicians (RCP), *Smoking and Health*, published in 1962, included in its section on preventive measures the removal of harmful substances from tobacco smoke; filtration of smoke; modification of tobacco to reduce nicotine and tar; and the adoption of safer smoking habits. It was the cigarette that was the main source of health hazard. The aim was to switch to less hazardous forms of smoking. Switching to pipes and cigars could be encouraged by fiscal means such as differential taxation, i.e. taxation graded according to the hazard of the product.[10]

This was an idea that was taken up within the British tobacco industry. Here the main grouping was the Imperial Tobacco Group Limited (ITGL), which had been established in 1901 at the time of the 'great division' in tobacco marketing worldwide.[11] It consisted of a conglomerate of tobacco manufacturers such as Ogdens and Players. However, at the time of its formation the Bristol-based Wills company was the largest tobacco manufacturer within the group, and remained so in the 1960s and 1970s. Consequently, directors and managers at Wills dominated policy decisions within ITGL. Thus, when the 1962 RCP report reaffirmed the links between smoking and lung cancer it was the directors at Wills who took the lead in formulating ITGL's reaction. They decided to adopt what they believed to be a responsible attitude towards the problem, and embarked on a policy of co-operation with the government. The RCP findings stressed the health risks associated with cigarette smoking rather than pipe tobacco and cigars. Subsequently the company stepped up its production of the latter products and the cigar trade boomed. The smoking public had also responded to the report by purchasing filter cigarettes in preference to ordinary cigarettes. To some extent Wills had predicted this trend, and by 1965 the company was the largest producer of tipped cigarettes in the country. Thus it was well placed to take advantage of the 'swing' in public preference.

Wills began to experiment with different types of cigarette filters in an attempt to make cigarettes 'safer'. In addition, large sums of money were invested in new machinery and research in order to produce a filter cigar. Code named 'Pongo', the filter cigar was supposed to appeal to members of the public who were concerned about the health and smoking issue by offering a dual safeguard. In the event, despite the considerable investment, 'Pongo' did not really get past the drawing board. As an experimental product 'Pongo' was probably the most expensive, but by no means the only, failure.[12]

However, further research that concentrated on the development of a low-tar and low-nicotine cigarette blend was more successful. The research began almost as soon as the RCP report was published, though it was considered to be a long-term project. Code named 'Wallflower' the research was shrouded in secrecy and information with regard to developments was only available on a 'need to know' basis. The product was considered to be a pre-emptive measure against further adverse publicity with regard to smoking and health. As the marketing minutes explained on 10 January 1966, 'The project is under development to provide for the possibility that further smoking and health publicity may awaken consumer interest in cigarettes with low tar characteristics.'[13]

Thus 'Wallflower' as the name suggested was laying in wait for the right 'health climate' in order to be launched. Even five years after the publication of the 1962 report the company believed that, 'smokers were not predisposed to seek out low tar and low nicotine cigarettes.'[14]

A relatively long time span elapsed before 'Wallflower' reached the market, during which time Wills conducted 'acceptability' experiments with the help of its workforce. By January 1966 internal tests were completed and a public relations firm, William Schlackman Ltd, were commissioned to carry out further consumer research. The fee for the research was estimated to be between £7,000 and £8,000, and the cost of the samples £6,600. A proportion of smokers were selected to smoke the experimental 'Wallflower' blend for a period of four weeks while a 'control' group smoked another brand, Embassy, for the same period.[15]

In the meantime Wills employees were set another 'assessment' task. The company wanted help in carrying out tests on experimental dual-filter versions of Woodbine Filter and Escort. These experimental cigarettes also provided lower tar and slightly lower nicotine in-smoke yields than the existing mono-filter versions of the same brand. For the Escort brand employees were asked to assess the following three types of cigarettes:

A   Existing Escort which has a 24% retention mono-acetate plug and which yields 13 mgm. tar and 1.68 mgm. nicotine per cigarette. (control cigarette).
B   The existing Escort blend fitted with a 32% retention dual plug which is expected to reduce yields to 11.7 mgm. tar and 1.5 mgm. nicotine per cigarette.
C   An experimental blend with a 48% retention dual plug. This cigarette is expected to yield 10 mgm. tar and 1.5 mgm. nicotine per cigarette.[16]

Employee assessment of cigarettes was considered to be 'phase one' in any test of new tobacco, cigar or cigarette blend. As usual the external tests were only carried out once these internal tests were completed. On the basis of the results of phase one William Schlackman Ltd carried out phase two, an external test on about 200 smokers.[17] Thus employees provided Wills with essential information in terms of consumer research on a regular basis, and were more than willing to do so.

While the smoking and health issue flared up from time to time Wills had not, at this stage, suffered any great economic loss as a result. Moreover the cigar trade was still booming in the late 1960s, and there was a quiet confidence amongst management personnel that new smoking materials would be found that would gain public approval. Like many other firms in the tobacco industry Wills had co-operated fully with the government's harm reduction policy and had invested large sums of money for research into smoking and health. But there were indications, too, that savings could be made as a result of health-prompted research. The production of low-tar/nicotine cigarettes saved the company money because the rag length of the cigarette was shorter than that which was used in normal cigarettes. There were problems with consumer research, however, and consequently with the overall development of the 'Wallflower' blend. Both in phase one and phase two of the 'Wallflower' tests, consumers had expressed dissatisfaction with the draw resistance of the cigarette and the level of tar/nicotine.

Eventually five different levels of tar and nicotine were tested, ranging from the Embassy cigarette, which was already on the market, down to the lowest 'Wallflower' blend. Some of this research ran parallel to a programme initiated in 1967 by the Tobacco Intelligence Department (TID). The object of the TID research was to compile a short list of acceptable levels of nicotine and tar in cigarettes, and measure as far as possible nicotine withdrawal tolerance by trying out twenty-seven permutations of tar, nicotine, sugar and draw-resistance levels.[18]

The results of consumer tests were not conclusive across the country, and, even in areas where they were, the results still posed a technical problem. In terms of the political climate that surrounded smoking and health, 'Wallflower' was ready to come off the shelf, since the government had announced its intention to publish tar and nicotine figures in the near future. Wills intended to use the 'Wallflower' blend to convert Embassy, its largest-selling cigarette, into a very low-tar/nicotine brand. But by this stage the sales of Embassy were already under threat from a proposed ban in coupon trading. Members of the Wills marketing committee were faced with yet another dilemma. In preparation for the publication of tar and nicotine yields they wanted to convert the Embassy blend in order for the brand to be competitive in the 'smoking and health climate'. Yet at the same time they believed that changes in the blend would have disastrous effects on sales when combined with a coupon ban.

> Concerning tar/nicotine yields, there is evidence from the recent 'Wallflower' tests that yields of 1.2mg and 9.5mg. would probably be acceptable to Embassy smokers. We cannot, however, achieve these yields even with a 16mm. plug without increasing the draw resistance of the cigarette above its present level. We do not know to what extent, if any, draw resistance could be increased without giving rise to adverse comment. It seems clear however, that within the limitations imposed by 15mm and 16mm. plugs the critical factor in terms of consumer acceptance will be draw resistance rather than absolute tar/nicotine levels.
>
> We therefore have to decide on the basis of judgement alone which will pose a greater risk to Embassy sales – a change in dimensions or tar and nicotine publicity....Our experience in the past has indicated that a change in the product is more likely to have an adverse affect on sales than smoking and health publicity.[19]

The Wills company was proceeding with product development round the safer smoking option, with both consumer preference and health risk on the agenda.

Differential taxation and safer smoking

The RCP report had raised the question of whether government fiscal policy could be used to encourage safer smoking. This was a crucial question that was to bring the scientific analysis of tobacco centrally on to the policy agenda. The question of differential taxation was taken up within government. A committee of civil servants reported to the Cabinet ministerial committee on smoking and health on 15 May 1962. The officials considered differential taxation and thought it would not be effective. Despite pressure on the Cabinet from the Lord President, Lord Hailsham, no action was taken. But the publication of the US Surgeon General's report on smoking in July 1964 revived interest. However, proposals from Members of Parliament for differential taxation were rejected by the Chancellor of the Exchequer in the Budget. The matter was discussed within the Treasury and a note prepared for the Economic Secretary in June 1964 pointed out that the introduction of differential rates would need a clear distinction between what was and was not harmful. Her Majesty's Customs was particularly opposed.

> While the Royal College of Physicians and the US Surgeon General have condemned conventional cigarettes but have given cigar and pipe tobaccos a cleaner if not entirely clean bill of health, they have at no time indicated what it is about cigarettes (such as the paper wrapper, the nature of the tobacco used therein, the method of manufacture, or the method of packing) which makes them more dangerous than the other categories. In the absence of knowledge concerning the factors which create greater risks to health, the distinctions which would have to be drawn in deciding whether a particular product was, say, a cigar or a cigarette could make it appear that the Government had reached conclusions about the causes of the danger to health whereas on the basis of present statistical and medical evidence the distinctions would in fact be arbitrary, misleading and wide open to criticism as being unfair between one smoker and another and between one section of the trade and another.[20]

There was clearly a need to define what was harmful. The differential taxation discussions opened up the issue of how a change in taxation policy could be justified scientifically. In effect, it brought together health, scientific and economic evidence at this stage in a way that anticipated the later alliances to be forged within the' new public health' of the 1970s. A twin-track strategy developed that was supported at this stage by government, industry and by some public health interests. This aimed to modify cigarettes in ways that removed the harmful cancer-causing components, or to replace them entirely by some new smoking product that would be risk free.

Tar and nicotine tables and safer smoking

Initially the question of how levels of harm could be scientifically defined was encompassed by discussion of the publication of tar and nicotine tables. The idea was that the provision of information about which cigarettes had the lowest tar and nicotine levels would provide a means of smokers making up their own minds. It was the tobacco companies who pushed initially for this strategy. Imperial Tobacco was pressing for tables in 1967 but no further action was taken then because of opposition from Gallahers and Carreras, the other main UK tobacco companies. At a meeting held in February 1968 chaired by Sir Arnold France, Permanent Secretary of the Ministry of Health, it was agreed that the scientific evidence was still inconclusive and so such tables should be available to research workers rather than to the public. But by 1971, when a second RCP report on smoking was published, scientific knowledge had solidified, and so the Secretary of State referred the matter to a new expert committee, a Standing Scientific Liaison committee.[21] The Consumers Association had also published its own tables in 1971. Chaired by Dr Dick Cohen, the Deputy Chief Medical Officer, the standing committee brought together scientists and industry representatives: it included Dr Herbert Bentley of Imperial Tobacco, Dr Colin Dollery, a clinical pharmacologist, and Geoffrey Rose of the London School of Hygiene and Tropical Medicine (LSHTM). Its first, and only, report was on tar and nicotine tables, whose publication it urged.[22] When the Department of Health, acting on this advice, published its first tables in 1973, there were ten brands whose tar and nicotine content was lower than the brand that had headed the Consumers Association table. Ten new lower-tar brands had been initiated within eighteen months. Clearly the industry could operate quickly when it had to.[23]

Safer smoking, the government enquiry of 1971 and the role of the Independent Scientific Committee on Smoking and Health

It was during the 1970s that this risk reduction strategy reached its peak and collaboration with industry was at its most optimistic point. In the early 1970s both the RCP and government initiated enquiries that looked into safer smoking. Subsequently, an expert committee with modification and replacement as its aims was established. Its history in that decade was that of the rise and decline of 'safer smoking' as a joint public health–industry–government objective. The second RCP report, *Smoking and Health Now*, published in 1971, in its section on 'less dangerous forms of smoking' included a reference to changing to pipes and cigars, but also addressed cigarettes with reduced nicotine and tar content in more detail. It wanted information on the packet and an authoritative medical statement on the significance of this analysis in relation to health risk. There should be a statutory upper limit for tar and nicotine. The production of 'less harmful' cigarettes was a more complex matter than at first envisaged, and so the MRC should sponsor some research.[24]

The taxation issue was also recognised as more complex; the RCP report called for an official inquiry into the economic consequences of a decrease in smoking. The RCP committee's own inquiry into the topic, published as an

Table 7.1 UK Committees investigating safer smoking, 1950s–1970s

1957–64	Cabinet committee on cancer of the lung
1958–62	RCP committee on smoking and air pollution
1962	RCP report, *Smoking and Health*
1971	RCP second report, *Smoking and Health Now*
1971–2	Standing Scientific Liaison committee (report published 1972)
1971	Interdepartmental committee of civil servants (report prepared 1971, not openly published, statistics published by DH 1972)
1973	Independent Scientific Committee on Smoking and Health (the Hunter committee). Reports in 1975 and 1979

appendix to its main report, was thin and had only two references. The government then commissioned its own inquiry, which was never officially published, although reference was made to it some nine years later, in a *Guardian* report and the statistics were published by the DH in 1972.[25] The unpublished report, along with its economic conclusions (which showed that there strong arguments for not reducing smoking, both in relation to demand management and because of the impact of reduction on social security payments), was also clear that there were twin objectives to smoking policy. It should aim to make smoking less dangerous and get people to smoke less. The report focused on the less dangerous objective. The tar yield of cigarettes had already been reduced, but a low-nicotine yield was a more difficult issue. These reduced yields should be publicised before statutory upper limits were imposed.[26]

The Standing Scientific Liaison committee appointed at this time to bring industry, scientists and government together was succeeded by another, the Independent Scientific Committee on Smoking and Health (ISCSH), appointed in the summer of 1973. Its chairman was Robert Hunter, vice chancellor of the University of Birmingham, a clinician who had also been involved in drug safety and public health policy initiatives.[27] The committee had a membership of public health scientists, including Walter Holland, a public health researcher at St Thomas', Peter Armitage, a statistician at LSHTM, David Poswillo, an oral surgeon, and Donald Ball, a physician who specialised in miners' chest diseases from Llandough Hospital, Penarth. Chief scientific adviser to the committee was Frank Fairweather, a Department of Health civil servant who was also involved in drug safety. It produced two reports in the 1970s that demonstrated the strength of the risk reduction initiative. In the first report, published in 1975, it stated that it had focused on the development of guidelines for the testing of cigarettes containing tobacco substitutes because a number of companies were planning to market these products and had undertaken smoke chemistry studies, animal tests and human studies. It was also developing guidelines on the testing and use of additives in tobacco products.[28] Prior to 1970, no additives had been allowed by Customs because of taxation issues. But the 1970 Finance Act had relaxed these restrictions. The report outlined the various stages of testing and also a future programme of work. There was hope that the remit of the committee would be expanded. It would need, so it reported, to continue to give attention to substitutes and to additives. It would be receiving submissions on tests and reports on tests from the companies for consideration and would be considering the form of long-term epidemiological studies. 'Nevertheless, the Committee hopes before making its next report to have been able to consider the wider range of problems on smoking and health that come within its terms of reference.'[29]

Tobacco was located in bureaucratic terms within the drug safety section of the Department of Health. The ISCSH was clearly planning to develop its role so that it became a body akin to the Committee on the Safety of Medicines (on which Hunter also served), which operated in a similar relationship, but with government and the pharmaceutical companies. The committee's terms of reference were widened after its first report had been published to make it clear that it advised both the government and the tobacco companies, although the industry representatives later claimed that they had never accepted this.[30] This stance came, however, after the failure of an initiative from David Owen as Minister of Health from 1974–6. Owen, as part of his negotiations with the industry in the mid-1970s, aimed to bring tobacco substitutes under the provisions of the 1968 Medicines Act; the ISCSH would operate with this statutory backing to bring independent medical and scientific advice to bear on tobacco products.[31] The objective of safer smoking would have been given greater weight through a joint initiative between government, industry and public health interests. But the initiative petered out after Owen's departure to the Foreign Office in 1976.

The second report of the ISCSH did not appear until the end of the 1970s; it was finally published, after much delay, in 1979.[32] The first part of the report gave an account of the work of the committee in relation to the inclusion of tobacco substitutes and additives in tobacco products; the second outlined progress towards the development of lower-risk cigarettes. In the first report, the manufacturers and importers had agreed to abide by the committee's guidelines for the testing of tobacco substitutes before they marketed them. Testing went on and, in 1977, Hunter had written to the health departments about the marketing of substitutes. Various provisos were agreed, including the monitoring of the long-term effects on smokers of cigarettes containing substitutes. The companies appointed a consultative advisory panel headed by the public health researcher Walter Holland, and an outline of a study protocol was prepared. But this could not be implemented because of the lack of market share of cigarettes containing substitutes. The development of lower-risk cigarettes, the other arm of the committee's work, also proved more difficult than at first envisaged. Tar yields continued to be reduced, but the issue of what should be done about nicotine and the carbon monoxide yield of tobacco remained unresolved. In the longer term, the second report stated, it might be necessary for manufacturers to modify the nicotine delivery of cigarettes or alter the factors that could influence the rate of absorption from inhaled smoke into the body tissues. The reduction of carbon monoxide levels was desirable.

The industry's response; the development of New Smoking Material (NSM)

What was the response from the industry point of view? Two testing submissions were made to the ISCSH: a consortium of Gallahers and Rothmans for a product called Cytrel 361 and from Imperial Tobacco for NSM14. This paper will concentrate on Wills' work on the latter product – New Smoking Material (NSM). In 1967 initial experiments into NSM were conducted at Wills no. 1 factory in Bedminster, Bristol. In the same year, ITGL joined forces with the Imperial Chemical Industry (ICI) and established a new offshoot company named Imperial Developments Limited (IDL). The sole purpose of IDL was to research, develop and produce a safe and economically viable alternative to tobacco.

According to ITGL, the smoking and health issue provided the strongest reason to develop NSM, but there were also economic considerations. If an alternative to tobacco could be found it would reduce the money the industry spent on import duty. Neither could it be argued that government concerns were entirely focused on the health aspects of NSM. From the government's standpoint the sale of NSM within the UK had the potential of saving foreign currency and sales of the material overseas held the possibility of improving the balance of payments. From the outset, therefore, the development of NSM was not merely health orientated. But it was anticipated that NSM would replace between 10 and 20 per cent of tobacco in cigarettes, and that the substance would provide the consumer with a healthier alternative to conventional cigarettes. As Dr Herbert Bentley, ITGL's research and development director, maintained,

> While no-one is making health claims for NSM, it follows the government's view that if people do smoke they should smoke brands with low tar and nicotine yields. NSM is a neutral substance and is tasteless. It delivers only a quarter of the tar in an equal amount of tobacco. And tar from NSM is five times less biologically active than tobacco tar. It does not contain any nicotine. It is based on cellulose which is present in all natural vegetable matter, including tobacco.[33]

NSM was actually obtained from wood pulp that had been subjected to heat treatment. The material was condensed into black sheets and known in the industry as HTC or heat-treated cellulose. It was then mixed with water and six secret components that gave the material a variety of different properties such as moisture retention and ash cohesion. The HTC was transformed into liquid form by this process and then travelled down an air-heated steel band. Eventually the NSM appeared from this band as a film and was sliced and diced into a conventional blending silo. The usual tar yield and moisture tests were applied to NSM in much the same way as for tobacco, and the material contained no less than the 10 per cent that was demanded by Customs regulations. Laboratory tests and development procedures, however, also included other biological tests such as mouse skin painting. Research was stepped up as a result of the 1971 RCP report and by 1973 over £3 million had been invested in the research and development of NSM. The director of IDL, Mr Malcolm Anson explained,

> This is of course a commercial project, but it is expected that the new material could make a substantial contribution to mitigating the smoking and health problem. Whether it does so will ultimately depend on the medical authorities. The tobacco industry has always taken the view that however good they are at making cigarettes or however painstaking their research, the medical assessment must come from the doctors and that decisions concerning the nation's health must rest with the government.[34]

Members of the ISCSH (the Hunter committee) quickly formed good working relationships with the directors of ITGL and the latter felt confident in the future of NSM. They had already invested over £3 million in the research and development of tobacco substitutes; they did not even bother to wait for the official outcome of the Hunter committee's assessment of NSM before they invested a further £13 million in a new NSM production factory, based in Ardeer, Scotland. They had invested large sums of money into the development of low-tar/nicotine cigarettes and continued to pour money into the research, development and production of tobacco substitutes. By the time that NSM cigarettes were launched the sum had reached over £26 million.

The first consumer tests of NSM were conducted 'in house' by Wills' own employees. Several had volunteered to take part in the testing of experimental cigarettes and volunteers were selected from a random cross-section of the workforce, ranging from factory workers to laboratory chemists. This policy did not represent any radical departure from the practice of previous years, since Wills had traditionally tested new brands and blends of tobacco on its workforce. Initially no scientific protocols were followed. Usually Wills simply gave away free samples to employees and hoped for a straightforward reaction. Responses tended to be in the form of one-word answers that described cigarettes as 'wonderful' or 'disgusting'. However, from 1970 onwards the testing became more methodical and scientific in its approach. Volunteer cigarette tasters were trained along the same lines as food tasters and rigorously instructed as to how to taste cigarettes through the mouth and then through the nose. They were prevented from wearing any deodorant, perfume or aftershave that could possibly interfere with the aroma of the cigarette, and expected to complete standardised forms that included descriptions of all the components of the blend and to grade them accordingly. When Wills moved its workforce to its highly publicised and very expensive new 45 acre site in Hartcliffe in 1975, purpose-built smoking booths were constructed to accommodate the cigarette tasters. Furthermore the volunteers were not restricted to testing Wills brands. Many brands that

> the panel savour come from competitors and others are experimental cigarettes which cannot be sold on the open market because of present laws. These include cigarettes made with Imperial Tobacco's NSM, other substitutes such as Cytrel, and cigarettes made with additives or cased tobacco.[35]

In 1974 the ISCSH (Hunter) committee permitted wider consumer tests and over 5,000 people across the country began to sample forty different kinds of NSM cigarettes containing between 10 per cent and 50 per cent NSM. The cigarettes were produced by Wills and Players, and consumers were asked to comment on flavour, aroma and cigarette satisfaction. IDL was renamed NSM in the same year and new headquarters were established in Manchester. The tobacco substitute was seen as a major breakthrough for the British tobacco industry and the first to gain official recognition. Dr Bentley of Imperial Tobacco pointed out 'We believe that NSM is the first substitute smoking material in the world to receive clearance from a government body'.[36]

The level of investment into NSM, however, was beginning to take its toll and 1974 was one of the worst trading years for ITGL since its formation. Group sales were actually higher than in previous years, but the increases in production costs, heavy duty and inflation combined to depress profits. The chairman of ITGL, Sir John Partridge, warned members of the group that future research might be curtailed:

> We have invested heavily in recent years, mainly out of profits, in the equipment and housing of our businesses with a view to safeguarding their future and to reducing costs. We planned to invest over £50 million in this way in 1974. This expenditure, a great part of it contracted in 1973 will not be significantly reduced. But given our present artificially depressed level of profitability and consequently smaller cash flow, the further substantial investment programme which we had hoped to implement in 1975 is now gravely threatened.[37]

In reality most of the profit loss was due to Imperial's other interests such as food, packaging and the brewery industry rather than tobacco sales. The group had diversified following the 1962 RCP report as a means of 'hedging its bets' over the smoking and health problem. The group even changed its name and dropped the word tobacco from its title in order to reflect this diversification. Imperial Tobacco Group Limited became Imperial Group

Limited, and Imperial Tobacco Limited became the umbrella name for the tobacco division of the group. Imperial Group Limited (IGL), however, still retained its faith in the potential of NSM, and despite a subsequent severe recession in 1975 invested a further £22 million in a new 'space age' factory at Ardeer, which was opened in 1977.

The Hunter committee had examined all the evidence with regard to tobacco substitutes and raised no objections to their use. Nevertheless the committee did demand assurances from the tobacco manufacturers and retained some control over the use of NSM. Manufacturers were obliged to inform the committee of the exact proportion of substitutes and other cigarette specifications. The rationale behind this obligation centred on the fact that the scientific evidence which had been accepted by the committee was directly related to certain cigarette specifications; sales of NSM could therefore be withdrawn if manufacturers deviated from the original specifications. The committee also wanted to have control over whether or not NSM was added to high-tar and high-nicotine cigarettes. A further condition was imposed whereby tobacco companies were required to agree on a date for the commencement of long-term health studies for NSM smokers.

The target date for the launch of NSM cigarettes was 1 July 1977, but the anti-smoking lobby was already pouring scorn on the whole concept of 'safer' smoking. Imperial Tobacco hit back by persuading eminent doctors to participate in a tribute film. The film was designed more for the company's employees than for the general public, but emphasised the long-standing responsible attitude of the tobacco industry, and Imperial in particular, towards the problem of smoking and health. A further RCP report also acknowledged the research efforts of tobacco manufacturers, and criticised the lack of government co-ordination in the area of research. Eventually NSM cigarettes left the warehouses on 28 July 1977.

The launch of NSM

There were increasing tensions between the industry and government policy, however, particularly around the issues of price controls, smoking and health, and cigarette advertising. Members of the industry accused the government of not understanding the stress relief value of smoking. Speaking in 1976 Mr John Pile, chairman of Imperial Group Limited, stated that, 'For many of us smoking provides considerable solace and the realistic course is not to attempt a sudden radical reduction in the habit'.[38] But whereas there were many who sympathised with John Pile's view in the mid-1960s, by the second half of the 1970s the context within which smoking policy was formed had changed. The launch of NSM in 1977 highlighted the new influences within smoking policy and the new players who had emerged. The new Minister of Health, David Ennals, acknowledged in a House of Commons statement that 'calls to legislate smoking out of existence would not work', and that 'it will not be banished quickly – but our long term aim must be its eventual disappearance'.[39] Ennals's speech was given a month before the Hunter committee gave the official go-ahead for the sale of NSM cigarettes and only four months before they were launched onto the open market.

The launch of NSM brought tensions to a head. There was a strong and organised lobby that opposed all smoking and the legitimacy of the industry. ASH, the new anti-smoking pressure group founded in 1971, took a more stringent position of opposition to safer smoking. The launch of NSM had upstaged, so anti-smoking campaigners argued, the launch of the third RCP report on smoking, *Smoking or Health,* whose title epitomised the new gulf widening over the issue of modified smoking.[40] The Health Education Council, relaunched in 1973, and an anti-smoking ally of ASH's, called smoking safer cigarettes the equivalent of jumping from the 36th instead of the 39th floor of a tall building. The financial position on tobacco substitutes had changed too. In January 1978 the taxation system was revised and statutory controls over substitutes ceased.[41] Manufacturers gave voluntary undertakings rather than be subject to statutory controls.[42] The Health Education Council had accused the tobacco industry of misleading the public and of making false health claims for its products. The directors at ITL were singularly unimpressed by what they believed to be an outright betrayal by the government. Indeed, such was the feeling of outrage that ITL chairman Mr Tony Garrett took out a full-page press advertisement to vent his anger, and accused the government of failing to support its own policy on smoking and health.

> By 1972 it had been established that a product could be used as a tobacco substitute in ways that showed every promise of reducing risks that had been associated by medical authorities with the smoking of cigarettes. Following its consultation with scientific and medical authorities, and of co-operation with the government, ITL started discussing the future of the product with the then Conservative government. The government, without compromising its long-term policy of discouraging smoking, agreed that this was an approach that should be pursued. The Hunter committee was set up, and following ITL's research with ICI, product testing and the building of the NSM factory at Ardeer, it concluded there would be no objection to the making and selling of cigarettes containing NSM. Accusations of misleading the public were sheer nonsense, Mr Garrett declared. The ITL chairman pointed out that accusations were made on behalf of a body (Health Education Council) that had been appointed by the same government with whom the policy leading to the introduction of NSM was agreed.[43]

This sense of outrage continued as NSM cigarettes failed to gain acceptance in the marketplace. Wills had prided itself on being the pacemaker within the tobacco industry and along with ICI had funded all the research into NSM. Their competitors such as Rothmans meanwhile had relied on Cytrel, a tobacco substitute produced by the American Celanese Corporation. These competitors also experienced losses but since they had not made any huge investment these were minimal in comparison to Wills and the Imperial Group. Evidently the latter had expected some government support for their new products, yet despite the initial endorsement of the concept of 'safe' smoking none was forthcoming. But although the IGL chose to blame the government and the negative effects of the Health Education Council's campaign, this was only one obstacle to the acceptance of tobacco substitutes. The issue of nicotine had been overlooked, and if smokers smoked to obtain nicotine they were not going to be enamoured with NSM. Since the Hunter committee had precluded manufacturers from adding NSM to cigarettes with a high nicotine content there was no incentive in terms of smoker satisfaction for consumers to buy the products. There was no financial incentive either, because the government had decided to tax NSM in exactly the same way as ordinary tobacco. The industrial policy of product modi-fication and 'safer' smoking had fallen foul of a major shift in health policy.

There were attempts to build bridges between government and industry following the failure of NSM. In 1979 the outraged Mr Tony Garrett was replaced by Mr Andrew Reid as chairman of Imperial Tobacco. Mr Reid defended the policy of product modification and the industry's responsible approach to the smoking and health controversy. He further stated:

> Our relations with the government, its advisory committee and medical authorities are generally good. We have taken account of the judgements of medical authorities and have modified our products. Our quarrel is with the extremists who are running an hysterical propaganda campaign against the social acceptability of smoking. We believe that the adult citizen must be free to make his or her own choice and any measures that seek to limit that freedom should be resisted. Of course, some people dislike tobacco smoke and some smokers were discourteous, but the views of extremists in relation to the effect on non-smokers of smoking by others have not generally been supported by medical authorities.[44]

In 1981 Mr Reid waxed lyrical about his faith in the future of Imperial Tobacco but the writing was already on the wall. A year later falling trade figures resulted in the closure of three factories at Bristol, Glasgow and Stirling, and numerous job losses at Newcastle, Nottingham, Liverpool, Swindon and Ipswich. On one level this situation arose because Wills and IGL had expanded furiously only to be caught out by unfavourable economic conditions. But changes in health policy and smoking had also played a role in the impending demise of Wills and IGL.

The launch of the second Hunter report in 1979 also underlined the new policy situation. Smoking researchers lambasted the report for the *naïveté* of its models of smoking behaviour. Low-tar and nicotine cigarettes might actually lead smokers to take in more rather than less tar because of 'compensatory smoking'.[45] The report was accompanied by a minority report from one of its members, the public health physician, Dr J. Donald

Ball, brother of Keith Ball, one of the founders of ASH. Donald Ball took a different line from that of the main committee, insisting on a greater sense of urgency in reducing tar and carbon monoxide yields; he wanted to see maximum levels set. But the main thrust of his argument exemplified the increasingly dominant anti-smoking argument. His view was that consumption should be reduced as well as toxicity, and the emphasis had to be on prevention. It was important to stop people smoking or prevent them starting, whereas the committee's main concern had been the health of persisting smokers.[46] Ball's stance was also founded on a change in smoking culture apparent by the end of the 1970s; for the first time, smoking was in decline, among men, and, to a lesser extent, among women as well.[47]

The later history of safer smoking. The 'invisible industrialist' and the history of smoking policy and public health

The end of the 1970s seemed to be a parting of the ways. The emergence of passive smoking as a 'scientific fact' in the early 1980s underlined the gulf between anti-smoking interests and the industry.[48] Government and industry meanwhile continued a close relationship, one in its turn underlined by the removal of a Conservative health minister, Sir George Young, who strongly opposed smoking, and his replacement by Geoffrey Finsberg, more sympathetic to industrial interests. The story could be written as one of the rupture of alliances and of opposition replacing co-operation for public health interests. The tripartite alliance of the 1950s–70s, it could be argued, was replaced by two opposing hostile camps. This was certainly the public image and also the analysis given in journalist history.[49]

Yet, behind this public image, the harm reduction agenda continued. It continued to bring together government, industry and public health scientists. This is the not the place to take that history further in detail. It involved the continuance of ISCSH and its successor in the 1990s, SCOTH (Scientific Committee on Tobacco and Health). Through those committees, work was carried out with research funding provided by the industry; this was administered at arms length through a research funding body, the Tobacco Products Research Trust.[50] Its work entailed the reformulation of the scientific harm reduction agenda through work on the role of nicotine[51] carried out by leading public health researchers.[52] It also ultimately brought a change of industrial alliance through the rise of a replacement product, nicotine replacement therapy (NRT) that, unlike tobacco substitutes, was subject to medicines control. This was the new government–industry–public health alliance that began to emerge in the 1990s and attained policy significance with health measures introduced by the Labour government elected in 1997. The pharmaceutical industry replaced the tobacco industry in an alliance with government to develop the twin harm reduction–elimination agenda.

The story of 'safer smoking' in the 1970s underlines the historical myopia or truncated vision of contemporary public health in its policy discussions. Harm or risk reduction as a policy objective has a history that has been forgotten. Drawing attention to the close involvement of public health interests with the tobacco industry and with government from the 1950s to the 1970s is neither an exposé nor a justification of those relationships. What is needed is the type of critical distance that is often absent from the discussions, even the historical ones, of such connections. Reinstating this different history enables us to reflect about the process whereby the objective of reducing harm or risk as an aim of policy, which was central from the 1950s to the 1970s, has come back on to the agenda since the 1990s, although in rather different ways. The industrial alliances that have been cemented in more recent times have been with the pharmaceutical industry. In forging those alliances public health researchers have forgotten the earlier history of co-operation, or framed it through concepts of betrayal and corruption that have not helped clear analysis of current options. The relationship of public health with industrial interests draws our attention to the changing nature of the public health enterprise.

Another framework for analysis of these relationships comes from the work of historians of science, who have begun to bring the 'invisible industrialist' into the historical picture. Work by Gaudillière and Lowy, for example, has shown how industry entered into the laboratory world. The generalisability of scientific knowledge and the replication of local results was dependent on industrially produced items, such as laboratory animals or kits for analysis. This is the industrialist as the producer of instruments and research materials, as part of the process of health technology development. The twentieth century saw the growth of networks linking research, academics and industry in these areas.[53,54] Most of this historical assessment has concentrated on the links between academics and industry, without drawing out the input into government policy. Edgerton's work on the 'warfare state' traces that process effectively but from the perspective of science, industry and government connections stimulated by defence interests.[55] Neither of these strands of historical analysis has examined health policy. This chapter has looked at science–industry–public health and health policy developments. Here industry and the market have been, and are, important mediators of policy agendas. The role of the tobacco industry has not been absent from analyses of smoking policy. But the role of the industry has indeed been invisible so far as the significance of the changing content of public health agendas is concerned. Throwing light on the role of 'the invisible industrialist' in smoking policy is a central part of the historical reassessment of industrial relationships in health and of the relationships between public health, government and industry interests in smoking policy.

Notes

1 Text on ASH website www.ash.org.uk, accessed January 2003.
2 P. Taylor, *The Smoke Ring. Tobacco, Money and Multinational Politics*, London: Sphere Books, 1985.
3 P. Pringle. *Dirty Business – Big Tobacco at the Bar of Justice*, London: Aurum Press, 1998.

4 'The Smoke Screen' in *Yes, Prime Minister*, series one. First transmitted 23 January 1986, www.yes-minister.com/episodes.htm.

5 S.A. Glantz , J. Slade, L.A. Bero, P. Hanauer and D.E. Barnes, *The Cigarette Papers*, Berkeley: University of California Press, 1996.

6 J.-P. Gaudillière and I. Lowy, *The Invisible Industrialist. Manufacturers and the Production of Scientific Knowledge*, London and Basingstoke: Macmillan, 1998.

7 B.W.E. Alford, *W.D. and H.O. Wills and the Development of the UK Tobacco Industry, 1786–1965*, London: Methuen & Co., 1973, p. 399.

8 Ministry of Health papers, MH55/1011, 18 December 1953. Letter from Sir Alexander Maxwell, Chairman of TAC, to Dr. Goodman at Ministry of Health enclosing copy of memo sent to Himsworth.

9 Ministry of Health papers, MH 55/1011. Letter from John Boyd Carpenter to Marquess of Salisbury, Lord President of the Council.

10 Royal College of Physicians, *Smoking and Health,* London: Pitman, 1962.

11 H. Cox, *The Global Cigarette. Origins and Evolution of British American Tobacco, 1880–1945*, Oxford: Oxford University Press, 2000.

12 Bristol Record Office, Wills Archive. 38169. M/11/C Marketing Minutes, 13 February 1967, minute no. 3316; 15 May 1967, minute 3378, and 18 July 1967, minute 3402.

13 Bristol Record Office, Wills Archive. 38169. M/11/C Marketing Minutes, 10 January 1966, minute no. 3081.

14 Bristol Record Office, Wills Archive. 38169. M/11/C Marketing Minutes, 22 February 1967, minute no 3326.

15 Bristol Record Office, Wills Archive. 38169. M/11/C Marketing Minutes, 3 January 1966, minute no. 3070.

16 Bristol Record Office, Wills Archive. 38169. M/11/C Marketing Minutes, 23 May 1967, minute no. 3379.

17 Ibid.

18 Bristol Record Office, Wills Archive. 38169. M/11/C Marketing Minutes, 18 July 1967, minute no. 3403.

19 Bristol Record Office, Wills Archive. 38169. M/11/C Marketing Minutes, 17 October 1967, minute no. 3426.

20 Treasury papers. T 320/371. Customs and Excise brief, 26 June 1964.

21 Department of Health papers. MH 154/1013 contains a resume of this history, '1972–77 health hazards of carbon monoxide from cigarettes'.

22 Department of Health and Social Security. (DHSS) *Report of the Standing Scientific Liaison Committee (on the Scientific Aspects of Smoking and Health) to the Secretary of State for Social Services on the Publication of Tar and Nicotine Yields of Packeted Cigarettes*, London: DHSS, 1972.

23 Department of Health papers. MH 154/1013 contains a copy of a letter from Michael Russell of the Institute of Psychiatry in the *British Medical Journal* that makes this point.

24 Royal College of Physicians, *Smoking and Health Now*, London: Pitman, 1971.

25 M. Phillips, '"Curb smoking" call unheeded', *Guardian*, 6 May 1980, pp. 1 and 2.

26 Cabinet Office. *Cigarette smoking and health. Report by an interdepartmental group of officials.* Confidential report. October 1971.

27 Hunter was also chair of the DHSS working party on medical administration in health services and of the working party on community medicine, appointed in 1970.

28 Independent Scientific Committee on Smoking and Health. (ISCSH) *First Report. Tobacco Substitutes and Additives in Tobacco Products: Their Testing and Marketing in the United Kingdom*, London: HMSO, 1975.

29 Ibid.

30 Department of Health papers. MH 148/1473, Minutes of the Independent Scientific Committee on Smoking and Health, 30th meeting, 16 November 1978.

31 Department of Health papers,.MH154/1013, Minutes of ISCSH 15th Meeting, 28 November 1975.
32 DHSS/DHSSNI/SHHD/WO, *Second Report of the Independent Scientific Committee of [sic] Smoking and Health. Developments on Tobacco Products and the Possibility of 'Lower-risk' Cigarettes*, London: HMSO, 1979.
33 Bristol Record Office, 38169/E/14/4, 'Now public gives verdict on NSM', *Wills World*, 22 August 1974, p. 7.
34 Bristol Record Office, 38169/E/14/4, 'NSM stands on the threshold', *Wills World*, 28 June 1973, p.3.
35 Bristol Record Office, 38169/E/14/4, 'Course is in good taste', *Wills World*, 20 November 1975, p.3.
36 Bristol Record Office, 38169/E/14/4, 'Now public gives verdict on NSM', *Wills World*, 22 August 1974, p.7.
37 Bristol Record Office, 38169/E/14/4, 'Sir John warns on profits', *Wills World*, 25 July 1974, front page.
38 Bristol Record Office, 38169/E/14/4, 'Price code must go', *Wills World* (supplement on trade), 25 March 1976, front page.
39 Bristol Record Office, 3816/E/14/4, 'Minister outlines strategy', *Wills World*, 24 March 1977, p. 8.
40 Royal College of Physicians (RCP), *Smoking or Health*, London: Pitman Medical, 1977.
41 These had been established under the Tobacco Substitutes regulations of 1970 after the 1970 Finance Act and had provided for tobacco duty to be charged on additives and substitutes used in the manufacture of smoking products.
42 DHSS, *Second Report of the Independent Scientific Committee.*
43 Bristol Record Office, 38169/E/14/4, 'IMPS accuse government on NSM policy', *Wills World*, 27 October 1977, p. 3.
44 Bristol Record Office, 38169/E/14/4, 'The way I see it', *Wills World*, 27 September 1979, p 3.
45 M.J. Jarvis and M.A.H. Russell, 'Comment on the Hunter committee's second report', *British Medical Journal* 280, 1980: 994–5.
46 J.D. Ball, minority report, pp. 49–55 in *Second Report of the Independent Scientific Committee.*
47 V. Berridge, 'Constructing women and smoking as a public health problem in Britain 1950–1990's', *Gender and History* 13(2), 2001: 328–48.
48 V. Berridge, 'What I would most like to know' (series), 'Why have attitudes to industry funding of research changed?' *Addiction* 92(8), 1997: 965–8.
49 For example, Taylor in *Smoke Ring.*
50 V. Berridge, 'Voluntarism and policy making networks: ASH, the Tobacco Products Research Trust and UK smoking policy', in V. Berridge, *Making Health Policy*, Amsterdam: Rodopi, 2005.
51 This had been initiated in the tobacco industry's own laboratories at Harrogate in the 1960s.
52 Berridge, 'Voluntarism'.
53 Gaudillière and Lowy, *Invisible Industrialists*, pp.1–15.
54 J.V. Pickstone, *Ways of Knowing. A New History of Science, Technology and Medicine*, Manchester: Manchester University Press, 2000, Ch. 7.
55 D.E.H. Edgerton, *Science, Technology and the British Industrial 'Decline', 1870–1970*, Cambridge: Cambridge University Press, 1996.

Recommended further reading

B.W.E. Alford, *W.D. and H.O. Wills and the Development of the UK Tobacco Industry, 1786–1965*, London: Methuen & Co., 1973.

V. Berridge, 'What I would most like to know' (series), 'Why have attitudes to industry funding of research changed?' *Addiction* 92(8), 1997: 965–8.

H. Cox, *The Global Cigarette. Origins and Evolution of British American Tobacco, 1880–1945*, Oxford: Oxford University Press, 2000.

J.-P. Gaudillière and I. Lowy, *The Invisible Industrialist. Manufacturers and the Production of Scientific Knowledge*, London and Basingstoke: Macmillan, 1998.

J.V. Pickstone, *Ways of Knowing. A New History of Science, Technology and Medicine*, Manchester: Manchester University Press, 2000.

8 Drug regulation and the Welfare State

Government, the pharmaceutical industry and the health professions in Great Britain, 1940–80

Stuart Anderson

Introduction

There has been increasing interest in recent years in the development of drug regulatory systems, and in locating them in a broader political, economic and social context. Some of this interest has taken the form of comparative analysis, particularly between developments in Great Britain and the USA. Abraham's account has done much to take this debate forward,[1] and others have drawn attention to the similarities and differences in the British and US responses to a number of therapeutic challenges. For example, Marks has reviewed the development of the birth control pill in this context,[2] and Goodman and Walsh have offered a similar interpretation in relation to the anti-cancer drug taxol.[3] Others have examined the impact of the emergence of new diseases on drug regulation, such as Edgar and Rothman's account of the challenge that AIDS presented for the drug regulatory process in the USA.[4]

These comparative accounts demonstrate both similarities and differences in the way in which drug regulation developed in Great Britain compared to the USA, responding to different political, economic and social factors at different times. In Britain drug regulation had its origin in concerns about the levels of poisoning, both accidental and deliberate.[5] Early developments in the USA were largely in response to concerns about the adulteration of imported drugs.[6] Adulteration was also a problem in Britain, but action against it in the early years of the twentieth century followed that to control poisons. Abraham notes that 'the initial legislation passed to control drug adulteration in this period was very similar in Britain and the US'.[7] He observes that the main difference between British and US drug control at that time was in the institutional approach to enforcement: the Americans had a centralised bureau to carry out investigations and test drugs, while the British depended entirely on routine sampling by local inspectors; government only became involved when problems arose.

During the first half of the twentieth century both the British and US governments became much more involved in the regulation of drugs. There was a steady flow of legislation on both sides of the Atlantic, in response to international, national and technological developments. Both governments enacted legislation in the light of international agreements such as the Hague Convention of 1912, concerning the control of narcotics; both responded to the discovery of new, more potent drugs from the 1930s onwards by the passage of new laws.

Yet there was one important difference in the national contexts in which drug regulation developed in these two countries, and that was the establishment of a Welfare State in Britain but not in the USA. This difference was to have a crucial impact on the nature of drug regulation, and particularly on the roles played by their respective governments. For example, Marks has demonstrated that Britain and the USA monitored and secured the safety of the oral contraceptive pill between 1960 and 1970 in very different ways.[8] She explored the reason for this difference in policy, showing that it was shaped by the research orientation of each country, and by the specific legal, medical, social and political traditions within Britain and the USA. Marks further suggests that one of the key differences between the regulation of the contraceptive pill in Great Britain and the USA during the 1960s was the impact that the National Health Service (NHS) had on the relationship between the government, health professions and the pharmaceutical industry.

But what was the nature of these relationships, and how had they been formed? What combination of social, political and economic factors had converged for the NHS to dominate the exchanges between the parties? And what was their impact on drug regulation? This chapter explores the relationships between the government, the health professions and the pharmaceutical industry in Great Britain from before the introduction of the NHS in 1948, to after the enactment of the Medicines Act in 1968. It demonstrates that introduction of the NHS caused the British government to focus almost exclusively on the cost of drugs at the expense of drug safety, and that it took a major regulatory disaster, the Thalidomide tragedy in 1961, for drug safety to become the primary consideration.

This chapter is in five main parts. I begin with a brief review of medicines regulation in Britain up to the time the NHS was introduced in 1948. I then give a brief account of the key players in this drama – the Ministry of Health, the pharmaceutical industry and the doctors – and the nature of the relationship between them at that time. This is followed by a review of the drug-related issues of concern to the parties during the period from 1948 to 1961. I return to the regulation of medicines during the period 1948 to 1968, and conclude with an analysis of the impact of the NHS on both the relationship between the players and on drug regulation.

Regulation of medicines in Britain before 1948

Drug regulation in Britain has its origins in the mid-nineteenth century. In Britain before 1851, there was no control of any kind over any substance, however lethal.[9] But the late 1840s saw a growth in public concern about the unrestricted availability of poisons. Reports from the Registrar General's office began to draw attention to the large number of deaths resulting from poisoning, both accidental and deliberate. More than a third resulted from the use of arsenic.[10] In 1849 the Pharmaceutical Society found that its members were heavily involved in the sale of poisons, and succeeded in persuading the government that the safe use of arsenic could be achieved by restricting its retail sale to pharmacies. The result was the Arsenic Act of 1851.[11]

The next step in the regulation of poisons came with the 1868 Pharmacy and Poisons Act. The 1868 Act effectively extended the arrangements made for arsenic to twenty commonly used medicinal poisons, including opium, strychnine and prussic acid, by restricting their sale to pharmaceutical chemists, who would be able to exercise professional judgement and control.[12] There was however another drug-related problem of concern to the state, and that was adulteration. Following a number of highly publicised incidents, such as the Bradford tragedy in 1858 (in which a large number of people died after taking peppermint lozenges that had been inadvertently adulterated with arsenic)[13] a Drug Adulteration Act was passed in 1872. This appointed public analysts to test medicines prior to sale.

A new Poisons and Pharmacy Act in 1908 gave pharmacists additional responsibilities in relation to the control of poisons. The Pharmaceutical Society retained its powers to deem a substance a poison, to decide which compounds should be available for sale, and to decide who should be allowed to become both authorised and listed sellers of poisons. This legislation still had many gaps. It placed no control over the manufacture or possession of narcotics. Both opium and cocaine were freely available in unregulated quantities without prescription. This omission was rectified in 1920 with the Dangerous Drugs Act, following Britain's signing of the Hague Convention in 1912.[14]

Developments in the field of bacteriology in the late decades of the nineteenth century led to the availability of a wide range of biological products, such as vaccines and sera. Following several incidents in the USA (where a number of people died following errors in the manufacturing or testing of biological products) there was recognition of the need for regulation of these products in Britain. They were substances used for medicinal purposes that could not be tested chemically; they could not easily be regulated as poisons, and some other definition was needed. A Therapeutic Substances Act was eventually passed in 1925, which controlled by licence the manufacture, but not the sale or supply, of a range of preparations, the potency or purity of which could not be tested chemically.[15] These included vaccines, sera and antitoxins. With these two Acts (for dangerous drugs and therapeutic substances) the boundaries between medicinal preparations and drugs were being redrawn.

The introduction of the barbiturates in the early 1930s accelerated this shift, although new drugs continued to be treated as poisons. The Pharmacy and Poisons Act of 1933 contained a fourth schedule, which listed a number of poisons that could only be sold to the public in accordance with a prescription written by a doctor, dentist or veterinary surgeon. These included barbiturates and digitalis preparations. The creation of this schedule represented a major increase in the medical profession's control of the supply of drugs to the general public. Following introduction of the sulphonamides in the late 1930s a new Pharmacy and Medicines Act was passed in 1941. Despite its title this confirmed that these new medicines would be regulated under poisons legislation. The development of penicillin at the end of the Second World War led to further difficulties. The response was a separate Penicillin Act, passed in 1947, designed to control the sale and supply of penicillin.

These developments illustrate the fact that the state only became interested in medicines once they were generally available. The state had little interest in the inherent safety of medicines, provided they were not adulterated and their supply was in the hands of responsible people; how they were developed, and what testing had been done on them, were not its concern. Even when serious side-effects became apparent with some of the early therapeutic advances there was little interest in official circles. The attitude to side-effects was summed up by Leo Schindel, a leading pharmacologist. 'Until the 1930s there had been little need to worry about side effects. It was understood that an overdose might be lethal, but there was practically no such thing as an unexpected reaction to a particular medicament'.[16] The prevailing view was that, although they were unpleasant, side-effects were acceptable as a small price to pay for the advantages derived from the drugs that caused them.

By the late 1940s concerns about the safety of some of the new drugs emerging were being expressed, but the government had more pressing matters to attend to, not least the introduction of its NHS. In its early years the supply, and particularly the cost, of medicines were both to loom large, but before I consider the impact this had on drug regulation I need to briefly describe developments up to this point concerning the principal actors in the debate, the pharmaceutical industry, the medical profession and the Ministry of Health.

The industry, the ministry and the medical profession before 1948

Although pharmaceutical manufacturers had been in existence in Great Britain since before the start of the nineteenth century[17] most were relatively small, were not research-based, and viewed their competitors with suspicion. With the introduction of mass production in the second half of the nineteenth century many more companies entered the market, including manufacturers of proprietary medicines such as Beecham and Holloway. Further manufacturers emerged to meet the demand for sera and antitoxins at the end of the century, and yet others emerged to supply the needs for vitamins and other fine chemicals with medicinal uses.

By 1930 there was general agreement amongst pharmaceutical manufacturers of the need to speak with a common voice: a Wholesale Drug Trade Association (WDTA) was formed to represent them.[18] In the late 1930s sulphanilamide (the first of the sulphonamides) was introduced. This stimulated a search for other antibacterial substances, and other agents having a variety of pharmacological activities. By the late 1930s the industry was becoming more research-based, effective drugs were becoming available but only on the prescription of a doctor, and the customer was increasingly the government itself.

After the Second World War, and with talk of a Welfare State available to all, the WDTA took on new members, and in 1948 it changed its name to the Association of the British Pharmaceutical Industry (ABPI). The fact that this was the year that the NHS was established was no coincidence. The industry needed to be in a strong position to argue the case to the government for expenditure on medicines.

The medical profession had long had a body to represent its members, with extensive experience of lobbying government to get the best deal for its members. The British Medical Association (BMA) had its origins in the Provincial Medical and Surgical Association (PMSA), formed in 1832.[19] It became the BMA in 1856, rapidly becoming a powerful lobbyist on behalf of doctors. The PMSA had worked with the Pharmaceutical Society in submitting the proposals to government to restrict the supply of poisons that had resulted in the Arsenic Act of 1851.

This was to be the start of what became a permanent interest in medicines and prescribing. From the 1880s the medical profession began campaigning for legal controls on proprietary medicines.[20] In 1909 it published *Secret Remedies*, and in 1912 *More Secret Remedies* followed. These books presented results of analysis of hundreds of proprietary medicines, demonstrating that most contained virtually worthless ingredients of no therapeutic value. Many of these were sold by well-known companies. The BMA thus had early experience of challenging pharmaceutical manufacturers.

The BMA's experience of negotiating with government during the second half of the nineteenth century placed it in good stead to strike a hard deal with the government at the time of introduction of the National Health Insurance Scheme in 1913.[21] The deal included incentives to minimise prescribing. Under the 'floating sixpence' rule doctors received a payment that included the cost of any drug they prescribed. If the actual cost of the drug did not reach this limit the doctor could retain the difference up to a maximum of sixpence. Negotiations concerning the terms of service of doctors under the National Insurance Scheme continued throughout the period between the two world wars, and formed a crucial part of the negotiations to create the NHS.[22]

Of all the key players in the medicines arena the government itself was perhaps the most fragmented. The Ministry of Health had only been formed in 1919. Negotiations with the doctors concerning introduction of the National Health Insurance Scheme had been conducted directly by the Chancellor of the Exchequer, Lloyd George. In getting agreement with the doctors for its plans for the NHS the Ministry was cutting its negotiating skills teeth against a formidable and experienced opponent. At the same time it had very little interest in drugs: responsibility for the regulation of medicines and poisons fell to the Home Office, whilst responsibility for the testing of medicines fell to local authorities. Its contact with the pharmaceutical industry was limited to a concern for the supply of essential drugs when these became available, such as insulin and penicillin.

Thus, by the time the NHS was introduced in 1948, the BMA already had extensive experience of dealing with the government, and it had some experience of dealing with the pharmaceutical industry. The government had recent dealings with the medical profession, but very limited contact with the pharmaceutical industry. The supply of drugs under the NHS came to change the relationship between them all.

The triumph of economics over risk management, 1948–61

In the immediate postwar period, and in parallel with the introduction of the NHS, the pharmaceutical industry began the search for new therapeutic substances in earnest.[23] In this it was very successful. Between 1952 and 1960 some 1,000 new pharmaceutical products came on the market. There was a steady stream of antibiotics: chloramphenicol appeared in 1951, oxytetracycline in 1954, and tetracycline in 1955. Hormone research resulted in the launch of prednisone in 1957, and work on the cardiovascular system resulted in the development of chlorothiazide in 1958.[24]

However, of these only 118 were new chemical entities; all the others were new formulations of old drugs, or else combinations of old and new ones.[25] Of the 1,000, some 130 were still in use in 1987. These new products would inevitably be more expensive than the drugs they replaced, and, together with extension of the provision of free medicines to all, would place an enormous financial burden on the NHS.

Drugs, money and the NHS

But in the early days of the NHS there were still relatively few active drugs available. Loudon and Drury identified only twenty-five drugs and vaccines available to medical practitioners before 1950 that were likely to be judged 'effective' if subjected to a modern randomised trial.[26] Most medicines supplied under the National Insurance Scheme were mixtures intended to relieve symptoms rather than cure disease.

The steady outpouring of new therapeutic agents during the 1950s, so soon after introduction of the NHS, had not been anticipated, and had certainly not been budgeted for. The original estimate for the pharmaceutical service for the part year 1948/9 was based on the costs incurred under National Insurance, extrapolated to the wider population. In 1947 the total cost of the

Table 8.1 Current expenditure on Family Practitioner Services, UK, 1948–80

Financial year	General medical service	Pharmaceutical service	General dental service	Ophthalmic service
1948/9	33.8	17.9	20.7	12.8
1949/50	48.2	36.6	49.3	24.6
1950/1	48.9	40.5	46.6	22.4
1951/2	48.8	52.5	36.3	9.6
1952/3	87.3	49.7	25.2	6.8
1953/4	59.9	46.4	24.5	7.6
1954/5	61.0	49.7	26.9	8.3
1955/6	63.7	51.6	32.8	9.0
1956/7	67.8	60.6	36.0	9.6
1957/8	72.6	61.7	39.0	10.1
1958/9	76.5	67.2	42.4	10.1
1959/60	76.7	74.9	46.9	11.3
1960/1	103.5	83.5	49.8	11.6
1961/2	87.7	77.4	52.0	10.1
1962/3	88.6	79.8	52.9	9.8
1963/4	93.0	114.0	66.0	19.0
1964/5	95.0	133.0	68.0	20.0
1965/6	104.0	155.0	70.0	22.0
1966/7	112.0	163.0	80.0	23.0
1967/8	130.0	179.0	82.0	24.0
1968/9	138.0	186.0	85.0	25.0
1969/70	148.0	204.0	92.0	28.0
1970/1	181.0	222.0	110.0	31.0
1971/2	196.0	249.0	122.0	28.0
1972/3	212.0	285.0	132.0	31.0
1973/4	228.0	313.0	147.0	35.0
1974/5	265.0	440.0	204.0	51.0
1975/6	341.0	485.0	239.0	76.0
1976/7	384.0	618.0	265.0	79.0
1977/8	406.0	745.0	273.0	80.0
1978/9	463.0	880.0	330.0	90.0
1979/80	574.0	1,004.0	395.0	109.0

Notes:

For dates before 1963/4 no separate information is supplied in the AAS tabulation about capital expenditure, but the amount of capital investment before this date was negligible.

Source: Annual Abstract of Statistics, 1964, 1972, 1980.

pharmaceutical service had been £6.8 million. The estimate for 1948/9 was £11.5 million; the actual cost was £17.9 million, an overshoot of 52 per cent.[27]

This was to set the pattern for spending on the pharmaceutical service over the next thirty years. Within a year it had more than doubled, to £36.6 million. Within ten years it had doubled again, to £74.9 million in 1959/60. It doubled again within another six years, to £155.0 million in 1965/6, and yet again in eight years to £313.0 million in 1973/4. Six years later it had exceeded £1 billion. Table 8.1 presents the relative costs of the various family practitioner services between 1948 and 1980.

The cost of the pharmaceutical service under the NHS was viewed as a problem right from the beginning. On top of greater coverage of the service, and the costs of new drugs, there was another problem. Aneurin Bevan, who had been the principal architect of the NHS, and who was Minister of Health from August 1945 until January 1951, readily admitted that the service was subject to abuse.[28] In his view the bottle of medicine was 'generally a routine item, whose value was often questionable'. 'I shudder to think' he said 'of the ceaseless cascade of medicine which is pouring down British throats at the present time'.[29] It was Bevan who set in motion consideration of prescription charges by accepting the principle that patients should pay a container charge. His view was that such a charge was a 'useful deterrent to unnecessary resort to medication'.

Yet the warning signs that the cost of pharmaceuticals would rise rapidly during the 1950s and early 1960s were already clear in the late 1940s. During the early 1930s annual output from the British pharmaceutical industry was below £20 million. The £100 million mark (a five-fold increase) was reached at the start of the 1950s.[30] A significant proportion of this was exported, and the value of pharmaceutical exports increased steadily, rising rapidly during the 1970s. The value of the balance of trade in pharmaceuticals between 1950 and 1980 is illustrated in Figure 8.1. Thus by the early 1950s the pharmaceutical industry was already a large and important player; it could not easily be brushed aside by any government.

Towards the end of 1951 the Labour government was replaced by a Conservative one. This was as much concerned with rising costs in the NHS as had been Labour. Attention shifted from concern with overall NHS spending in general to the cost of drugs in particular. Macleod, the new Minister of Health, admitted that expenditure on pharmaceutical products caused him 'more concern than any other item, including the hospitals'.[31] The overall drug bill and the cost per prescription climbed unremittingly. In 1947 the cost per prescription had been just 24 pence; by 1955/6 it had more than doubled to 58 pence.

The health ministers described this trend as 'frightening', and a range of options to control it were examined. But Webster notes that 'none of the methods adopted during the early years of the NHS for containing these costs was more than trivially successful'.[32] The greatest effort went into prescription charges, which had the double attractions of a deterrent effect

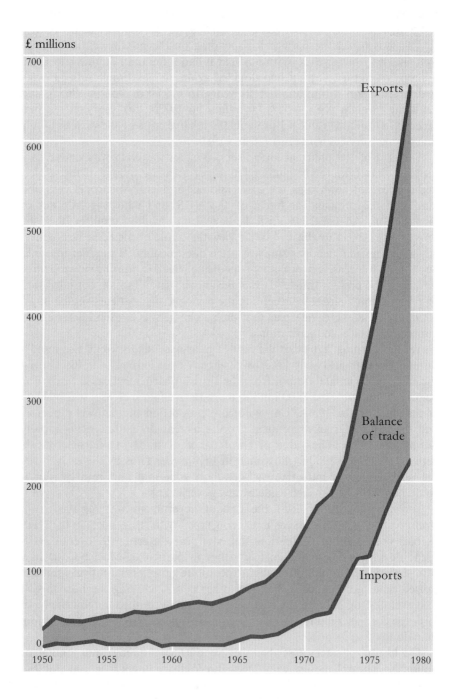

Figure 8.1 Pharmaceuticals: export and imports, 1950–78

and a direct contribution to revenue. Their introduction in 1952/3 produced a temporary slow down in total expenditure, but the deterrent effect proved only temporary. It was politically difficult to raise the charge, and difficult to maintain it at an economic level.

The failure of such blunt approaches persuaded the government to try more direct approaches in an attempt to control the drugs bill. Some limited attempts were made to educate patients to use the service more sensibly.[33] These proved unsuccessful and were quickly abandoned. Attention shifted to the doctors who wrote the prescriptions. But it proved equally impossible to reduce the bill by educating or disciplining the doctors. Macleod blamed the 'wholly improper pressure put upon doctors by patients on the one hand, and more seriously by manufacturers on the other'. Efforts were made to provide doctors with more balanced information about these medicines, and the machinery designed to discipline doctors who prescribed excessively was refined. But neither of these initiatives made any difference to the relentless increase in the cost of the pharmaceutical services.[34]

In November 1952 the Treasury decided to refer the problem to a small independent enquiry. Its terms of reference were agreed only after protracted discussions; the government did not want to be accused of embarking on the destruction of the welfare state.[35] Eventually it was agreed that the committee should consider how 'rising charge' upon the Exchequer might be avoided. It was formally announced on 1 April 1953, to be chaired by an economist, Claude Guillebaud. The Guillebaud Report was eventually published in January 1956. It provided a glowing endorsement of the NHS during its first seven years, and rejected any suggestion of inefficiency. 'Any charge that there is widespread extravagance in the NHS,' it concluded 'whether in respect of the spending of money or the use of manpower, is not borne out by our evidence.'[36] The committee was unable to suggest any sources for major economies, and was not in favour of additional charges. No solution to the rising drugs bill was offered.

Drugs, the government and the pharmaceutical industry

The existence of the inquiry was a convenient excuse to defer many crucial decisions relating to health service expenditure, not least those relating to medicines. The health ministers were reluctant to force a resolution in the informal discussions they had recently entered into with the pharmaceutical companies concerning alleged excessive profits made from proprietary drugs, and the government's intention to introduce a limited list of drugs.[37] It had become clear that pharmaceuticals were the most profitable sector of all, a large part of which was at the expense of the government. By 1957 the rate of return after taxes for the industry was over 5 per cent ahead of its nearest rival. The rates of return of selected sectors in 1957 are illustrated in Figure 8.2.

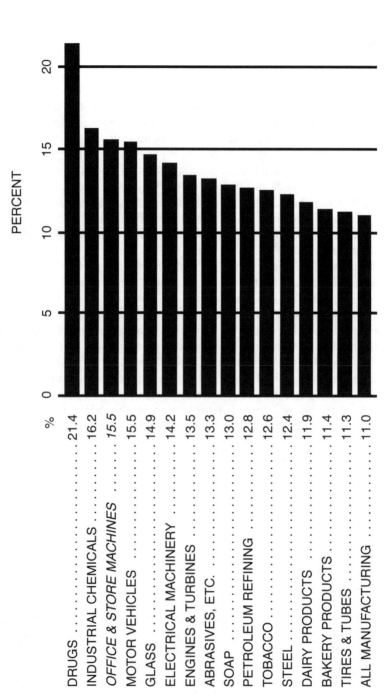

Figure 8.2 Comparison of rates of return after taxes in selected industries, 1957

The Guillebaud Report contained little in the way of concrete proposals for the achievement of economy in the health service. The Treasury was particularly annoyed at its failure to sanction either prescription charges, or mechanisms for controlling the cost of proprietary medicines.[38] It was soon realised by the government that the problem of rapidly rising expenditure on drugs would have to be tackled head-on, by scrutiny of the prices charged by the pharmaceutical companies.

The reasons for the endless increase in drug expenditure were now clear: the discovery and marketing of new and expensive drugs; the increased use of proprietary (branded) rather than non-proprietary (generic) drugs; the overall levels of profit in the pharmaceutical companies; and the promotion of drugs to the medical profession. In 1947 branded medicines accounted for only 5 per cent of National Health Insurance prescriptions; by 1953 they accounted for 25 per cent in number but about 50 per cent by cost of NHS prescriptions. The proportion by number of branded versus generic medicines dispensed during the course of the twentieth century is illustrated in Figure 8.3.

Branded medicines accounted for 50 per cent by number of all NHS prescriptions by 1957. The proportion continued to increase until 1977, after which it began to fall, most notably in 1985 when the limited list was eventually introduced, and it has continued to decrease. It passed the 50 per cent mark again in 1993. But the proportion of total cost accounted for by proprietary medicines was even higher. By the end of 1954 they accounted for 60 per cent of the NHS drugs bill, and by 1959 the proportion was 75 per cent.

The trigger for health department action against the pharmaceutical companies had been a report from the Public Accounts Committee. This concerned negligence in determining fair levels of profit made by suppliers. The committee could not 'view with equanimity the continued payment of prices which...include a profit margin substantially in excess of that hitherto accepted as appropriate for government contracts'.[39] Under Treasury pressure the Ministry of Health entered into discussions with the ABPI with a view to considering how costs might be controlled. Working parties were established to look at the cost of basic drugs, and also the earnings of firms packing drugs manufactured by others, and wholesalers. The impact of these inquiries was negligible, although some minor price reductions were negotiated following an investigation into the production of bulk drugs.

The government had made some attempt to limit the availability of drugs under the NHS at the time of its introduction. The Standing Joint Committee on the Classification of Proprietary Preparations (the Cohen Committee) had been established in 1949 to advise on what drugs should be available. It created a six-part classification system for drugs then in use. It suggested that two classes of preparation should not be prescribed under the NHS: those that were advertised directly to the public; and some 900 items that were judged to be of no proven therapeutic value.[40] There nevertheless remained some 4,000 proprietary products on the list that the committee

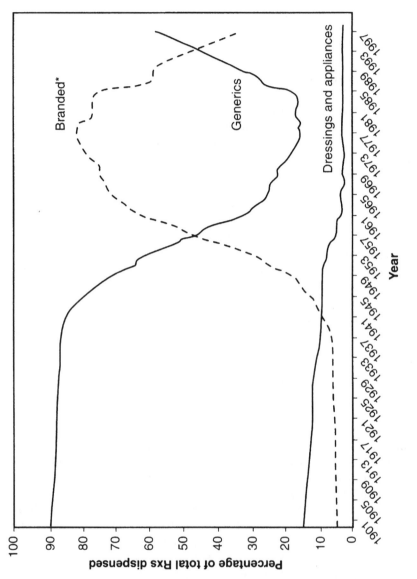

Figure 8.3 Branded or generic? Proportion of medicines prescribed, 1900–97

agreed could be prescribed 'subject to satisfactory arrangements for price being made between the Health Departments and the manufacturers'.

It was the prices of these 4,000 drugs that became the focus of attention. In July 1954 the ABPI submitted its own scheme for agreeing acceptable prices for drugs. This was always likely to be unacceptable to the ministry because the formulae failed to disclose any information about profits. However, negotiations did take place, and a number of options were considered.[41] With nothing else likely to succeed Treasury objections to the ABPI proposals were dropped, and a Voluntary Price Regulation Scheme was accepted for a trial period of three years from 1957. But the impact of the voluntary scheme was extremely limited. It was calculated that it resulted in savings of around £250,000 in the first year, and £400,000 in the second, at a time when the drug bill was around £70 million per year. At the end of the trial period the arrangement became formalised as the Prescription Price Regulation Scheme.[42]

Drugs, the government and the medical profession

Nothing the government did seemed to make any impact on the relentless growth in drug expenditure. Between 1957/8 and 1963/4 the cost of the pharmaceutical service almost doubled, from £61.7m. to £114.0m.[43] At the start of the NHS, expenditure on general medical services was about twice that on the pharmaceutical service; by 1963/4 the pharmaceutical service cost more than the medical service. Even so, its cost as a proportion of total NHS expenditure remained fairly constant, at around 10 per cent.

The idea of a limited list was raised again. This proposal had been deferred in 1953 in the expectation that the Guillebaud Committee would support it. The plan this time was to set up a joint working party between representatives of the doctors from the General Medical Services Committee, and the ministry. The intention had been to have a single inquiry covering England, Scotland and Wales, but this was rejected by the Scottish GMSC, and a separate Scottish enquiry was established. The terms of reference for the enquiries were agreed in October 1956, and the chairmen appointed early in 1957. The English committee was chaired by Sir Henry Hinchcliffe, an industrialist, and the Scottish committee by James Boyd Douglas, a farmer who was chairman of the Scottish Milk Board.

Both the Hinchcliffe and Douglas reports were published in May 1959. Neither came up with any new ideas for containing drug costs. Both rejected coercion and statutory regulation, which they viewed as impracticable and counterproductive. Instead they proposed the use of exhortation, peer pressure and education.[44] The committees were more concerned with improving standards of professional practice than with economy.

Both committees heard a great deal of evidence about the incompetence of general practitioners and wasteful prescribing in hospitals.[45] The Douglas committee concluded that 'there is, in fact, unnecessary and excessive expenditure on drugs and dressings under the NHS attributable to prescribing practice'.[46] The Hinchcliffe committee, on the other hand, concluded that there was only a minor problem of waste in the current system. 'While there is no evidence of widespread and irresponsible extravagance in general practitioners' prescribing, there is scope for economy.'[47]

Both committees rejected the idea of only a limited list of drugs being available on the NHS, or the introduction of a black list of drugs, which would only be available on a private prescription. The Hinchcliffe committee was more enthusiastic about introducing a limit on the quantity of drugs that could be prescribed on any one occasion: it wanted a two-year trial period of limiting quantities to one week's supply or less, except in chronic cases.[48] There were other differences: the Douglas committee was not in favour of abolition of the prescription charge; the Hinchcliffe committee wanted the government to abolish the prescription charge at the earliest opportunity.

The Treasury were not surprisingly dismayed by the two reports. They both presented damning evidence about waste and inefficiency but failed to make any significant recommendations for action to reduce it. Nevertheless, they were not without impact. They contained a great deal of information, which was used by the Joint Committee on Classification of Proprietary Preparations to produce a technical report on equivalence between unbranded and proprietary drugs. This was circulated to GPs for guidance. In 1960 the Ministry of Health produced a loose-leaf Handbook on Prescribing. In 1961 its *Prescribers' Notes* was replaced by the more influential *Prescribers' Journal*. The role of government in trying to influence the prescribing of doctors was now well established.

The pharmaceutical industry, the medical profession and the state

Disputes over the use of brand names persisted between the government and the pharmaceutical industry. Pharmaceutical companies invested heavily in persuading doctors to prescribe by brand name rather than by generic name. The government has been keen to promote the prescribing of generic drugs, since these are usually far cheaper than the branded version. The agreement reached at the inception of the NHS was that if a branded product was prescribed by a general practitioner, that brand must be supplied. If a generic name was used, the cheapest available version could be supplied.

The decade up to the mid-1960s witnessed a struggle between the industry and the government for the ears of the medical profession.[49] The doctors were, with their prescribing rights, the final arbiters in this dispute. The industry was determined not to lose the battle, since its profits depended on doctors prescribing by brand name. The problem for the government was how to persuade the doctors to change their prescribing habits. Again it was the Committee of Public Accounts that prodded the Ministry of Health into action. The Ministry was persuaded that if doctors were asked by other doctors to always prescribe a generic drug they would respond.

In 1961 the Cohen Committee issued a list of drugs that were available in generic form and that, in its opinion, were sufficiently identical to the branded products to justify substitution. If this were to be done it would result in a potential saving of £800,000 a year to the NHS in England and Wales.[50] But the battle was extremely one sided. On the one side doctors were bombarded with advertisements, literature and sales talk from drug company representatives that the new proprietary medicine did all that was claimed for it; on the other was a half-hearted plea from the ministry to prescribe generics to save it some money. The ministry conceded that the results of the appeal to the better judgement of the doctors were 'disappointing'.

The ministry decided to try again. It would concentrate on just five drugs, which accounted for potential savings of £600,000 a year. An article was inserted in the *Prescriber Journal*, sent to all doctors. But again the effect was marginal. The reasons became all too evident when Sir Bruce Fraser, permanent secretary at the Ministry of Health, appeared before the Committee of Public Accounts. 'You are not suggesting,' asked one of the members, 'that the average doctor in this country pays no attention to the cost of the drugs he supplies?' In a classic piece of understatement Sir Bruce replied: 'I am bound to say, that I do not think they pay as much attention as they might.' The reality was that doctors had no incentive to prescribe cheaper rather than more expensive drugs, and preferred to accept the drug companies' claims at face value.[51]

The regulation of medicines in Britain, 1948–61

In Britain in the 1950s, then, the main focus of attention concerning medicines was their cost. The system for regulating pharmaceuticals within which the therapeutic revolution unfolded was that which had been designed for the regulation of poisons in the nineteenth century. Additional legislation was only enacted if poisons regulations proved inappropriate, or supplementary controls were needed. A number of such developments did take place. Following introduction of the NHS a Drug Testing Scheme was introduced, to test the quality of medicines at the point of issue.[52] The development of antibiotics necessitated changes in relevant legislation. In 1953 the Therapeutic Substances (Prevention of Misuse) Act was enacted to include therapeutic substances that were not covered by poisons legislation.[53] In 1955 a Food and Drugs Act imposed new controls over standards of manufacture and adulteration.[54] And in 1956 another Therapeutic Substances Act was necessary to take account of pharmacological advances relating to hormones and other natural substances.

By the end of the 1950s the focus of pharmaceutical regulation in Great Britain was still firmly on the sale and supply of medicines. The legislative framework underpinning it was a complex patchwork, based on the control of substances as 'poisons' or 'therapeutic substances'. There was no legal definition of a medicine. The first time that new chemical entities came to the attention of the authorities was at the Poisons Board, who had to decide in which schedule to include it.[55] This was usually the fourth schedule, such that the new drug would only be available on a doctor's prescription. But there was no licensing of the manufacturer, no review of the tests carried out, no monitoring of its use. Once approved for the fourth schedule it was available for general use.

During the 1950s a few concerns began to be voiced about the inherent safety of medicines. Letters concerning lack of adequate testing of the new 'wonder drugs' began to appear in the medical press.[56] And serious side-effects from a number of these drugs began to be reported.[57] In 1961 the world was shaken by the Thalidomide disaster. During that year a number of physicians in different parts of the world began to see a sudden increase in cases of phocomelia, a condition in which babies are born without properly formed limbs.[58] Before Thalidomide, it was a recognised but rare condition. But in Germany in 1961 there was a three-fold increase: a paediatrician, Widukind Lenz, noted that 50 per cent of patients giving birth to such babies had taken Thalidomide during pregnancy.[59]

On 20 November 1961 Lenz reported his findings at a meeting of the Society for Paediatric Medicine in Düsseldorf. Under pressure from the German Federal Health Office the manufacturer, Chemie Grumenthal, withdrew the drug from the German market, on 26 November 1961. The story was picked up immediately and reached the front pages of newspapers across the world. In Britain a crisis meeting was held at the Ministry of Health, and on 28 November 1961 a statement was issued telling patients not to take the drug. Lenz made his findings available to the medical profession in January 1962.[60] By the time Thalidomide was identified as the culprit some 10,000 deformed children had been born around the world. Over 4,000 of these births occurred in Germany, but up to 5,000 deformities were reported in the UK.[61]

Medicines and the rise of risk management, 1961–8

The Thalidomide tragedy and the 'drug revolution' brought about new relationships between the government, the pharmaceutical industry and the medical profession, through an apparatus of drug regulation based on monitoring by the state. Prior to Thalidomide the main issue of contention between the government and the industry was the price of medicines; following Thalidomide the government was equally concerned with drug safety. Whilst concern for the cost of drugs did not diminish, there was now recognition that medicines were not without risks, and these needed to be managed by the state.

Drug regulation following Thalidomide

The Thalidomide tragedy, and the extensive publicity that surrounded it, produced a flurry of activity unprecedented in the history of medicines.

Over the months that followed the government, the industry and the medical profession all came under scrutiny in the search for someone to blame. Investigative journalists reported on the processes by which new drugs reached the market.[62] More than anything Thalidomide drew attention to the hopeless inadequacy of existing arrangements for the testing, approval and monitoring of new and potent medicines.

It was clear that a new arrangement would have to be developed for the reporting and monitoring of adverse reactions. The various representative bodies were all anxious not only to be seen to be doing something, but also to determine what those arrangements should be. In July 1962 the College of General Practitioners set up a Register of Unexpected Toxicity, a voluntary scheme in which GPs reported any unexpected effects of drugs to their own professional body.[63] In August 1962 the ABPI set up an expert committee on Drug Toxicity, with Dr R. Hennessey of the Wellcome Foundation as its chairman.[64] In the same month the Standing Medical Advisory Committee set up a joint subcommittee on the safety of drugs, under the chairmanship of Lord Cohen.[65]

The Cohen Committee set about its work immediately. Within three months, in November 1962, it had made three interim recommendations: that responsibility for testing should remain with manufacturers; that testing should not be the responsibility of government; and that a permanent expert body on the safety of medicines should be set up.[66] Not to be outdone the ABPI produced its own proposals, also in November 1962. The industry made two key proposals: that an independent advisory centre on drug safety should be established under a trust; and that an early warning system for drug safety should be set up.[67] Lord Cohen was already very familiar with the complexities of regulating and controlling medicines through his chairmanship of the Joint Committee on the Classification of Proprietary Preparations.[68] Some of the functions of the Cohen Committee were subsequently absorbed by the Dunlop Committee.[69]

The government's response was to wait for publication of the full Cohen Report in March 1963.[70] This recommended that all new drugs and preparations should be submitted to a Committee on the Safety of Drugs. This committee should have four subcommittees: on toxicity, clinical trials, therapeutic efficacy, and adverse reactions. But the report also expressed concern about areas of drug safety that were not covered in the committee's remit: the control of the quality of drugs, control of over-the-counter sales of medicines, the use of approved names of medicines, and the regulation of therapeutic claims made for new drugs by manufacturers.[71]

The recommendations of the Cohen Committee were accepted in full by the government.[72] A Committee on the Safety of Drugs was established under the chairmanship of Sir Derrick Dunlop, which began work on 1 January 1964. It was concerned with the assessment of new drugs submitted to trials, their safety in relation to efficacy before release onto the market, and considered evidence about the adverse effects of any drug in

Table 8.2 Research and development expenditure by the British pharmaceutical
         industry, 1960–1969

Year	£m	Year	£m
1960	7.5	1970 *	29.0
1961	7.8	1971 *	35.0
1962	8.3	1972 *	41.9
1963	NA	1973	44.1
1964	10.4	1974	50.0
1965	11.6	1975 *	82.6
1966	13.0	1976 *	120.0
1967	16.4	1977 *	150.0
1968	18.9	1978 *	190.0
1969	24.2		

Notes:
* Estimated.

Source: *IMS Pharmaceutical Marketletter*, 17 September 1979.

use. The scale of innovation in the pharmaceutical industry was apparent
from the volume of submissions handled by the Dunlop Committee, which
soon reached around 1,000 a year.[73] Yet in 1964 the total expenditure on
research and development by the British pharmaceutical industry was just
over £10 million; within fourteen years it had increased nineteen times
(Table 8.2).

Thereafter the pace of change in drug regulation quickened. In January
1965 a Directive from the European Union on the free movement of
medicines was published.[74] The government established a committee of
inquiry to consider the concerns raised in the Cohen Report that were
outside its remit. In September 1967 a White Paper *Forthcoming Legislation
on the Safety, Quality and Description of Drugs and Medicines* recommended
the establishment of a Medicines Committee to operate a licensing system
for all medicines.[75] In October 1968 a new Medicines Act became law,
bringing with it a new era in drug regulation in Great Britain.[76]

In November 1969 a Medicines Commission was established under the
chairmanship of Sir Derrick Dunlop.[77] A Licensing Authority was created
in 1971 with a nominated 'appointed day' after which only licensed products
could be marketed in the UK.[78] The Authority was to have three divisions,
each with its own chief: administration, medicine and pharmacy. 'Licenses
of right' were issued for products that were already on the market. In 1989
the system was changed, with the creation of a Medicines Control Agency,
again with three divisions: licensing, post-licensing, inspection and enforcement.[79] This time the agency had a single chief. By 1991 all the licenses of
right had been reviewed, and hence only licensed products could be
supplied. A system of drug regulation through licensing had triumphed as
the means of managing risk.

Drug costs following Thalidomide

Whilst the Thalidomide tragedy galvanised the government into reviewing its drug regulatory framework it remained no less concerned about the cost of drugs, particularly new ones. The Hinchcliffe Committee had concluded that 'the discovery and large-scale production of valuable but expensive drugs has been the main factor contributing to the rise in the cost of prescriptions'.[80] Between 1957–8 and 1963–4 the cost per prescription rose by 122 per cent, and the ingredient cost by 170 per cent.[81] Much of the excessive cost continued to be due to unrestrained profiteering by the pharmaceutical industry.[82]

In 1967 the government established a committee of inquiry under the chairmanship of Lord Sainsbury to consider the question. Its terms of reference were:

> to examine the relationship of the pharmaceutical industry in Great Britain with the National Health Service, having regard to the structure of the industry, to the commercial policies of the firms comprising it, to pricing and to sales promotion practices, to the effects of patents and to the relevance and value of research, and to make recommendations.[83]

The committee began work in 1965, and reported two years later, in September 1967.

The Sainsbury Report concluded that some of the existing arrangements for sales promotion, including the extensive employment of medical representatives, was wasteful, and lacking in appropriate responsibility.[84] It recommended the abolition of brand names, a requirement that therapeutic classifications appear on all medicines, and the establishment of a new independent regulatory body, to be known as the Medicines Commission.[85] This was an extension of the proposal for a body of the same name that had already appeared in planning documents circulating within the health departments.[86]

In the event the Sainsbury Report exerted little influence on policy. Critics of the industry judged the recommendations too timid, whilst the industry itself was scathing in its criticism.[87] This was both general and specific. It criticised the report's lack of understanding and judgement, and viewed it as damaging interference by government in a very successful industry. It contested the recommendations on brand names, was opposed to any reduction in the length of patent protection, and defended its profits on the need to invest in research.

The government was disappointed with the report. The Department of Health was disappointed with the 'general wooliness in substantiating the findings about excessive profits'. The Treasury found the report 'pretty disappointing and inadequate'.[88] The report was not something that the government could implement without extensive revision. It announced that the report would 'be studied further'.[89]

Conclusion

The Sainsbury Report was to be the last attempt by government to achieve a degree of order in relationships between itself, the pharmaceutical industry and the medical profession by means of an expert committee. Just as the Thalidomide tragedy had shown that the historical incremental approach to drug regulation was totally inadequate for the task of risk management in an age of highly potent medicines, so the Sainsbury Report finally convinced government that expert committees were simply not up to the job of putting the brakes on drug expenditure.

Excessive profits were however only one dimension of what was increasingly being seen as 'a drug problem'. The tragedy of Thalidomide alerted the public not only to laxity of controls over the safety of drugs. There was also increasing awareness of the opportunities for drug misuse and addiction. Despite the increase in legal constraints the market was becoming flooded with habit-forming drugs that were outside the framework of legal prohibitions.[90] It was being recognised that the issues extended far beyond the safety and costs of prescription medicines, and encompassed a broad range of social, political and economic factors.

In this paper I have argued that, in Britain in the decades following introduction of the NHS in 1948, the relationship between the Ministry of Health, the pharmaceutical industry and the medical profession was dominated by concern over the cost of drugs, and that as a result scant regard was taken of the adequacy of the drug regulatory framework to deal with the increasingly potent and effective medicines reaching the market. I have also argued that introduction of the NHS distorted the regulatory framework, resulting in it being very different during this crucial period from that in the USA.

But it would be wrong to suggest that concern with the cost of branded drugs was restricted to Britain, with its rapidly rising expenditure on the NHS. The same arguments were taking place in the USA. There, one of the key arguments used in defence of brand names was that these were a guarantee of purity and safety. Pfizer used this argument to justify the company's patent and price maintenance arrangements before the Federal Trade Commission.

The reasons why doctors in the USA were reluctant to change their prescribing habits were no different from those of their British counterparts. The Kefauver Committee, which inquired into drug prices, spent some time asking doctors about their prescribing habits.

> To a man, they explained that they didn't have the time to look into the reputations of the various small concerns and chose to play it safe. Also, several of them pointed out that most detail men hinted darkly at the sub-standard quality of drugs put out by the small companies.[91]

In both countries the state continued to promote the use of generic over branded drugs, but it was a losing battle. The pharmaceutical companies developed other techniques to avoid direct comparison between branded and generic drugs. One of the most successful was the marketing of mixtures of two or more drugs. This gave doctors a single short brand name to remember, and ensured that the drugs concerned were premixed in the 'correct' proportions. In Britain it was again a member of the Committee of Public Accounts who questioned this tactic. When questioned about giving mixtures of generic drugs a single generic name, Sir Bruce Fraser admitted that this was outside the Ministry's control.[92]

Politics played an important part in the ineffectiveness of the Ministry of Health in dealing with the pharmaceutical companies. A Conservative government was in power between 1951 and 1964. It traditionally had a more favourable attitude to private industry than did the Labour Party. It had long accepted that any move to reform or rationalise the purchase of drugs could be seen as the thin end of the nationalisation wedge.[93] Any action taken against the industry produced an enormous backlash.

There was another reason why the Ministry's relationship with the industry was very one-sided. A significant proportion of the pharmaceutical industry was foreign-owned. It was much more difficult for the Ministry to deal with companies based in the USA and Switzerland than those in the UK. Britain was only a very small part of their global market for the product. If lower prices were offered in Britain other countries would demand the same. It was better to lose the British market than to risk a drop in the price elsewhere. For the government, it was one thing to regulate drugs; it was another thing to regulate the market.

The proposal in the UK for a Medicines Commission to act as the overall regulatory authority for medicines mirrored the creation of the Food and Drugs Administration in the USA some thirty years earlier. The legislative responses of the US and British governments to the Thalidomide tragedy were quantitatively and qualitatively different. The USA effectively tightened its existing system: it passed and implemented additional federal regulations. Despite the actions of a vigilant medical officer in preventing the marketing of Thalidomide, the FDA ultimately increased its authority over both doctors and drug companies. In Britain, on the other hand, the response was the wholesale overhaul of the entire regulatory framework.

Perhaps the most telling postscript to the Thalidomide tragedy, to the state of drug regulation in the period following introduction of the NHS, and of the government's many failed attempts to control drug expenditure during this period, is a quote from Kenneth Robinson, the then Minister of Health, who addressed the House of Commons on the issue in 1963. 'The House and the public,' he declared, 'suddenly woke up to the fact that any drug manufacturer could market any product – however inadequately tested, however dangerous – without having to satisfy any independent body as to its efficacy or safety.'[94]

Notes

1 J. Abraham, *Science, Politics and the Pharmaceutical Industry: Controversy and Bias in Drug Regulation*, New York: St Martin's Press, 1995, pp. 36–86.

2 S. White Junod and L. Marks, 'Women's trials: the approval of the first oral contraceptive pill in the United States and Great Britain', *Journal of the History of Medicine and Allied Sciences* 57(2), 2002: 117–60.

3 J. Goodman and V. Walsh, *The Story of Taxol: Nature and Politics in the Pursuit of an Ant-cancer Drug*, Cambridge: Cambridge University Press, 2001.

4 H. Edgar and D.J. Rothman, 'New rules for new drugs: the challenge of AIDS to the regulatory process', in D. Nelkin, D.P. Willis and S.V. Parris (eds), *A Disease of Society: Cultural and Institutional Responses to AIDS*, Cambridge: Cambridge University Press, 1991, pp. 84–115.

5 S.C. Anderson and V.S. Berridge, 'Drug misuse and the community pharmacist: a historical overview', in J. Sheridan and J. Strang (eds), *Drug Misuse and Community Pharmacy*, London: Taylor & Francis, 2003, pp. 17–35.

6 Abraham, *Science, Politics and the Pharmaceutical Industry*, p. 42.

7 Abraham, *Science, Politics and the Pharmaceutical Industry*, p. 45.

8 L. Marks, 'Not just a statistic: the history of USA and UK policy over thrombotic disease and the oral contraceptive pill, 1960s–1970s', *Social Science and Medicine* (Special Historical Issue), 1999: 1139–55.

9 Anderson and Berridge, 'Drug misuse and the community pharmacist', p. 20.

10 S.W.F. Holloway, *Royal Pharmaceutical Society of Great Britain 1841–1991: a Political and Social History*, London: The Pharmaceutical Press, 1991, p. 221.

11 Holloway, *Royal Pharmaceutical Society of Great Britain*, p. 180.

12 Holloway, *Royal Pharmaceutical Society of Great Britain*, p. 242.

13 I.F. Jones, 'Arsenic and the Bradford poisonings of 1858', *Pharmaceutical Journal* 265, 2000: 938–9.

14 S.C. Anderson and V.S. Berridge, 'Opium in twentieth century Britain: pharmacists, regulation and the people', *Addiction* 95(1), 2000: 23–36.

15 Holloway, *Royal Pharmaceutical Society of Great Britain*, p. 374.

16 B. Inglis, *Drugs, Doctors and Disease*, London: Mayflower-Dell, 1965, p. 116.

17 J. Liebenau, G.J. Higby and E.C. Stroud, *Pill Peddlers: Essays on the History of the Pharmaceutical Industry*, Madison, WI: American Institute of the History of Pharmacy, 1990.

18 Abraham, *Science, Politics and the Pharmaceutical Industry*, p. 53.

19 P. Bartrip, *Themselves Writ Large: the British Medical Association 1832–1966*, London: BMJ Publishing Group, 1996, p. 1.

20 Bartrip, *Themselves Writ Large*, p. 177.

21 A. Digby, *The Evolution of British General Practice 1850 to 1948*, Oxford: Clarendon Press, 1998.

22 C. Webster (ed.), *Aneurin Bevan on the National Health Service*, Oxford: University of Oxford, Wellcome Unit for the History of Medicine, 1991.

23 G.J. Higby and E.C. Stroud, *The Inside Story of Medicines: a Symposium*, Madison, WI: American Institute of the History of Pharmacy, 1997.

24 M. Weatherall, *In Search of a Cure: a History of Pharmaceutical Discovery*, Oxford: Oxford University Press, 1990.

25 M. Hodges and G.E. Appelbe, 'Control of the safety of drugs, 1868–1968 (part 1)', *The Pharmaceutical Journal* 239, 1987: 121.

26 I. Loudon and M. Drury, 'Some aspects of clinical care in general practice', in I. Loudon, J. Horder and C. Webster (eds), *General Practice under the National Health Service 1948–1997*, London: Clarendon Press, 1998, p. 100.

27 C. Webster, *The Health Services since the War, Volume I: Problems of Health Care, The National Health Service before 1957*, London: Her Majesty's Stationery Office, 1988, pp. 222–3.

28 Webster, *The Health Services since the War, Volume I*, p. 144.
29 Webster, *The Health Services since the War, Volume I*, p. 145.
30 N. Wells, *Medicines: 50 Years of Progress 1930–1980*, London: Office of Health Economics, 1980, p. 50.
31 Webster, *The Health Services since the War, Volume I*, p. 222.
32 Webster, *The Health Services since the War, Volume I*, p. 223.
33 Webster, *The Health Services since the War, Volume I*, p. 223.
34 Webster, *The Health Services since the War, Volume I*, p. 224.
35 Webster, *The Health Services since the War, Volume I*, p. 204
36 *Report of the Committee of Enquiry into the Cost of the National Health Service*, Command 9663, London: Her Majesty's Stationery Office, 1956, p. 725 (the Guillebaud Report).
37 Webster, *The Health Services since the War, Volume I*, p. 205.
38 Webster, *The Health Services since the War, Volume I*, p. 210.
39 Webster, *The Health Services since the War, Volume I*, p. 224.
40 *Report of the Joint Committee on Prescribing on Form EC10*, London: Her Majesty's Stationery Office, 1954.
41 Webster, The Health Services since the War, Volume I, p. 226.
42 *The Pharmaceutical Price Regulation Scheme*, 2002, London: The Department of Health.
43 C. Webster, *The Health Services since the War, Volume II: Government and Health Care, the National Health Service 1958–1979*, London: Her Majesty's Stationery Office, 1996, appendix 3.19, p. 809.
44 Webster, *The Health Services since the War, Volume II*, p. 143.
45 Webster, *The Health Services since the War, Volume II*, p. 144.
46 *Report of the Scottish Committee on Prescribing Costs*, Edinburgh: Her Majesty's Stationery Office, 1959 (the Douglas Report).
47 *Final Report of the Committee on the Cost of Prescribing*, London: Her Majesty's Stationery Office, 1959 (the Hinchcliffe Report).
48 Webster, *The Health Services since the War, Volume II*, p. 145.
49 Inglis, *Drugs, Doctors and Disease*, p. 191.
50 Inglis, *Drugs, Doctors and Disease*, p. 194.
51 Inglis, *Drugs, Doctors and Disease*, p. 195.
52 Holloway, *Royal Pharmaceutical Society of Great Britain*, p. 343.
53 H.W. Fowler, *Aids to Forensic Pharmacy*, 5th edn, London: Bailliere, Tindall & Cox, 1960, pp. 146–56.
54 Fowler, *Aids to Forensic Pharmacy*, pp. 173–9.
55 J.R. Dale and G.E. Appelbe, *Pharmacy Law and Ethics*, 3rd edn, London: The Pharmaceutical Press, 1983, pp. 175–6.
56 W. Gainsford, 'Associations of achrodynia', *Practitioner* 163, 1949: 282.
57 G. Discombe, 'Drug idiosyncrasies', *British Medical Journal* 1, 1952: 1270.
58 W. McBride, 'Thalidomide and congenital abnormalities', *Lancet*, 1961: 1358.
59 A. Daemmrich, 'A tale of two experts: Thalidomide and political engagement in the United States and West Germany', *Social History of Medicine* 15(1), 2002: 137–58.
60 W. Lenz, 'Thalidomide and congenital abnormalities', *Lancet*, 1962, p. 45.
61 M.L. Burstall and B.G. Reuben, *Critics of the Pharmaceutical Industry*, London: REMIT Consultants Ltd, 1990, pp. 20–4.
62 T. Mahoney, *The Merchants of Life*, New York: Harper & Brothers, 1959; L. Lasagna, *The Doctors' Dilemmas*, New York: Harper & Brothers, 1962.
63 M. Hodges and G.E. Appelbe, 'Control of the safety of drugs, 1868–1968 (part 2)', *The Pharmaceutical Journal* 239, 1987: 151.
64 Abraham, *Science, Politics and the Pharmaceutical Industry*, p. 45.
65 M. Hodges and G.E. Appelbe, 'Control of the safety of drugs, 1868–1968 (part 2)', p. 152.

66 M. Hodges and G.E. Appelbe, 'Control of the safety of drugs, 1868–1968 (part 2)', p. 152.
67 M. Hodges and G.E. Appelbe, 'Control of the safety of drugs, 1868–1968 (part 2)', p. 152.
68 'Classification of Proprietary Preparations', *Report of the Standing Joint Committee*, London: Her Majesty's Stationery Office, 1965.
69 Webster, *The Health Services since the War, Volume II*, p. 216.
70 'Safety of Drugs', *Final Report of the Joint Subcommittee of the Standing Medical Advisory Committees*, London: Her Majesty's Stationery Office (the Cohen Report), 1963.
71 Abraham, *Science, Politics and the Pharmaceutical Industry*, p. 57.
72 Webster, *The Health Services since the War, Volume II*, p. 216.
73 Committee on Safety of Drugs, *Report for the Year Ended 31 December 1965*, London: Her Majesty's Stationery Office, 1967.
74 M. Hodges and G.E. Appelbe, 'Control of the safety of drugs, 1868–1968 (part 2)', p. 153.
75 *Forthcoming Legislation on the Safety, Quality and Description of Drugs and Medicines*, Command 3395, London: Her Majesty's Stationery Office, 1967.
76 Webster, *The Health Services since the War, Volume II*, p. 223.
77 Dale and Appelbe, *Pharmacy Law and Ethics*, pp. 123–46.
78 R.J. Harman, 'The structure and functions of the Medicines Control Agency', *The Pharmaceutical Journal* 269, 2002: 574–8.
79 K. Holland, 'The Medicines Control Agency', *The Pharmaceutical Journal* 258, 1997: 28–31.
80 *Final Report of the Committee on the Cost of Prescribing*, London: Her Majesty's Stationery Office, 1959 (the Hinchcliffe Report).
81 Webster, *The Health Services since the War, Volume II*, p. 148.
82 Webster, *The Health Services since the War, Volume II*, p. 149.
83 *Report of the Committee of Enquiry into the Relationship of the Pharmaceutical Industry with the National Health Service 1965–1967*, Command 3410, London: Her Majesty's Stationery Office, 1967 (the Sainsbury Report).
84 Abraham, *Science, Politics and the Pharmaceutical Industry*, p. 69.
85 *Report of the Committee of Enquiry into the Relationship of the Pharmaceutical Industry with the National Health Service 1965–1967*, p. 329.
86 Webster, *The Health Services since the War, Volume II*, p. 219.
87 Webster, *The Health Services since the War, Volume II*, p. 222.
88 Webster, *The Health Services since the War, Volume II*, p. 220.
89 Webster, *The Health Services since the War, Volume II*, p. 220.
90 Abraham, *Science, Politics and the Pharmaceutical Industry*, p. 56.
91 'Administered Prices: Drugs', *Report of the Committee on the Judiciary*, US Senate, Made by Its Sub-committee on Anti-trust and Monopoly, Washington, 1961 (the Kefauver Committee).
92 Committee of Public Accounts Report 1962/63, cited in Inglis, *Drugs, Doctors and Disease*, p. 197.
93 Hansard, 26 February 1963, cited in Inglis, *Drugs, Doctors and Disease*, p. 198.
94 Hansard, 8 May 1963, cited in Inglis, *Drugs, Doctors and Disease*, p. 199.

Recommended further reading

J. Abraham, *Science, Politics and the Pharmaceutical Industry: Controversy and Bias in Drug Regulation*, New York: St Martin's Press, 1995.
S.C. Anderson and V.S. Berridge, 'Opium in twentieth century Britain: pharmacists, regulation and the people', *Addiction* 95(1), 2000: 23–36.

S.W.F. Holloway, *Royal Pharmaceutical Society of Great Britain 1841–1991: a Political and Social History*, London: The Pharmaceutical Press, 1991.

J. Liebenau, G.J. Higby and E.C. Stroud, *Pill Peddlers: Essays on the History of the Pharmaceutical Industry*, Madison, WI: American Institute of the History of Pharmacy, 1990.

M. Weatherall, *In Search of a Cure: a History of Pharmaceutical Discovery*, Oxford: Oxford University Press, 1990.

Part IV

Changing models and different national styles

9 Cleansing the air and promoting health

The politics of pollution in postwar Britain

Mark Jackson

Introduction

In April 1956, Anthony Eden's Conservative government successfully steered the Clean Air Bill through its third reading in the Commons. The resultant Clean Air Act, which received the Royal Assent in July that year, introduced a number of measures designed to substantially reduce urban air pollution in Britain: the Act encouraged the creation of 'smoke control areas' by local authorities, established the Clean Air Council responsible for monitoring and regulating levels of air pollution, and created a tariff of financial penalties for non-compliance with local and national standards of air purity.[1] Although not the first legislation to tackle the growing problems of urban air pollution, the 1956 Act contained two novel features: first, it aimed to control domestic, as well as industrial, smoke production; and, second, the Act enforced compliance with predetermined standards of air quality and smoke production rather than relying on a plaintiff to demonstrate that smoke was causing a nuisance, as previous legislation had done. As a result, the 1956 Clean Air Act constituted a significant milestone in the evolution of modern clean air and environmental policies in Britain.

At one level, the Clean Air Act can be seen as the outcome of a relatively simple sequence of events. In December 1952, a deep smog settled over London bringing the capital to a standstill and causing the death of several thousand people from respiratory and cardiac diseases. This calamity precipitated a national panic, in the wake of which the government set up a Committee on Air Pollution (the Beaver Committee) to consider the social, economic and medical effects of pollution and to make recommendations for improvements based on expert advice. This process of careful scientific review of the evidence generated the policy initiatives enacted in the Clean Air Act of 1956.[2]

There is clearly some truth in this focused narrative. The 'great smog' of 1952 undoubtedly served as a catalyst for reform and the recommendations of the Beaver Committee provided the blueprint for subsequent legislation. However, the story is immediately more complicated. A deeper analysis of the political, socio-economic, medical and cultural contexts in which clean air policies were formulated is required to explain, for example, why a national policy became possible only in the 1950s even though both the links between air pollution and respiratory disease and death and the economic cost of pollution had been recognised by clinicians and politicians alike since the late nineteenth century. In addition, it is unclear from brief historical surveys of air pollution control precisely how concerns about health, environmental protection and economic constraints combined to frame either the recommendations of the Beaver Committee or subsequent legislative responses to air pollution.

In spite of several more recent broad surveys of the 1952 smog and its aftermath,[3] Roy Parker's exemplary study of the 'struggle for clean air', published in 1975, and Eric Ashby and Mary Anderson's account of the 'politics of clean air', published in 1981, remain the most insightful analyses of the social and political context in which a national clean air policy was formulated.[4] However, while these studies provide comprehensive coverage of the political background to the introduction of new policies, they do not closely address the manner in which debates about air pollution control in postwar Britain were shaped by, and in turn served to mould, modern concerns about the impact of the environment on public health. The aim of this chapter, therefore, is to explore events surrounding the London smog of 1952 from this perspective, focusing in particular on debates about the relation between atmospheric pollution and health, and on the processes and politics of health policy formation. The first section briefly surveys the perceived problems of, and responses to, rising levels of air pollution before 1952. The second section explores events during and after the smog of 1952, examining in detail the major concerns, particularly about the impact of smog on respiratory health, expressed by the Beaver Committee, Members of Parliament and the press. The third section of the chapter examines more closely the context in which such concerns were effectively converted into an innovative policy that combined contemporary economic pressures with shifting medical and environmental imperatives. In the final main section, I shall argue that, by fusing public health and environmental concerns, the Clean Air Act of 1956 constituted an early form of modern environmentalism, one that both anticipated and informed the ecological and environmental turn in public health discourse that emerged in the late twentieth century.

Air pollution and its control in the nineteenth and early twentieth centuries

Although the economic and medical problems associated with excessive smoke production had been regularly discussed since the seventeenth century (and indeed sporadically for much longer),[5] it was only during the Industrial Revolution of the late eighteenth and early nineteenth centuries that urban smoke was identified as a major and spreading problem. Industrial expansion and urbanisation led to the increased consumption of coal and a rapidly rising production of smoke, particularly in London and large provincial industrial centres such as Manchester.[6] Significantly, the problem was a consequence not only of greater industrial productivity but also of rising domestic fuel consumption in this period.

During the middle decades of the nineteenth century, doctors and politicians expressed growing concerns about the impact of atmospheric smoke on health. As Bill Luckin has shown in a number of seminal articles on air pollution in the late nineteenth and early twentieth centuries, the reports of the Registrar-General regularly attributed the excess deaths in the capital from bronchitis, asthma, pneumonia and whooping cough to a combination of London fog and pollution.[7] In addition, writers around the turn of the nineteenth century noted, and pursued research into, the impact of diminished sunlight on health.[8] These concerns persisted into the early decades of the twentieth century, underwriting contemporary interest in open-air colonies for tuberculosis and open-air schools for children with tuberculosis, bronchitis and asthma,[9] and fuelling the fashion for taking holidays in coastal 'respiratory resorts', where the air was supposedly cleaner and more invigorating than the polluted urban atmosphere.[10] Of course, open-air colonies and schools offered patients with respiratory disorders much more than merely cleaner air; improvements in health were also attributed to better diets, physical exercise and removal from the pressures and stresses of home. Nevertheless, the promotion of clean air as both preventative and therapeutic testifies to contemporary concerns about the impact of urban air pollution on public health.

During the late nineteenth and early twentieth centuries, anxieties about the economic and medical repercussions of rising levels of air pollution stimulated tentative legislation, government inquiries and the formation of pressure groups advocating greater state intervention. In the 1840s, advocates of smoke abatement (such as W.A. Mackinnon) had attempted unsuccessfully either to introduce specific bills aimed at reducing smoke pollution or to incorporate smoke abatement clauses in other legislation such as the Public Health Bill in 1846. Several years later, however, a smoke clause was included in the City of London Sewers Act 1851 and the Smoke Nuisance Abatement (Metropolis) Act was passed in 1853. Following renewed pressure from leading public health experts, such as John Simon, Medical Officer of Health for the City of London, legislation designed to control the emission of gases from the alkali industry was passed in 1863 and clauses aimed at reducing smoke production were included in the Sanitary Acts of 1858 and 1866, and in the Public Health Act of 1875.[11]

In general, these early legislative provisions, and the subsequent Public Health (Smoke Abatement) Act of 1926, proved ineffectual, hampered both by magistrates' reluctance to impose fines on local industries and by the absence of any reliable information about the levels and effects of air pollution. During the early years of the twentieth century, the government attempted to remedy this latter problem. After occasional sporadic investigations into the levels of impurities in the air and into the relationship between smoke particles and mortality rates, an Advisory Committee on Atmospheric Pollution was established in 1912 as the result of a meeting of municipal authorities and local smoke abatement societies at an international smoke abatement conference and exhibition held in London that year. In the 1920s, the Committee's responsibilities for monitoring levels of air pollution and for co-ordinating local investigations were taken over by the Department of Scientific and Industrial Research.[12]

Both legislative measures relating to smoke abatement and government interest in air pollution were driven largely by the endeavours of local activists and smoke abatement societies. Local societies promoting cleaner air and agitating for a reduction in smoke pollution had been established in the late nineteenth century in Manchester (the Noxious Vapours Abatement Association, known after 1910 as the Smoke Abatement League) and London (initially the Smoke Abatement Committee, later the Coal Smoke Abatement Society). In 1929 the two societies merged to form the National Smoke Abatement Society (later the National Society for Clean Air), which was originally based in Manchester but which relocated to London in 1937.[13] These societies had continuously campaigned for the establishment of 'smokeless zones' (the first of which was officially created in Manchester in 1946), for more rigorous enforcement of smoke abatement laws, for greater regulation and monitoring of heating appliances, and for greater government intervention. Aware that their efforts were often defeated by public apathy, members of the Society continued to exert pressure on successive governments, waiting for a propitious moment to achieve their ends. As one of the delegates at the Society's Annual Conference noted in 1949:

> To educate these authorities and the lukewarm mass of the general public entails a very long-term policy of snail-like progress. Few reforms have come about by waiting for public opinion to express its approval; indeed, many benefits enjoyed by mankind today have been brought about in spite of adverse public opinion and opposition....The Society could be more militant in its policy, and even though the present time may not be favourable for action on these lines, preparation could proceed so as to be ready immediately the situation is ripe for positive action.[14]

Although, as it happened, advocates of cleaner air did not have to wait long for public opinion to shift in their direction, in the decades prior to the 1950s, legislation, government inquiries and local activism made little overall impact on levels of smoke production, and did not promote the formation of a national clean air policy. The reasons for this are multiple. In the first instance, central government and local authorities were reluctant to interfere with, and possibly limit, industrial interests, preferring to operate a *laissez-faire* approach to the regulation and restriction of fuel consumption and smoke production.[15] Second, although there was growing concern about the impact of pollution on health, the evidence was equivocal. Indeed, according to many commentators, soot possessed bactericidal properties that served to 'disinfect the urban atmosphere' and boost immunity to infectious diseases.[16] Sufferers from non-infectious respiratory diseases, such as asthma, were sometimes also thought to benefit from the atmospheric conditions in London.[17]

Smoke also carried ideological connotations that effectively thwarted attempts to remove it completely from the urban scene. As Mosley has pointed out in his incisive survey of smoke pollution in Victorian and Edwardian Manchester, 'a factory chimney and, for that matter, a domestic chimney belching out black smoke symbolised the creation of wealth and personal well-being'. As an inevitable consequence of industrial productivity, smoke thus constituted 'a barometer of economic success and social progress', an image that was not only utilised by politicians during the 1930s to portray the National Government as one of prosperity, but which was also mobilised in popular songs and poems, a process that in turn served to 'naturalise and rationalise the relationship between wealth and air pollution'.[18] From a domestic perspective, smoke also signified wealth and comfort. The open coal fire and hearth had become a central British institution (where friends met and hearts were warmed),[19] and an 'extravagantly smoking chimney pot visibly demonstrated to onlookers that a family was doing well economically'.[20] As a result, attempts to limit smoke production, by changing from burning coal to smokeless coke for example, were resisted as vigorously by the public as by industrial manufacturers and politicians.

It may also be the case that deaths from pollution had become too frequent to attract public and political attention. In 1947, in his book on the problems of coal in the atmosphere, Arnold Marsh, honorary secretary to the National Smoke Abatement Society, issued a warning along these lines:

> Because death in this way has become a commonplace in industrial Britain it has ceased to excite any comment or cause any alarm, whereas if a period of hitherto harmless fog suddenly caused such results there would be a sensation of the first order, with great newspaper headlines, questions in the House, a call for drastic action, and so on.[21]

Marsh's comments proved prescient. In postwar Britain, not only did an unexpected air pollution episode dramatically increase the mortality rate in London and indeed raise public alarm, but the ideological and economic props tacitly condoning pollution of the atmosphere also began to crumble. In the years following the Second World War, smoke production increased as both industrial and domestic consumption of cheap coal rose in the wake of economic expansion, contributing to the atmospheric conditions that produced the 'great smog' in 1952. At the same time, the scientific links between cleansing the air and promoting health had been clearly demonstrated by the increased mortality associated with occasional air pollution episodes such as those in the Meuse Valley in Belgium in 1930, in Donora, Pennsylvania, in 1948, and indeed in various London smogs during the 1930s and 1940s.[22] Such episodes served to undermine ideological attachments to smoke and to foster the opinion that controlling air pollution constituted a major step towards promoting public health. As Marsh pointed out in 1947, 'any local or national policy to raise the general level of health must, if it is fully to achieve its objective, include measures that will restore to our towns that primary and fundamental element of healthy life: clean air'.[23]

The great smog and its aftermath

During the 1930s and 1940s, a combination of climatic conditions and pollution had periodically generated dense 'smogs' (a term first coined in Britain in 1905 to describe the combination of smoke and fog) with a concomitant rise in morbidity and mortality from respiratory and cardiac diseases.[24] However, between 5 and 9 December 1952, a thermal inversion trapped a particularly deep and impenetrable layer of smog over London. As visibility decreased dramatically, transport in the capital became virtually impossible and accidents multiplied. In addition, both hospital admissions and mortality rates rose sharply, with most patients admitted for (and dying from) heart and respiratory problems.[25] The situation prompted extensive public alarm, and newspaper editorials and correspondence and speakers in parliament argued vehemently for an immediate government inquiry and more effective legislation before another severe winter smog plunged the country into further turmoil.[26] Although the government attempted to delay intervention, claiming that there were more pressing priorities (such as the growing housing crisis),[27] a Committee on Air Pollution was eventually appointed in July 1953, partly as a public relations exercise in response to mounting public pressure.[28]

The Committee was chaired by Sir Hugh Beaver (1890–1967), a prominent chemical engineer who at that time was Managing Director of Arthur Guinness, Son & Co. Ltd, chairman of the British Institute of Management, and Director of the Colonial Development Corporation.[29] Beaver, who became a frequent advocate of the campaign for clear air,[30] was joined on the Committee by two doctors, both of whom worked in the field of public health,[31] and a range of scientists, a housing manager from Rotherham, an economist from Cambridge, and the Director of the Meteorological Office. Recognising the value of previous work both by public authorities and by the National Smoke Abatement Society, the Committee's remit was to 'examine the nature, causes and effects of air pollution and the efficacy of present preventive measures; and to consider what further preventive measures are practicable; and to make recommendations'.[32] Although it reviewed information from a variety of sources and drew on its own expertise, the Committee took little formal evidence, an approach that facilitated the rapid production of an *Interim Report* in December 1953 and a final *Report* in November 1954.[33]

The *Interim Report* came to a number of conclusions about the impact of the smog on health. First, it acknowledged that the smog had been 'accompanied by an immediate and sudden rise in both illness and mortality', and that approximately 4,000 people had died as a result of the smog during the first three weeks of December 1952.[34] In addition, it presented evidence demonstrating that at the height of the smog deaths from bronchitis had increased nine-fold, deaths from pneumonia four-fold, and deaths from other respiratory diseases in the region of five to six-fold,[35] figures which suggested that the smog in 1952 was far more severe than previous episodes.[36] Illness rates, measured by hospital admissions, also increased dramatically for patients with respiratory and heart diseases.[37] Although the Committee expressed some reservations about accurately identifying the precise pollutants responsible for increased morbidity and mortality, and stressed the need for further research, the *Interim Report* suggested that there was a 'clear correlation between the pollution by smoke and sulphur dioxide, and the daily death rate in Greater London at that time'.[38] Arguing that pollution not only contaminated the air that people breathed but also 'deprives them of sunlight and makes their surroundings dirty and dark', the *Report* identified urban air pollution as 'one of the most urgent problems today in the field of environmental hygiene'.[39]

In addition to addressing the immediate impact of the 'great smog' on health, the *Interim Report* also considered the on-going economic burden of air pollution. The direct costs of smoke in the atmosphere included bills for cleaning, repairing and renewing 'soiled or damaged buildings, materials, clothing and other articles'. Indirect expenses included 'the cost of damage to health and its consequences, the extra cost of artificial lighting due to the reduction of daylight, and the loss of efficiency of all forms of transport in town "smogs"', as well as the waste of fuel through incomplete combustion.[40] Estimating that the total economic losses incurred by continuing atmospheric pollution were in the region of £100–150 million per year, the *Report* concluded that 'the expenditure of many millions of pounds a year in eliminating smoke would be a most profitable national investment'.[41]

The Committee's full *Report*, published just under a year later in November 1954, added little to the analysis presented in the *Interim Report*, except to provide evidence accentuating concerns about atmospheric pollution and public health. In relation to the impact of air pollution on respiratory health, for example, the full *Report* pointed out that the death rate from bronchitis in Britain was fifty times higher than the death rate in Denmark and that mortality rates from pneumonia and bronchitis were far higher in urban than in rural areas. Although the urban–rural gradient was less marked for other respiratory diseases, and although the Committee acknowledged that factors other than air pollution (climate or housing, for example) contributed to these comparative figures, the *Report* concluded that there was 'a clear association between pollution and the incidence of bronchitis and other respiratory diseases', and stressed the need for urgent remedial action.[42]

The work of the Beaver Committee was not the only formal investigation into air pollution and health following the smog. In 1953, the Medical Research Council (MRC) formed a subcommittee of its Social and Environmental Health Committee to study the composition and clinical effects of atmospheric pollution, and subsequently established research units at St Bartholomew's Hospital in London and at the University of Sheffield.[43] And in 1954, the Ministry of Health published a report summarizing the health consequences of the 1952 smog.[44] Nevertheless, it was the publication of the final *Report* of the Beaver Committee that prompted extensive media and parliamentary agitation for legislative intervention. The first concrete sign of parliamentary attention to the problem came on 15 December 1954 (almost exactly two years after the great smog) when Gerald Nabarro, Conservative MP for Kidderminster, introduced a Private Member's Bill ostensibly aimed at 'securing in all connections the abatement of atmospheric pollution and smoke',[45] but also with the purpose of stimulating government action. Nabarro's bill was read a second time in February 1955 but withdrawn once Duncan Sandys, the Minister of Housing and Local Government, promised to draft a more comprehensive government bill.[46] The government's Clean Air Bill was introduced later that year, committed, read a third time in April the following year, and became law in July 1956.

The Clean Air Bill was warmly received in principle by all parties. As Duncan Sandys asserted during the second reading of the government bill, most Members of Parliament were united in their 'determination to eradicate what is a great social and economic evil; what is a menace to the health of our people and a source of disgraceful waste and destruction'.[47] Sandys's belief that air pollution legislation attracted support from all parties is sustained by other evidence. In 1955, during the run up to the General Election, the Conservative Manifesto accepted the need for a national clean air policy and promised that 'comprehensive legislation on smoke abatement' would be introduced.[48] Although speakers at the annual Labour Party conference held in Margate later the same year criticised the government bill for being 'hopelessly inadequate, as you would expect of Tory legislation', they nevertheless supported a resolution that 'the policy of the next Labour Government shall include the provision of an Act of Parliament to end all air pollutents [*sic*] which are injurious to the health and economy of the nation'.[49]

Sandys's emphasis on the bill's significance from a public health perspective was also echoed regularly elsewhere in the debates. According to Dr Barnett Stross, a doctor and MP for Stoke-on-Trent Central, for example, the bill constituted an important and exciting 'piece of preventive medicine' designed to combat 'misery and death, to say nothing of squalor and disease'.[50] There was also an apparent consensus, expressed most forcibly by MPs from heavily industrialised areas (such as the Black Country, Warrington, Sheffield and Newcastle) that air pollution was a particularly potent cause of morbidity and mortality from respiratory diseases such as bronchitis, pneumonia and asthma. During the debate on Nabarro's bill in 1955, for example, Arthur Blenkinsop (a Labour MP for Newcastle-upon-Tyne East who had served as Parliamentary Secretary at the Ministry of Health between 1949 and 1951, and who was a junior shadow health minister throughout the 1950s) made particular reference to the health aspects of the bill, pointing out that, although it is 'difficult to get accurate and detailed facts about the relationship between air pollution and health, it is true that there is close link between bronchitis and other chest complaints and air pollution'.[51] In later debates on the government bill, Blenkinsop's opinions were supported by other MPs eager to provide evidence of the particular health and pollution problems faced by their own constituencies. Having stressed the high incidence of bronchitis in Warrington, Dr Edith Summerskill (Labour MP for that town and a Labour spokesperson on health) insisted that, although bronchitis could appear anywhere, 'an individual who is exposed to a smoky atmosphere might well develop it whereas he might be free if he lived in a smokeless atmosphere'.[52] John Leavey, Conservative MP for Heywood and Royton, similarly highlighted the significant problems experienced in industrial parts of Lancashire:

> For many years in that part of the country we have suffered from the disagreeable effects of air pollution. Indeed in company with many other industrial parts of the country we have suffered from air pollution since the Industrial Revolution. It is a district where the incidence of bronchial disease is very high, and although air pollution is, perhaps, only a contributory factor, I am sure that medical opinion would support the view that it is a serious menace to health.[53]

However, in spite of evident agreement on the public health impact of the proposed legislation, and indeed of the urgency of remedial action, there were several aspects of the legislative measures (and particularly the evident limitations of the legislation) that stimulated considerable debate. Although Members of Parliament were anxious in principle to reduce the economic burden of air pollution, for example, they also recognised the importance of appeasing the financial concerns of industrial manufacturers, who would be responsible in large part for introducing and financing smoke reduction measures and who would be vulnerable to fines for defying clean air regulations. Along the same lines, contributors to the debates were undecided about the relative significance of controlling industrial over domestic smoke production. In addition, speakers debated the relative merits of local and central authority responsibility for monitoring air pollution and imposing fines, opting eventually for a mixed system in which standards were set by a central Clean Air Council but in which smokeless control areas (rather than smokeless zones)[54] were to be introduced and supervised by local authorities.

Doubts were also expressed about the legislative preoccupations with visible smoke rather than other less perceptible pollutants, such as sulphur dioxide, diesel particulates, carbon monoxide and other fumes. In 1955, during the debate on Nabarro's bill, for example, Ronald Bell, Conservative MP for Buckinghamshire South, reminded his colleagues in the Commons not to forget

> the pollution of the atmosphere from road traffic. Diesel fumes and carbon monoxide of the ordinary motor car exhaust reach a fantastic concentration in certain atmospheric conditions in streets in central London. There is nothing more damaging to the general health and vitality of the human being than a consistent breathing of a fair concentration of carbon monoxide in the air.[55]

Although such concerns about rising pollution from motor vehicles had also been voiced by the Beaver Committee, they failed to be accommodated in the new legislation. Echoing Bell's concerns about invisible pollutants, Somerville Hastings (a Labour MP for Barking, a doctor and a prominent figure in the Socialist Medical Association) quoted leaders in the *British Medical Journal* and the *Lancet* to support his view (and indeed to some extent that of the Beaver Committee) that it was 'the sulphur oxides which do the harm' and that smoke was important largely because 'sulphur dioxide on particles of smoke be more easily oxidised into sulphur trioxide and formed into sulphuric acid'.[56]

In spite of reservations about the failure of either Nabarro's bill or the government bill to tackle these issues with sufficient clarity and force, the Clean Air Bill was read for the third time in April 1956 and passed. The Clean Air Act, which became law in July that year, contained a number of innovative features. The act prohibited the emission of 'dark smoke' from chimneys, required that new furnaces should be as smokeless as possible and emit only minimal grit and dust, and set down regulations for the erection of new chimneys carrying smoke, grit, dust and gases. It also granted local authorities the power to declare certain districts 'smoke control areas', to contribute to the expense of adapting industrial furnaces and domestic hearths in such areas (subsidised by funds from central government), and to penalise the occupiers of any building that emitted smoke within a smoke control area.[57] The prevention of pollution in England and Wales, and progress in abating air pollution under the terms of the act, were to be monitored by a Clean Air Council, chaired by the Minister of Housing and Local Government. By setting predetermined standards of air purity and by authorising the punishment of domestic as well as industrial smoke producers, the Clean Air Act constituted a significant milestone in the evolution of environmental, and indeed public health, policies in Britain. As an article in the *Chest and Heart Bulletin* commented in 1963, the Clean Air Act 1956 may well have been 'the only good result' that emerged from the 'calamity' of the great smog in the winter of 1952.[58]

The regulatory politics of pollution

Death and disease during the great smog and the subsequent recommendations of the Beaver Committee to minimise atmospheric pollution undoubtedly proved the catalyst for the formation of a national clean air policy. However, the emergence of a national policy in 1956 was not simply the product of unequivocally humanitarian concerns about the impact of air pollution on morbidity and mortality rates. Successive governments had suspected a close relationship between air pollution and respiratory diseases since the mid-nineteenth century without attempting to remedy the problems in a comprehensive manner. The key to understanding the formulation of new policies lies instead in the particular constellation of political, medical, socio-economic and cultural factors that combined to form the context in which a national policy became possible in postwar Britain.

Although public health issues certainly figured fairly strongly in the Beaver Committee reports and in parliamentary debates, both Members of Parliament and the Committee also spent considerable time and effort gauging the socio-economic impact of air pollution. Indeed, when illness and death were discussed, they were often framed in economic terms, that is in terms of 'national loss'. As the Committee's full *Report* explained in 1954:

> But we are confident that our proposals, if carried out, will secure happier and more healthy living conditions for millions of people, and that on all accounts the cost of the cure will be far less than the national loss in allowing the evil to continue.[59]

Greater morbidity and mortality from pollution drained the domestic economy in a number of ways: demand for hospital beds; drug treatments; doctors' time; the loss of human efficiency; days away from work; and increasing National Insurance claims after the smog.[60] For most commentators on the perils of air pollution, a greater economy was to be achieved by investing in controlling pollution and, thereby, promoting health and efficiency.

The economic argument was persuasive. Although Anthony Eden's Conservative Party had been returned with an increased majority (of sixty) in the general election in May 1955, partly as a result of economic growth, the government remained anxious about the state of the domestic economy and about the cost of rearmament following the Korean War (1950–3), and ironically continued to contribute to the problems of pollution by generating funds by selling high-quality coal abroad and leaving low-quality coal for domestic consumption. More particularly, however, the government was concerned about the rapidly escalating cost of the National Health Service, a problem that had been only partially offset by the introduction of prescription charges.[61] In addition to being seen as a humane response to a specific human catastrophe, the emergence of a national clean air policy in 1956 should therefore also be regarded as a measured response to these political and economic contingencies.

Legislation should also be seen against a backdrop of rising medical interest in the environmental determinants of respiratory diseases, driven by growing concerns about the role of smoking in the aetiology of bronchitis and about rising asthma mortality, but more notably of course by the link elaborated in the early 1950s between smoking and lung cancer. However, it would be a mistake to assume that there was a clear consensus about the impact of pollution on respiratory health during this period. In the first instance, as Roy Parker has suggested, 'there was no cohesive and well-developed medical interest group concerned primarily with the consequences of atmospheric pollution' at the time of the smog.[62] More particularly, although the Beaver Committee and Members of Parliament appeared convinced of the role of air pollution in the pathogenesis of bronchitis, pneumonia, asthma and cancer, the evidence was equivocal and contested by some commentators throughout the 1950s, 1960s and 1970s. In debates on Nabarro's bill in 1955, for example, Michael Higgs (a lawyer and Conservative MP for Bromsgrove who retired at the 1955 general election) pointed to flaws in the Beaver Committee's arguments about the impact of urban pollution:

> In the section which deals with the effect of atmospheric pollution upon health, a conclusion is drawn that pollution has a considerable effect in causing bronchial diseases, pneumonia, and similar diseases. When we study it, we find the main fact which leads to that conclusion is that more people who live in towns suffer or die from those diseases than people who live in the country....There are many reasons why people who live in towns might get diseases of that kind more than their cousins in the country. It may be because they spend more time indoors and get less fresh air, or take less exercise and use their lungs less, or it may be because those in the towns see less of the sun. I am even naughty enough to suspect that it is because they suffer more from central heating and electric fires, which do not promote ventilation as the good old-fashioned open fire does. It is a very big jump from the fact that more people die in towns than in the country to the assumption that it may be due to smoke; it may be petrol fumes.[63]

Over the following decade or so, Higgs's concerns were taken up enthusiastically by scientists, epidemiologists and clinicians in a spate of surveys, symposia and publications exploring both the nature of the link between atmospheric pollution and health, and the efficacy of implementing the Clean Air Act, a development that provides a clear example of the manner in which policy can generate research rather than *vice versa*. In 1964, for example, the problems of precisely identifying the aetiology of respiratory diseases formed the focus of many contributions to a Royal Society of Medicine symposium on the medical and epidemiological aspects of air pollution. While contributors acknowledged the possible link between the social environment and exacerbation of respiratory diseases, they were more concerned with the relationship between smoking and health, and repeatedly stressed the difficulties of establishing with any certainty the role of air pollution in bronchitis, asthma or pneumonia, pointing instead (like the Beaver Committee a decade earlier) to the need for further studies.[64] The continuing equivocacy of experts on this issue and the growing interest in cigarette smoking as harmful were neatly summed up by Dr Ian Gregg, a general practitioner and senior lecturer at the Brompton Hospital in London, speaking at a symposium on the environment and the respiratory system chaired by Richard Doll in 1970. Although he insisted that the eradication of air pollution constituted 'an urgent public health measure', Gregg emphasised the responsibility of individuals to reduce their risk of respiratory disease by giving up smoking and outlined the evidential problems facing epidemiologists:

> The importance of this low-grade, insidious pollution of the atmosphere as a cause of respiratory disease is very difficult to assess. It is important to note that while there is a good prima facie case for incriminating air pollution as one factor in the pathogenesis of chronic bronchitis, the evidence upon which it is based is entirely circumstantial.[65]

While clinicians and epidemiologists continued to express doubts about the precise role of air pollution in determining disease, in the wake of 1952 the public and the media were unimpressed by what was regarded as official apathy. From the public's perspective, the facts spoke for themselves: thousands of Londoners had suffered and died during and after the great smog, which was itself becoming a potent popular image symbolising the perils of pollution. Accordingly, there was intense media and public activism for legislative intervention, evident in the columns and correspondence of the daily newspapers, the publications of the National Smoke Abatement Society, and indeed the general medical press,[66] and creeping into and influencing parliamentary debates. In May 1953, when Norman Dodds (Labour MP for Dartford and a publicity manager by profession) challenged the government to expedite an inquiry into events during the preceding winter (which he later referred to evocatively as the 'December massacre'),[67] he contrasted the 'apathy of the Government' with the interest shown both by the public and by the national press, quoting liberally from the *Evening Standard*, the *Daily Sketch* and the *Star*, applauding the 'grand job of work' done by the National Smoke Abatement Society, and citing correspondence from his constituents and his observations of respiratory problems amongst the general public while he was out canvassing for the imminent local elections.[68] In response to Dodds's arguments, Ernest Marples, parliamentary secretary to the Ministry of Housing and Local Government, disputed Dodds's diagnosis of the cause of death during the great smog, and challenged the need to satisfy the *Star* rather than the public and parliament.[69] Nevertheless, it may well have been persistent pressure from Dodds and his associates in parliament, supported as Roy Parker has suggested by public and media demands, that prompted the government to set up the Beaver Committee later that year.[70] It may also have been a desire to appease public concerns that prompted both the Beaver Committee and the legislature to focus in the first instance on reducing smoke, that is a visible form of pollution, rather than on tackling other, less visible, pollutants such as carbon monoxide and sulphur dioxide that excited less attention.[71]

The vivid involvement of the media in provoking public and parliamentary debate is not surprising. It was during the 1950s and 1960s that producers of both print and visual media began to develop a stronger interest in medical topics and themes, creating films and television programmes (such as *Your Life in Their Hands*, first screened in 1958), and running leading articles and editorials on health-related issues.[72] In addition, the medical press at this time was becoming increasingly active in health education, for example advertising the link between smoking and health during the 1950s. While media portrayals of health matters and medicine were designed primarily to be educational and, in the case of television, entertaining, they may well also in this instance have contributed to the public pressure that eventually precipitated a government inquiry and legislation.

The creation of a national clean air policy in 1956 may also have been driven to some extent by national pride. British politicians and members of the Beaver Committee confronted by the smog of 1952 were clearly aware not only of air pollution episodes elsewhere but also of legislative initiatives to combat pollution in the USA, for example. They were also conscious of the fact that British mortality statistics for respiratory diseases (not only during smogs but also at other times) were far worse than those of most of their international neighbours and competitors in the industrialised world.[73] In particular, members of the Committee and Members of Parliament compared Britain unfavourably with Scandinavian countries, which were rapidly attracting attention not only because they appeared less polluted but also because they offered possible blueprints for more efficient council schemes to resolve the housing crisis, another strident political concern for successive British governments and local authorities during the 1950s.[74] Such comparisons meant that Britain's unenviable international reputation as 'one of the countries where pollution is most serious'[75] could not be easily concealed and may have been a contingent consideration for legislators eager not only to appease the voting public at home but also to boost the country's international standing on increasingly politicised environmental issues of this nature.

Civic, as well as national, pride may also have motivated Members of Parliament to argue for greater regulation of smoke production and, indeed, to assert support for alternative energy sources, such as nuclear fuel. In Sheffield, for example, both civic leaders and members of the public were anxious to fashion a new image for the city and eagerly supported the movement for a national clean air policy.[76] It was Richard Winterbottom, Labour MP for Sheffield Brightside, for example, who had moved the resolution to introduce legislation tackling air pollution at the Labour Party conference in 1955, complaining that 'the children of Brightside have to go into the green belt of Sheffield to smell what they call "that peculiar smell", which is fresh air'.[77] Significantly, at the same time as speaking in parliament in support of clean air legislation, Winterbottom also advocated the use of nuclear energy as a means of alleviating air pollution and was keen to situate a power station in Sheffield.[78] Winterbottom was not alone in his support for such supposedly cleaner energy sources. Gerald Nabarro was also interested in the potential benefits of nuclear fuel, serving as vice-chairman of the Atomic Energy Committee and joint secretary to the Conservative Fuel and Power Committee. Although such support for nuclear power was shaken by the accident at the Windscale nuclear power station in 1957, the potential for nuclear energy to provide cleaner alternatives to solid fuel combustion clearly appealed to both local and national activists committed to creating and maintaining a less polluted and more healthy environment.

Pollution, public health and modern environmentalism

According to many environmental historians, the modern environmental movement did not emerge with any force until the 1960s. When it did, it appeared as 'a fusion of public health and preservation concerns'.[79] Initiated in particular by the publication of Rachel Carson's *Silent Spring* in 1962,[80] it had developed rapidly into an international movement by the 1970s.[81] In 1970, *Time* magazine declared 'the environment' the issue of the year, Greenpeace and Friends of the Earth were founded in 1971, and the 1970s was labelled the 'environmental decade' by *Life* magazine.[82] In 1975, the Green Party was first formulated and, by the 1980s, was attracting votes in European elections.[83] In Britain, the creation of the Department of the Environment in 1970 perhaps marked the official start of the gradual greening of British politics, a process that accelerated, but was also deeply contested, during the 1980s and 1990s. Motivated in part by international disputes about the apparent conflict between economic development and environmental protection, and, in particular, about the limits of sustainability,[84] the evolution of modern environmentalism was also shaped by greater recognition of the impact of environmental change on health at individual, national and global levels.[85]

However, it is important to recognise that environmental sensitivity was not new in the 1960s but had been evident in some form in Britain at least from the middle years of the eighteenth century.[86] Since the last decades of the nineteenth century, the National Smoke Abatement Society and its various precursors had been campaigning for greater protection of both the built and the natural environment, for limiting the ill-health caused by air pollution, and for reducing the wasteful incomplete combustion of coal. During the twentieth century, political attention to environmental issues was also prominent well before the emergence of the modern environmental movement, not only in the rise of urban planning (regulated, for example, by the Green Belt Act of 1938 and by the Town and Country Planning Acts of 1932, 1944 and 1947) but also in the establishment of areas of national beauty (under the Countryside Act of 1949) and the creation of national parks from 1951.[87]

Equally, a close link between environment and health had been an integral feature of public health campaigns from the mid-nineteenth century, infusing sanitarian approaches to urban health problems, shaping attitudes to slum clearance, and directing the work of Medical Officers of Health.[88] Although environmental approaches to health and disease were strongly challenged in the late nineteenth and early twentieth centuries by the emergence of the germ theory of disease (in which specific causes – germs rather than social conditions – were held responsible for the manifestations of diseases such as tuberculosis) and by a growing commitment to hereditarian theories of disease, environmental approaches to public health persisted. In the early decades of the twentieth century, Medical Officers of Health, such as James Niven in Manchester (and later proponents of 'social medicine'), continued to emphasise a close relationship between the health of populations and the environment in which people lived (including housing conditions and smoke pollution), and to confirm the importance of an environmentally sensitive public health profession.[89]

Although clean air legislation in 1956 constituted a specific response to a specific catastrophe and to a particular constellation of political contingencies, it can also be regarded as consistent with the traditional interest of public health doctors in the environmental determinants of disease. At the same time, however, the Clean Air Act can be construed as a seminal moment in the history of environmental health, constituting an early example of modern environmentalism in which both environmental and health concerns were fused within a novel framework of regulatory legislation. The Clean Air Act thus not only drew on an older version of public health environmentalism but also served to promote a new wave of concern about the impact of environmental change on health.

In the first instance, as the Beaver Committee had hoped, publication of the *Report* and subsequent legislation triggered renewed interest in mapping the impact of pollution on respiratory health. During the 1960s and 1970s, a variety of government inquiries and international symposia (especially those convened by the World Health Organization) attempted to chart patterns and levels of air pollution more carefully and to elucidate the precise connection between specific pollutants and diseases such as bronchitis, lung cancer and asthma.[90] Although recognition of a close aetiological link between smoking, on the one hand, and bronchitis and cancer, on the other hand, deflected attention away from the role of atmospheric smoke and fumes in those diseases, air pollution emerged as a major suspect in the search for explanations of rising trends in asthma, and indeed other allergic diseases.[91] In the closing decades of the twentieth century, growing professional and public concerns that rising asthma morbidity and mortality might be related to shifting patterns of pollution contributed to a resurgence of government interest in the impact of atmospheric pollution on public health. During the 1990s, for example, both the Department of Health and the Medical Research Council established advisory groups and committees, convened workshops and published surveys devoted to exploring the possible links between air pollution and respiratory health in particular.[92]

Second, by setting the agenda for future research and policies aimed at regulating pollution and promoting health, the Clean Air Act of 1956 anticipated, and perhaps served to shape, the environmental and ecological turn in public health that emerged during the 1990s. Anxious to reverse a trend towards accounts of disease that focused almost exclusively on the importance of individual behaviour and lifestyle (such as diet and smoking), proponents of the new public health and the new field of 'health promotion' have attempted to re-establish the role of the environment and the notion of ecological balance in debates about the aetiology and pathogenesis of disease.[93] Significantly, however, in reasserting the impact of indoor and outdoor, built and natural, and work and domestic environments on patterns of morbidity and mortality, and in prioritising environmental regulation as a means of preventing disease, the new public health movement has aligned itself with a traditional approach to public health that was well-established in the late nineteenth and early twentieth centuries, and that, in the context of air pollution, was crystallised in the Clean Air Act of 1956.

Conclusion

According to the final report of the Beaver Committee published in 1954 the objective of their recommendations was 'that by the end of ten to fifteen years the total smoke in all heavily populated areas would be reduced by something of the order of 80 per cent'.[94] While the precise figures might be debated, it is evident that during the years following the passage of the Clean Air Act in 1956 (and a supplementary act in 1968),[95] urban air did become less polluted by smoke. Although subsequent scientific inquiries continued to debate the links between air pollution and health, it is possible that a gradual reduction in urban smoke (in conjunction with other factors, such as the introduction of new antibiotics) did contribute to the declining morbidity and mortality from chronic bronchitis. At the same time, however, it is evident that other forms of pollution (sulphur dioxide, carbon monoxide and diesel particulates) remained stable, or indeed increased, possibly contributing to the rapidly rising trends in asthma and other allergic diseases in the closing decades of the twentieth century.

Both the historical determinants and the historical legacies of the first Clean Air Act are complex. Official inquiry and eventual legislation were driven partly by concerns about disease and death rates precipitated by the great smog in the winter of 1952. However, government intervention was also shaped by a national, and indeed global, socio-economic and political context which ensured that both environmental protection and the promotion of public health were becoming increasingly conspicuous, and closely related, political imperatives. In addition, while the Clean Air Act fitted a traditional public health interest in the environmental causes of disease and death, it also constituted a milestone in modern regulatory policies. By effectively fusing public health and environmental concerns within a single national policy, the Clean Air Act of 1956 constituted a nascent form of modern environmentalism, one that both anticipated and informed the ecological and environmental turn in public health discourse that emerged in the late twentieth century.

Notes

1 'An Act to make provision for abating the pollution of the air [Clean Air Act]', 4 & 5 Eliz. 2, c. 52, 1956.
2 This is the way the story has often been told, generally convincingly, by environmental historians. See, for example: J. McNeill, *Something New under the Sun: an Environmental History of the Twentieth Century*, London: Penguin, 2000; P. Brimblecombe, *The Big Smoke: a History of Air Pollution in London since Medieval Times*, London: Methuen, 1987; B.W. Clapp, *An Environmental History of Britain since the Industrial Revolution*, London: Longman, 1994. These broad overview texts do not provide more detailed study of the particular context in which national, and in particular health, policies were forged.
3 See for example: Brimblecombe, *The Big Smoke*; McNeill, *Something New under the Sun*; Clapp, *An Environmental History*; J. Sheail, *An Environmental History of Twentieth-Century Britain*, Basingstoke: Palgrave, 2002. A conference commemorating the impact of the 1952 smog was convened by the London School of Hygiene and Tropical Medicine in December 2002. See www.lshtm.ac.uk/history, also V. Berridge and S. Taylor (eds), *The Big Smoke: Fifty Years after the 1952 London Smog*, London: Centre for History in Public Health, 2005. See also various websites either recounting events surrounding the smog or providing overviews of air pollution control: www.npr.org/display_pages/features/feature_873954.html; www.met-office.gov.uk/education/historic/smog.html; www.eih.uh.edu/air/tfors/history.htm; www.epa.gov/region2/epa30/timeline.htm.
4 R. Parker, 'The struggle for clean air', in P. Hall, H. Land, R. Parker and A. Webb (eds), *Change, Choice and Conflict in Social Policy*, London: Heinemann, 1975, pp. 371–409; E. Ashby and M. Anderson, *The Politics of Clean Air*, Oxford: Oxford University Press, 1981.
5 For an account of interest in both indoor and outdoor air pollution from the thirteenth century through to modern times, see Brimblecombe, *The Big Smoke*.
6 See: Brimblecombe, *The Big Smoke*; S. Mosley, *The Chimney of the World: a History of Smoke Pollution in Victorian and Edwardian Manchester*, Cambridge: White Horse Press, 2001.

7 B. Luckin and G. Mooney, 'Urban history and historical epidemiology: the case of London, 1860–1920', *Urban History* 24, 1997: 37–55; B. Luckin, 'Review essay: versions of the environmental', *Journal of Urban History* 24, 1998: 510–23; B. Luckin, 'Death and survival in the city: approaches to the history of disease', *Urban History Yearbook*, 1980: 53–62; B. Luckin, 'Town, country and metropolis: the formation of an air pollution problem in London, 1800–1870', in D. Schott (ed.), *Energy and the City in Europe: from Preindustrial Wood-shortage to the Oil Crisis of the 1970s*, Stuttgart: Franz Steiner, 1997, pp. 77–92.

8 For an analysis of the links between sunshine and mortality rates between 1881 and 1920, see N. Shaw and J.S. Owens, *The Smoke Problem of Great Cities*, London: Constable, 1925, pp. 63–74.

9 L. Bryder, '"Wonderland of buttercup, clover and daisies": the open-air school movement, 1907–1939', in R. Cooter (ed.), *In the Name of the Child: Health and Welfare, 1880–1940*, London: Routledge, 1992, pp. 72–95; M. Worboys, 'The sanatorium treatment for consumption in Britain, 1890–1914', in J.V. Pickstone (ed.), *Medical Innovations in Historical Perspective*, London: Macmillan, 1992, pp. 47–71; F. Wilmot and P. Saul, *A Breath of Fresh Air: Birmingham's Open Air Schools 1911–1970*, Chichester: Phillimore, 1998.

10 J. Hassan, *The Seaside, Health and the Environment*, Aldershot: Ashgate, 2003; J. Beckerson, 'Selling air: marketing the intangible at UK resorts', unpublished paper presented at 'Good airs and bad: historical perspectives on the atmosphere in relation to health and medicine', a conference held at the UEA in November 2000.

11 See the discussion in Brimblecombe, *The Big Smoke*, pp. 102–8.

12 For more detailed discussion of these developments, see: Shaw and Owens, *The Smoke Problem of Great Cities*, pp. 75–102; C.V. Malcolm, 'Smokeless zones – the history of their development: part 1', *Clean Air*, autumn 1976: 14–20; C.V. Malcolm, 'Smokeless zones – the history of their development: part 2', *Clean Air*, spring 1977: 4–10.

13 The Society's records are kept at its headquarters in Brighton and are catalogued in P. Bassett, 'A list of the historical records retained by the National Society for Clean Air' (Centre for Urban and Regional Studies, University of Birmingham and Institute of Agricultural History, University of Reading, 1980).

14 Quoted in Malcolm, 'Smokeless zones: part 2', p. 7.

15 Mosley, *The Chimney of the World*. See also an awareness and discussion of this issue by the World Health Organization in 'Air pollution', *WHO Chronicle*, 14, 1960, 426–31.

16 See: Mosley, *The Chimney of the World*, pp. 78–84; A. Marsh, *Smoke: the Problem of Coal and the Atmosphere*, London: Faber & Faber, 1947, pp. 69–70.

17 'Asthma Research Council', *Lancet*, 17 March 1928: i, 561–2.

18 Mosley, *The Chimney of the World*, pp. 69–78. I am grateful to Andrew Thorpe for alerting me to the manner in which Neville Chamberlain in particular employed the image of the 'smoking chimney' in the early 1930s.

19 Ibid., p. 76.

20 Ibid., pp. 74–8.

21 Marsh, *Smoke*, p. 74. A similar point about the 'apathetic acceptance' of such deaths was made by the National Smoke Abatement Society shortly after the smog – see the quote from 1953 in Parker, 'The struggle for clean air', p. 378.

22 For accounts of the Meuse Valley and Donora episodes, see: R.C. Ziegenfus, 'Air quality and health', in M.R. Greenberg (ed.), *Public Health and the Environment: the United States Experience*, New York: The Guilford Press, 1987, pp. 139–72; L.P. Snyder, 'The death-dealing smog over Donora, Pennsylvania: industrial air pollution, public health, and federal policy, 1915–1963', Ph.D. thesis, University of Pennsylvania, 1994.

23 Marsh, S*moke*, p. 80.

24 Brimblecombe, *The Big Smoke*, pp. 165–6; McNeill, *Something New under the Sun*, pp. 64–75.

25 A particularly evocative portrayal of the smog is provided in 'Killer Fog', a television documentary made for the Channel 4 *Secret History* series first broadcast in 1999. See also the semi-fictional account of the smog in W. Wise, *Killer Smog: the World's Worst Air Pollution Disaster*, Chicago: Rand McNally & Co., 1968.

26 *The Times*, 12 December 1952, p. 9e; *The Times*, 6 February 1953, p. 7d; *Parliamentary Debates*, 515 (1953), col. 845; *Parliamentary Debates*, 518 (1953), col. 202.

27 Parker, 'The struggle for clean air', pp. 380–1, 408.

28 According to an internal memo in 1952, Harold Macmillan admitted that setting up the committee was simply a convenient way of looking busy – see F. Pearce, 'Darkness at noon', *New Scientist* 2371, 30 November 2002: 48–9.

29 Papers relating to Sir Hugh Beaver's personal and professional life have been catalogued by the Contemporary Scientific Archives Centre (CSAC 40/4/76) and are deposited in the British Library of Political and Economic Science in the London School of Economics.

30 Examples of some of Beaver's addresses to a variety of audiences on clean air and pollution control are contained in his professional papers.

31 The two doctors were Dr. J.L. Burn, Medical Officer of Health for Salford, and Professor T. Ferguson, Chair of Public Health and Social Medicine at Glasgow University.

32 *Committee on Air Pollution – Interim Report*, London: HMSO, 1953, Cmd. 9011, pp. 4–5.

33 *Committee on Air Pollution – Report*, London: HMSO, 1954, Cmd. 9322. On the speed with which the Committee conducted the inquiry, see Parker, 'The struggle for clean air', p. 384.

34 The statistics suggest that mortality rates in fact remained higher than usual for nearly three months after the initial smog, bringing the total death toll to approximately 12,000.

35 *Interim Report*, para. 36.

36 Ibid., para. 37.

37 Ibid., para. 38.

38 Ibid., paras 39 and 40.

39 Ibid., para. 41.

40 Ibid., para. 44.

41 Ibid., para. 45.

42 *Report*, paras 12–18. Interestingly, the final *Report* also highlighted early concerns about rising pollution from motor vehicles – see *Report*, paras 64–7.

43 'Studies of urban air pollution', *Current Medical Research*, London: HMSO, 1962, pp. 35–40.

44 Ministry of Health, *Reports on public health and medical subjects No. 95: mortality and morbidity during the London fog of December 1952*, London: HMSO, 1954.

45 *Parliamentary Debates*, 535 (1954–5), col. 1776. It is not clear precisely why Nabarro became involved with the air pollution issue in the first instance, but it would appear that he was a member of a cross-party group of twelve MPs who each agreed to introduce a Private Member's Bill aimed at regulating pollution if any of them were chosen – see Wise, *Killer Smog*, pp. 171–2.

46 *Parliamentary Debates*, 536 (1954–5), cols 1426–514.

47 *Parliamentary Debates*, 545 (1955), col. 1337.

48 F.W.S. Craig, *British General Election Manifestos, 1918–1966*, Political Reference Publications, 1970, p. 172.

49 *The Labour Party: Report of the 54th Annual Conference*, London, 1955, pp. 120–1. I am grateful to Andrew Thorpe for providing this reference.

50 *Parliamentary Debates*, 551 (1956), col. 148.

51 *Parliamentary Debates*, 536 (1954–5), col. 1486. See also the comments of Ellis Smith, M.P. for Stoke-on-Trent South, in ibid., col. 1456.

52 *Parliamentary Debates*, 545 (1955), col. 1239.

53 *Parliamentary Debates*, 551 (1955–6), cols 140–1. Leavey was also a Director of Smith & Nephew Associated Companies Ltd.

54 There was also considerable discussion about the relative merits of 'smokeless zones' (as advocated by the National Smoke Abatement Society) and the less rigorous 'smoke control areas'.

55 *Parliamentary Debates*, 536 (1954–5), col. 1508. Bell's concerns about diesel fumes were echoed by Sir L. Plummer during debates on the government Bill – see *Parliamentary Debates*, 545 (1955), col. 1303–4.

56 *Parliamentary Debates*, 536 (1954–5), col. 1510.

57 Summary conviction under the act could result in a fine ranging from £10 to £100 depending on the precise offence.

58 Anon., 'Light through smog', *Chest and Heart Bulletin*, February 1963: 16–17.

59 *Report*, para. 6.

60 See: Clapp, *An Environmental History*; R. D. Webster, 'Bronchitis 1900–1965: the social construction of the "British disease"', undergraduate dissertation, Sheffield Hallam University. I am grateful to Mick Worboys for alerting me to this thesis.

61 See Tony Cutler's paper in this volume. Prescription charges had been introduced in 1951 to defray the rising costs of the NHS.

62 Parker, 'The struggle for clean air', p. 392.

63 *Parliamentary Debates*, 536 (1954–5), cols 1469–70.

64 See in particular the papers by Reid, Ferris and Anderson, and Goldsmith in 'Symposium number 6: medical and epidemiological aspects of air pollution', *Proceedings of the Royal Society of Medicine* 57, 1964: 965–1040.

65 I. Gregg, 'The effects of air pollution as seen in general practice', in Chest and Heart Association, *Human Environment and the Respiratory System*, London: Health Horizon Limited, 1970/1, pp. 25–32.

66 See, for example: *The Times*, 12 December 1952, p. 9e; *The Times*, 20 December 1952, p. 3c; *The Times*, 6 February 1953, p. 7d; J. Pemberton, 'Air pollution and bronchitis', *British Medical Journal*, 4 September 1954; J. Fry, 'Chronic bronchitis in general practice', *British Medical Journal*, January 1954; W.P.D. Logan, 'Mortality from fog in London January 1956', *British Medical Journal*, March 1956.

67 *Parliamentary Debates*, 518 (1953), col. 202.

68 *Parliamentary Debates*, 515 (1953), cols 845–56.

69 Ibid., cols 852–6.

70 Dodds challenged the government to outline their plans for an inquiry again in July 1953 – *Parliamentary Debates*, 518 (1953), cols. 201–4. See the discussion in Parker, 'The struggle for clean air'.

71 See the comments in *Report*, para. 7. According to the Channel 4 programme, 'Killer Fog', Harold Macmillan admitted in government memoranda that many measures adopted during the smog, such as distributing gas masks, had been intended primarily merely to placate public concerns and had not been based on scientific evidence of efficacy.

72 For a discussion of these developments and the politics surrounding media representations of medicine, see: K. Loughlin, '"Your Life in Their Hands": the context of a medical-media controversy', *Media History* 6, 2000: 177–88; K. Loughlin, 'The history of health and medicine in contemporary Britain: reflections

on the role of audio-visual sources', *Social History of Medicine* 13, 2000: 131–45; A. Karpf, *Doctoring the Media: the Reporting of Health and Medicine*, London: Routledge, 1988. Films had already been used to expose the problems of pollution during the interwar years. See T. Boon, 'The smoke menace: cinema, sponsorship and the social relations of science in 1937', in M. Shortland (ed.), *Science and Nature: Essays in the History of Environmental Sciences*, Oxford: Oxford University Press, 1993, pp. 57–88.

73 For evidence of Britain's position in a 'league table', see the standard mortality rates given in M. Alderson, *International Mortality Statistics*, London: Macmillan, 1981.

74 For a discussion of how these concerns framed responses both to smoke pollution and the housing crisis in the heavily polluted area of Sheffield, for example, see W. Hampton, 'Optimism and growth 1951–1973', in C. Binfield, R. Childs, R. Harper, D. Hey, D. Martin and G. Tweedale (eds), *The History of the City of Sheffield, 1843–1993: Volume I Politics*, Sheffield: Sheffield Academic Press, 1993, pp. 119–49.

75 'Air pollution', *WHO Chronicle* 14, 1960: 426–31.

76 Hampton, 'Optimism and growth', pp. 129–31.

77 *The Labour Party: Report of the 54th Annual Conference*, p. 120.

78 Hampton, 'Optimism and growth', p. 130.

79 S.R. Lichter and S. Rothman, *Environmental Cancer – a Political Disease*, New Haven: Yale University Press, 1999, p. 9.

80 R. Carson, *Silent Spring*, Boston: Houghton-Mifflin, 1962.

81 See the discussion of this in Lichter and Rothman, pp. 1–22.

82 Ibid., p. 9. I am grateful to Katy Walker for digging out some of the information on the emergence of the modern environmental movement.

83 J. Black, *Modern British History since 1900*, Basingstoke: Macmillan, 2000, p. 64.

84 For a discussion of some of these debates, see T. Jackson, *Material Concerns: Pollution, Profit and Quality of Life*, London: Routledge, 1996.

85 See, for example, World Health Organization, *Health Hazards of the Human Environment*, Geneva: WHO, 1972.

86 F. Walter, 'The evolution of environmental sensitivity 1750–1950', in P. Brimblecombe and C. Pfister (eds), *The Silent Countdown: Essays in European Environmental History*, Berlin: Springer-Verlag, 1990, pp. 231–47.

87 See Black, *Modern British History*, pp. 61–5.

88 For overviews of the history of public health, and of the place of environmentalism, see: C. Hamlin, *Public Health and Social Justice in the Age of Chadwick: Britain, 1800–1854*, Cambridge: Cambridge University Press, 1998; J.M. Eyler, *Victorian Social Medicine: the Ideas and Methods of William Farr*, Baltimore: Johns Hopkins University Press, 1979; D. Porter (ed.), *The History of Public Health and the Modern State*, Amsterdam: Rodopi, 1994; S. Szreter, *Fertility, Class and Gender in Britain 1860–1940*, Cambridge: Cambridge University Press, 1996.

89 J. Niven, *Poverty and Disease*, London: John Bale, Sons & Danielsson, 1909; J. Niven, *Observations on the History of Public Health Effort in Manchester*, Manchester: John Heywood Ltd, 1923. On the emergence of social medicine in the middle decades of the twentieth century, see J. Stewart, *'The Battle for Health': a Political History of the Socialist Medical Association, 1930–51*, Aldershot: Ashgate, 1999.

90 See, for example: 'Symposium number 6: medical and epidemiological aspects of air pollution', *Proceedings of the Royal Society of Medicine* 57, 1964: 965–1040; WHO, *Air Pollution*, Technical Report Series, no. 157, Geneva: WHO, 1958; WHO, *Atmospheric Pollutants: Report of a WHO Expert Committee*, Technical Report Series No. 271, Geneva: WHO, 1964.

91 See: H.R. Anderson, 'Air pollution and trends in asthma', in D.J. Chadwick and G. Cardew (eds), *The Rising Trends in Asthma*, Chichester: John Wiley & Sons, 1997, pp. 190–207; A. Wardlaw (ed.), 'Air pollution and allergic disease: report of a working party of the British Society for Allergy and Clinical Immunology', *Clinical and Experimental Allergy* 25, 1995, Supplement 3.

92 The Department of Health established an Advisory Group on the Medical Aspects of Air Pollution Episodes in 1990 and a Committee on the Medical Aspects of Air Pollutants in 1992, the latter of which has a subgroup on asthma. The MRC has a Working Group on the Environmental Determinants of Asthma and an Institute for Environment and Health. In 1994, the Institute sponsored workshops on air pollution and health, and air pollution and respiratory disease. For some of the publications generated by these committees, see: Department of Health, *Asthma and Outdoor Air Pollution*, London: HMSO, 1995; Department of Health, *Handbook on Air Pollution and Health*, London: The Stationery Office, 1997.

93 See, for example: D. Blane, E. Brunner and R. Wilson (eds), *Health and Social Organisation: Towards a Health Policy for the 21st Century*, London: Routledge, 1996; A. Peterson and D. Lupton, *The New Public Health*, London: Sage, 1996; S. Griffiths and D.J. Hunter (eds), *Perspectives in Public Health*, Abingdon: Radcliffe, 1999; L. Adams, M. Amos and J. Munro (eds), *Promoting Health: Politics and Practice*, London: Sage, 2002.

94 *Report*, para. 7.

95 'An Act to make further provision for abating the pollution of the air', 1968, c. 62.

Recommended further reading

E. Ashby and M. Anderson, *The Politics of Clean Air*, Oxford: Oxford University Press, 1981.

P. Brimblecombe, *The Big Smoke: a History of Air Pollution in London since Medieval Times*, London: Methuen, 1987.

S. Griffiths and D.J. Hunter (eds), *Perspectives in Public Health*, Abingdon: Radcliffe, 1999.

B. Luckin and G. Mooney, 'Urban history and historical epidemiology: the case of London, 1860–1920', *Urban History* 24, 1997: 37–55.

A. Marsh, *Smoke: the Problem of Coal and the Atmosphere*, London: Faber & Faber, 1947.

S. Mosley, *The Chimney of the World: a History of Smoke Pollution in Victorian and Edwardian Manchester*, Cambridge: White Horse Press, 2001.

R. Parker, 'The struggle for clean air', in P. Hall, H. Land, R. Parker and A. Webb (eds), *Change, Choice and Conflict in Social Policy*, London: Heinemann, 1975, pp. 371–409.

A. Peterson and D. Lupton, *The New Public Health*, London: Sage, 1996.

N. Shaw and J. Switzer Owens, *The Smoke Problem of Great Cities*, London: Constable, 1925.

J. Sheail, *An Environmental History of Twentieth-Century Britain*, Basingstoke: Palgrave, 2002.

W. Wise, *Killer Smog: the World's Worst Air Pollution Disaster*, Chicago: Rand McNally & Co., 1968.

10 Americans and Pavlovians

The Central Institute for Cardiovascular Research at the East German Academy of Sciences and its precursor institutions as a case study of biomedical research in a country of the Soviet Bloc (*c.* 1950–80)

Carsten Timmermann

Introduction

This chapter deals with biomedical research in East Germany, a country of the Soviet Bloc during the era of the Cold War. It may help us revise some of the assumptions that have for a long time haunted our perceptions of socialist medicine in Eastern Europe, especially with a view to organisational matters and the role of epidemiology.[1] In Britain, a certain degree of fascination with medicine in the Soviet Bloc amongst left-leaning political and medical elites keen on modernising the health system has a long tradition and can be traced back to the interwar period.[2] Soviet medicine was seen as 'the other' of medicine under capitalism, a model case of socialist medicine where the most obvious shortcomings of health care in capitalist countries were resolved, and where medical research was reunited with health care under the banner of effective disease prevention.[3] Such expectations were fuelled, for example, by books on Soviet socialised medicine such as that by the eminent historian of medicine, Henry E. Sigerist.[4] Sigerist's book (with a Foreword by Sidney Webb), and the positive picture it drew of medicine in the USSR as an exciting experiment in the purposeful rationalisation of healthcare and medical research, may have played its part, for example, in drumming up support for a National Health Service in the UK.

Sigerist published his book five years after a volume dealing with medicine in the USA, which he found 'splendidly equipped technically' but 'backward socially'.[5] Soviet medicine, in contrast, embodied to him what was lacking in US medicine and medicine under capitalism more generally. Soviet medicine to Sigerist proceeded systematically, where its Western counterpart was haphazard. It followed definite, rational plans and used its limited resources carefully, where capitalist medicine was wasteful. More recent publications commissioned by the GDR government to advertise the

East German health system to Western audiences have argued along similar lines.[6] Studies, such as the recent work by Thomas Schlich on the uptake of an innovative, operative system of bone fracture treatment in the GDR, seem to support this notion.[7] My study, however, draws a different picture, at least for the realm of biomedical research.

I will tell the tale of an institution dedicated (at least partly) to research on cardiovascular disease and launched at a time when the focus of interest in public health, in the GDR as well as in most other industrialised countries, shifted away from acute, infectious disease towards the chronic disorders of old age. Cardiovascular diseases and the threats they posed became a central issue in GDR social hygiene textbooks and in the medical journals in the 1950s, towards the end of the so-called epidemiological transition, when this group of diseases replaced infections as the leading cause of death and disability in industrialised countries.[8] The rise of cancer and cardiovascular disease to public consciousness coincided with the rise of big science in biomedicine, in the West as well as in Eastern Europe. In 1954, health guidelines passed by the GDR Council of Ministers called for a large institute of cardiovascular research.[9]

Initially, as we will see, the Council's plans were only incompletely realised, resulting in the formation of the Laboratory for Circulatory Research (*Arbeitsstelle für Kreislaufforschung*), headed by Albert Wollenberger (1912–2000), whose work was mostly dedicated to the cell biology of the heart muscle. It took almost two decades before the Central Institute for Research on Cardiovascular Regulation (*Zentralinstitut für Herz-Kreislauf-Regulationsforschung*) was finally formed in 1972, as part of a large-scale reorganisation of the biomedical research campus of the Academy of Sciences in Berlin-Buch, by merging Wollenberger's laboratory with the Institute for Cortico-Visceral Pathology and Therapy, headed by Rudolf Baumann (1911–88).[10] This chapter traces the history of these two institutions in a context dominated by the GDR government's attempts to create a Soviet-style research academy and implement a particular model of utilitarian research, and by the very different relationships with national and international collaborators and audiences enjoyed by the two directors. The changing international status and policy priorities of the GDR government during the Cold War, dominated by the conflicting desires to create a Soviet-style system on the one hand (not only with regard to healthcare) and to be recognised by Western governments as a legitimate state on the other, also shaped the fortunes of the two institutes.

While in the 1950s the biological Academy institutes in Berlin-Buch were largely free from direct political pressures and their work was geared mostly towards basic research, from the 1960s there was increasing government pressure to redesign research programmes according to utilitarian principles. In a book that the government published to advertise the achievements of the East German health system to an English-speaking audience in 1974, the author, one of Baumann's former co-workers, praised the Central Institute for Heart and Circulation Research as an 'outstanding example of the smooth transition from purposeful basic research via applied and clinical research to the application of the results in practice'.[11] As I will attempt to show, the links between basic, clinical and laboratory research were not always quite as smooth. The main factors that informed and affected the development of Baumann's and Wollenberger's institutions and their research programmes were restrictions on travel that limited exchange with colleagues in the West, and increasing difficulties in purchasing state-of-the-art equipment due to a lack of Western currency reserves. There were also repeated demands from the authorities for direct relevance and utility of research, be it political or economical.

I will begin this chapter with a brief outline of science policy in the Soviet Occupied Zone and the GDR in the aftermath of the Second World War, with special attention to biomedical research within the Academy of Sciences. I will then look at the history of the two institutes in detail, which provides us with an interesting case study of an approach to biomedical research that was in many ways similar to contemporary developments in Western Europe. This applies especially to the early history of Wollenberger's laboratory. Looking at Baumann's institute, however, shows us that there were some major differences peculiar to East Germany. In the final section I will look at the place of epidemiology in GDR cardiovascular research at a time when new epidemiological approaches were developed in the West to deal with the increasingly visible problems of chronic disease. I will attempt to explain how the so-called risk factor approach, which since the 1960s has dominated Western thinking about heart disease, found its way into the research programme of the Central Institute. This only happened after the merger of the two precursor institutions in 1972, due to generational change and as a consequence of new priorities in GDR research and health policy.

The Academy of Sciences becomes a research institution

When Albert Wollenberger's laboratory took up its work as part of the newly founded *Arbeitsstelle für Kreislaufforschung* in 1957, the first phase in the development of the Academy of Sciences, from German-style *Gelehrtenakademie* (academy of sages) to Soviet-style socialist research academy was already completed.[12] The former Prussian Academy of Sciences had closed its doors in the summer of 1946, in order to be immediately reopened by the education authority in the Soviet Occupied Zone as German Academy of Sciences, with members in both East and West Germany. At this point, neither of the two German states existed (both the Federal Republic and the German Democratic Republic were founded in 1949), and it was far from clear what was going to happen to the German science landscape. It made sense, then, for the Soviet Military Administration (SMA) to keep all options open, encourage the membership of West Germans in the Academy, and be thus prepared for a possible reunification of the country.

According to its new statutes, the German Academy was to include research institutes and so provide an institutional home for former Kaiser Wilhelm Institutes (KWI) in the Soviet sector.[13] Amongst the first research institutes taken over by the Academy in 1947 was the famous former KWI for Brain Research in Berlin-Buch, whose work, following an order by the Soviet occupation authority, as Institute for Medicine and Biology was now to be dedicated to cancer research.[14] The Academy's new institute included a clinical department (opened in 1949) and employed 149 people in 1949, including twenty-seven scientists and medics. Two years later there were 248 employees, forty-three of whom were scientists or doctors.[15]

Until 1949 the leaders of the Socialist Unity Party had paid little attention to the future of the Academy. After the GDR was founded, they increasingly sought to gain control over the institution, whose membership still included many 'bourgeois' scientists, and to turn it into a socialist academy. In 1952 the SED leadership under its strong man, Secretary General Walter Ulbricht, announced that the GDR was going to be a Soviet-style, socialist state and asked the Academy Council what the institution would be willing to contribute to the building of socialism. A little later, the *Politbüro* of the Central Committee, the decision-making body in charge of policy decisions between party congresses, set up a commission for reorganising the institution.

While in the Prussian Academy there was parity between humanities and natural sciences, now increasingly the natural sciences and research and development concerns gained the upper hand. As the historian of the Academy, Peter Nötzold points out, the SED leadership under Ulbricht had high expectations of the ability of science to solve economic problems. Scientists nourished such expectations and used them to promote their disciplines, which led to a phase of rapid expansion in the Academy's research capacities in the 1950s.[16] Both Wollenberger's and Baumann's institutes were products of this phase. We will see, however, that their intended function was not only utilitarian. International prestige played a central role, and Baumann's institute was also designed as a model for a Soviet approach to medical science, based on the teachings of Ivan Pavlov, the Russian physiologist, and his followers in the Soviet Union.

The two institutes were opened just before the so-called *Forschungsgemeinschaft der naturwissenschaftlichen und technischen Institute* (Research Community of Institutes for Natural Science and Technology) was launched in 1957, the *de facto* autonomous head organisation of this group of institutes (by then thirty-nine) within the Academy. This consolidated the Academy's hybrid character as an academy of sages (dominated by distinguished and often old professors in the humanities, social and natural sciences) and research institutions. Almost simultaneously, the Council of Ministers set up its own 'Council for Natural-Scientific Research and Development' (the *Forschungsrat* or Research Council of the GDR). Cardiovascular disease, as we will see in the following section, had meanwhile become an important item on the research agenda in the medical sciences.

Cardiovascular research at the Academy of Sciences and Albert Wollenberger's laboratory

The official justification for the opening of Wollenberger's laboratory was two decisions of the GDR Council of Ministers. On 8 July 1954, the Council agreed guidelines for the future development of healthcare and disease prevention, which included the call for an institute of cardiovascular research.[17] On 5 May 1955, the Council decided on recommendations for the improvement of the work of the Academy of Sciences, including plans for a cardiovascular institute within the Academy. In the same year, an expert commission for cardiovascular research (*Arbeitskreis für Kreislaufforschung*) was launched. Wollenberger was one of the founding members of the *Arbeitskreis*, lobbying for the future institute to become part of the Academy.[18]

Wollenberger was not typical of East German scientists and doctors. While many established members of the scientific and medical communities left the Soviet Occupied Zone for the West, Wollenberger was a so-called *Westemigrant* who had moved from West to East.[19] The term *Westemigranten* (literally translated as West *émigrés*) describes the returnees from exile in Western countries rather than the USSR, which had hosted most of the GDR political leaders during the Nazi dictatorship. Wollenberger was born in 1912 in the small, southwestern university town of Freiburg.[20] He started to study medicine in Berlin in 1931, where he joined the Communist Student Association and the Communist Party. He left for Switzerland and France in 1933, and after a brief return to Germany, with the permission of the Communist Party leadership, he emigrated via Denmark to the USA in 1940. There he studied medicine and biology at Harvard, and completed his Ph.D. with the German biochemist Fritz Lipmann at the Pharmacological Institute headed by Otto Krayer, another *émigré*, working on the biochemistry of heart failure. Wollenberger stayed at Harvard until 1951. From 1951 to 1954 he worked as a guest scientist at the Carlsberg Laboratories in Copenhagen, at the University of London's Institute of Psychiatry and at the Biochemical Institute at Uppsala University. In 1954 he took up a position as *Oberassistent* at Humboldt University in East Berlin, on the understanding that this would be an interim solution, until an Academy institute for cardiovascular research was set up.

Some members of the Academy and researchers in Buch were doubtful about the plans for an institute of cardiovascular research: would not such an institute need a large clinic, and, if so, would the Academy be the right place for it? Other leading members of the *Arbeitskreis* had their institutional homes at the medical schools of the universities of Berlin and

Leipzig.[21] They possessed both the know-how and the facilities for clinical research on cardiovascular problems. Both the secretary of the Academy's class of medicine, Lohmann, and the director of the Institute for Medicine and Biology in Berlin-Buch, Friedrich, were opposed to the plans. As a consequence, the *Politbüro* had to intervene in favour of the institute.[22] In December 1955, Wollenberger was appointed Director of a new laboratory, the first one within the planned new institute for cardiovascular research, against the votes of Lohmann and Friedrich.[23] On 1 January 1956, the *Arbeitsstelle für Kreislaufforschung* was officially launched, and in May 1956 a number of rooms in the former KWI for Brain Research in Berlin-Buch were equipped so that the work could start.[24] In 1960, Wollenberger employed twenty-six people, seven of whom were scientists.[25]

The directions that Wollenberger's scientific work took can be explained partly with his experiences in the USA. *Westemigranten* like Wollenberger occupied a peculiar position in GDR society. Returned to the GDR in the late 1940s and 1950s, many of them to escape McCarthyism, they often found themselves suspected of espionage. However, returning scientists and artists also enjoyed many privileges, including, for example, housing in suburban estates, purpose-built especially for the cultural elite, and relative freedom to travel to Western countries.[26] Wollenberger's student and later successor, Ernst Georg Krause, remembers an occasion when Wollenberger returned from a trip to West Germany with his Mercedes, where somebody had fixed a note to his windshield wipers. The author of the note had identified the GDR licence plate and commented: 'Walter Ulbricht loves the Wall and the comrade loves his Mercedes'.[27] Wollenberger found this funny, but his co-workers, who were stuck behind that Wall, evidently had different feelings. The privileged West *émigrés* were often confronted with the envy of ordinary GDR citizens who dreamed about leaving the country for the West and did not understand why anybody would choose to move in the other direction, and with the ambivalent feelings of their co-workers and students who created the results that the boss presented at international conferences.[28]

Work in Wollenberger's laboratory was dedicated to what in 1983 he called 'molecular and cellular cardiology, a field at the boundary between molecular and cell biology on the one hand and clinical cardiology on the other'.[29] He is still seen internationally as one of the fathers of the biochemistry of the heart, and work in his laboratory focused mostly on biochemical processes in the heart muscle and the metabolism of heart failure, including the metabolic action of cardiac glycosides, important sugar molecules that are involved in the regulation of the heart. Wollenberger's student and co-worker, Ernst Georg Krause, was amongst the first, worldwide, working on a particular regulatory pathway. In 1983, Wollenberger showed satisfaction that the laboratory's results might have contributed to a better understanding of the role of adrenergic receptors and thus to the development of the beta-blockers, but the priorities of his laboratory were clearly on basic research.[30] He gained international recognition with a technical invention, the *Wollenberger-Zange*, a metal clamp that, cooled down to minus 196 degrees Centigrade, allowed the rapid freezing of tissue samples in order to determine the concentration of metabolites in the tissue at a fixed state of a metabolic process.[31]

Wollenberger was a cosmopolitan. He continued to correspond and collaborate with colleagues in the West, directed his publications to an international audience and was only marginally interested in the internal affairs of GDR science.[32] Krause, in fact, had come to Berlin to study biochemistry in the 1950s, when he heard that 'two Americans had arrived', Wollenberger and the biochemist Samuel Mitja Rapoport.[33] Once his laboratory was running, Wollenberger kept a low profile in GDR health and research politics (with one notable exception: he was a figurehead of the jogging movement). His memory is still held in high regard in the institution that succeeded the Academy institutes in Buch after the demise of the GDR, the Max Delbrück Centre for Molecular Medicine. While Wollenberger's group had to make do with 1950s laboratory technology until the Wall came down, their research programme remained in gear with what was going on in cell biology in the heart in the West.

Along with Wollenberger's laboratory, a working group for experimental cardiac surgery, headed by Petros Kokkalis, formerly professor at Athens University, was set up at Friedrichshain Hospital, to work on improved techniques of heart surgery. Together the two groups constituted the *Arbeitsstelle für Kreislaufforschung*, the first stage in the development of a large research institute, and it was planned to move them into a new building on the Buch campus in due time. Academy officials admitted that Wollenberger's and Kokkalis's work may not have represented cardiovascular research proper (especially the lack of epidemiological research was later often deplored) but starting the new research institute with only two groups working on pharmacology and surgery respectively was deemed necessary due to the lack of suitable candidates in other fields.[34] Once it was complete, according to Lohmann's plans, the institute was to work in four fields: physiology, chemistry, pharmacology and surgery, and also to draw on haematology, experimental pathology, histology, physics and biophysics, X-ray diagnostics and social hygiene. The work of the institute was going to be mostly dedicated to fundamental research, while a group based at Leipzig University would work predominantly clinically. Lohmann did, however, consider collaboration with the Municipal Hospital in Buch as desirable.[35]

When Kokkalis died in 1962, ironically from a heart attack, no successor was available and the work of the group lacked guidance and a sense of direction. The *Forschungsgemeinschaft* decided to restructure the *Arbeitsstelle*. The Friedrichshain group was taken over by Humboldt University and the HU cardiologist H.-J. Serfling was appointed acting director. Wollenberger was appointed director of the whole *Arbeitsstelle*.[36] In 1964 the Wollenberger group moved into a new, modern laboratory building. The original plans for a large, central institute for cardiovascular research that included more than just Wollenberger's laboratory for biochemistry of the heart were put on ice, only resurfacing in the late 1960s with the Academy Reform and the idea of the merger with Baumann's group.

Pavlov in the GDR and Rudolf Baumann's institute

In contrast with Wollenberger's, Rudolf Baumann's name has all but disappeared from the official histories of the Max Delbrück Centre, and he is generally seen as a controversial character. His research and publications were not addressed to an international, primarily Western audience, but to colleagues in the GDR and in the socialist countries of the Eastern Bloc. Baumann's interest in cardiovascular problems was only secondary in the 1950s, while one of his primary aims was to introduce the teachings of the Russian physiologist Ivan Pavlov to GDR medical science. Only gradually, cardiovascular problems came to play a more central role in his research programme. Baumann's Institute for Cortico-Visceral Pathology and Therapy was launched in 1956, the same year as Wollenberger's laboratory, but initially within the Municipal Hufeland Hospital in Berlin-Buch, where Baumann had been head of internal medicine since 1948 and medical director since 1951.[37] The complicated name of Baumann's clinic and institute was a tribute to Pavlov and his followers in the Soviet Union.[38] The brief but intense love affair with Pavlov in GDR academic medicine was the expression of an officially sanctioned attempt to promote a new, dialectical-materialist approach to medical science. Its promoters expected it to transform the medical landscape of East Germany by loosening old ties with the West and creating new alliances with Soviet medicine.[39]

The central doctrine of the new Pavlovian approach in all branches of the medical sciences in the Soviet Union was what his followers called the leading role of the cerebral cortex for the interaction between organism and environment. Pavlov's teachings were interesting for Soviet officials because they allowed the 'materialist' interpretation of all organic and psychological processes as chains of reflexes, controlled by a central power. The reception of Pavlov in the GDR followed the Soviet model and specifically attacked Western psychoanalytical and psychosomatic concepts. Starting in 1950, the medical journal published by the GDR Ministry of Health, *Das deutsche Gesundheitswesen*, printed a growing number of articles on Pavlov's teachings and their implications, partly by German authors and partly translations of texts originally published in Russian.[40] In 1952 the physiologist Emil von Skramlik organised a Pavlov workshop in Dresden. In the same year, the Central Committee of the SED founded a Commission for Questions of Medical Science, with the explicit goal of popularising Pavlov. Its chairman was Samuel Mitja Rapoport. In 1953, the health ministry launched its own Pavlov Commission, chaired by Maxim Zetkin. Baumann was one of its members. Pavlov conferences in 1953 and 1954 attracted large, international audiences.[41]

Like the institute for cardiovascular research, an 'institute for the physiology of higher nerve activity (Pavlov Institute)' was on the list of desiderata included in the 1954 Council of Ministers guidelines for the further development of the GDR health system.[42] The *Forschungsgemeinschaft* took over the Baumann institute from the municipal authorities in 1958, turning it into an Academy institute.[43] The Institute included a small clinic, whose work already in 1960 was predominantly dedicated to hypertension research.[44] Associated with the clinic (which grew substantially in later years) were laboratories for the study of the higher nerve activity of human beings, for electrophysiology, for blood circulation and haematology, for clinical physiology and patho-physiology, and for clinical psychology. A theoretical-experimental department included laboratories for electro-physiological basic research, for experimental physiology and patho-physiology of higher nerve activity, for physiological and patho-physiological studies of metabolism with radioactive isotopes, for radiochemistry, for experimental pharmacology, for biochemistry and clinical chemistry, for histology and histochemistry, and an electro-physical workshop. In 1959 the institute had 122 employees, including twenty-nine scientists; in 1961 there were 164, including fifty-one scientists.[45]

Even after being appointed as institute director within the Academy, Baumann continued to be head of internal medicine at the Hufeland hospital. In an article for the Academy's magazine, *Spectrum*, Baumann later characterised his work as neurobiology, and it may not be immediately obvious how he became the champion of hypertension research in the GDR.[46] He turned to research on hypertension in the 1950s, after initially working on the treatment of diabetes. Both high blood pressure and diabetes to him exemplified defects in the regulation of somatic processes by the brain, cortico-visceral or, as he preferred to call them later, cerebro-visceral interactions, due to insufficient adaptation of the organism to a stressful environment. In the 1960s, when the enthusiasm for Pavlov was fading, Baumann and his co-workers stressed the links between their work and then fashionable cybernetic theories.[47] In the 1970s Baumann no longer mentioned Pavlov but drew extensively on the stress theories of the Austrian-Canadian physiologist, Hans Selye.[48] The roots of the institute's work, however, remained visible, while the context of GDR research policy was changing.

Science as a 'productive force'

The 1960s were characterised by increasing pressure on the GDR scientific community to pursue research that was immediately applicable and would yield visible economical (and political) gains. This development was accompanied by a proliferation of new councils and workgroups (see Figure 10.1). In February 1960 a party health conference in Weimar discussed the necessity of long-term planning and agreed on a 'Perspective Plan for the

Development of Medical Science and the Health System in the GDR' for 1960–80, which was subsequently adopted by the Council of Ministers. The institutions that were active in medical research and healthcare were asked to develop their own long-term perspectives.[49] The aim was 'steady improvement, concentration and rationalisation' of medical research, centrally controlled and co-ordinated by the ministry of health.[50]

In 1962 a 'Council for Planning and Co-ordinating Medical Science' was constituted at the ministry (*Rat für Planung und Koordinierung der medizinischen Wissenschaft beim Ministerium für Gesundheitswesen*, see Figure 10.1) to translate health policy goals into medical research. The Council swiftly set up 'Problem Commissions' (*Problemkommissionen*) for various areas of medical research, whose role as expert commissions of the new Council was comparable to what the *Arbeitskreise* did for the *Forschungsrat*. In the case of cardiovascular research, in fact, the chairman of the problem commission, Harald Dutz, a professor at the Charité, was also chairman of the *Arbeitskreis*. In contrast with cancer research, where the Academy Institute was also home to the chairs of the respective scientific bodies, cardiovascular research continued to be co-ordinated from outside the Academy until 1985. This was a consequence of both Wollenberger's lack of interest in GDR research policy – his audience was an international one – and the complete absence of collaboration between Wollenberger's and Baumann's institutes before their 'forced marriage' in 1972.

In January 1963 the Sixth Party Congress of the SED declared science to be one of the central 'productive forces' (*Produktivkraft Wissenschaft*), besides industrial labour and farming. In June 1963, an economic conference of the SED and the Council of Ministers discussed new 'Guidelines for the New Economic System of Planning and Directing', adopted by the State Council in July. For the Academy researchers, this ultimately led to a further centralisation of decision-making. Institute directors increasingly held responsibility for decisions that were only partly their own. The government also experimented with different funding models. Towards the end of the 1960s, some direct government funding for the Academy institutes was withdrawn and research work had to be ordered (and paid for) by the nationalised GDR industries.

Parallel with the increasing centralisation of decision-making, there was a trend towards 'big science' within the Academy's research institutes. In 1961 the institutes on the Berlin-Buch research campus were joined together in the 'Medical-Biological Research Centre Berlin-Buch'.[51] The idea was to use synergies between laboratories to make research more productive. The *Akademiereform* that began in 1968 and ended with the restructuring of the Buch research campus in 1972 and the concentration of biomedical research in three large central institutes marked the endpoint of this process.

The division of labour between head and hands, academy and production industry, which the government intended, was ultimately unsuccessful. Companies neglected research and development, the communication between institutes and with the industry left a lot to be desired, and institute directors found imaginative ways to pursue their basic research projects, which often had little in common with the official function of their institution. Baumann and Wollenberger continued the work they had been doing since the 1950s. However, Baumann in particular did so under imaginative new labels, arguing for the work's relevance with reference to whatever was in fashion at the time and stressing its importance for the modernisation of the GDR health system and the standing of GDR science in the world. Especially the experiments with primates, involving elaborate and expensive computer

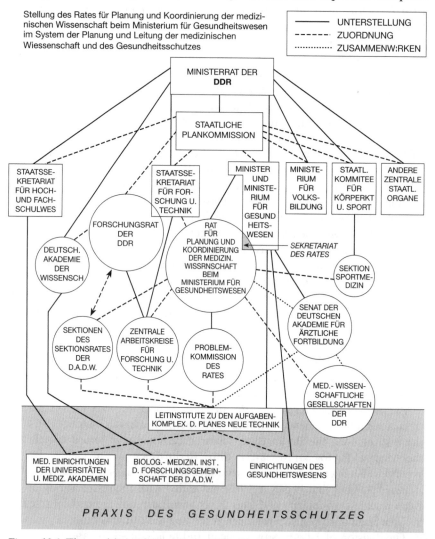

Figure 10.1 The position of the 'Council for Planning and Coordinating Medical Science' at the Ministry of Health within the GDR planning system for health and medical science. Source: BBAA, AKL 477, Beziehungen zu fremden Institutionen.

technology in the division of the institute headed by Baumann's wife, Hannelore, were sometimes suspected to be more show than substance.[52] That the claims of some medical researchers with regard to the clinical relevance of their work were occasionally exaggerated worried the Academy's Class of Medicine. In a confidential memorandum in 1964 the class warned that 'those institutes whose work is exclusively theoretical and experimental neglect clinical questions and turn to more interesting problems, which have only indirect relevance for the main problems of clinical research'.[53]

In cardiovascular research, university-based researchers continued to retain a much higher stake than, for example, in cancer research. We have already noted that the head of the *Arbeitskreis* for cardiovascular research, unlike for cancer research, was not based at the respective Academy institute. While Baumann's priorities increasingly moved away from Pavlovian approaches and towards cardiovascular problems, he was neither a member of the respective *Arbeitskreis* nor the *Problemkommission*. In 1963, this (in concert with Baumann's rather unfocused research programme) led to a conflict with the *Arbeitskreis*. In a meeting of the Council for Planning, Dutz suggested that Baumann's institute should lose twenty out of its forty academic staff and forty of its 150 non-academic employees, because the institute's work was 'only of minor importance for reaching our scientific and practical goals' and its staff 'not in all areas scientifically qualified'.[54] The savings should be used to set up decentralised research groups within university hospitals.[55] Baumann was able to maintain the size of his institute, but he may have felt compelled to move more towards cardiovascular research than he would have done otherwise. Nevertheless, his work was again severely criticised in 1965 as being not sufficiently relevant, this time from within the Academy.[56]

An analysis of cardiovascular research for the SED party leadership described the strained relations between HU and Academy researchers as one of the main obstacles for more efficient research in this field, but lauded the transformation of the institute from Pavlov institute into a centre of hypertension research.[57] Cardiovascular disease moved higher and higher on the agenda, not least in response to developments in the West, as we will see in the following section. The party leadership was concerned that work in the GDR could fall back further in terms of quality and significance behind that by Western competitors, with regard to laboratory research as well as epidemiology and the clinic.[58]

The Academy reforms and the status of epidemiology

With a view to such concerns in the *Politbüro*, let us take a brief look at the role of epidemiology in the GDR, before we turn to a brief outline of further developments at the Central Institute after the forced marriage in 1972. It is today often assumed, almost automatically, that epidemiological research featured strongly in the countries of the Eastern Bloc, as their health system was centrally organised and prevention-oriented.[59] However, epidemiological research on cardiovascular disease in the GDR in the 1950s and 1960s had no home at the prestigious Academy of Sciences. While Baumann's work did focus on hypertension, his group did not pursue any epidemiological work before the restructuring of the Buch campus. Nor was Wollenberger particularly interested in epidemiology, apart from a brief excursion in the 1950s, for which he was severely criticised by the social hygienist Kurt Winter.[60]

Epidemiology and preventive medicine in the GDR were originally the domain of social hygienists, who worked at the universities and medical academies, and who saw themselves as part of a tradition founded by Alfred Grotjahn.[61] Their brand of epidemiology was different from the new epidemiological approaches developed in the West, for example in the context of the US National Heart Institute's Framingham Heart Study. Social hygiene was geared towards a broader study of life conditions and the economics of health, while the so-called risk factor approach, which began to dominate epidemiological thinking about chronic disease in the West, was perceived as reductionist and more closely associated with clinical medicine than with social hygiene proper.[62]

Risk factors did find their way into GDR medicine (and into the new Central Institute for Cardiovascular Research), but not via social hygiene. A small number of clinicians working outside the Academy (some had trained with Harald Dutz), turned their interest to the incidence of heart disease in the 1960s and emulated US approaches. These clinicians included, for example, Karl-Heinz Straube, a hospital director in the Saxonian town of Zwickau, who had worked with Dutz in Rostock in the late 1950s and was a champion of the cardiological dispensary system in Saxony.[63] Straube combined his clinical work with an interest in medical research, taking advantage of his access to dispensary patients, as was in fact intended by health policy-makers, in line with the model of Soviet medicine that Sigerist presents in his book.

In the GDR, healthcare was provided by the state and by (state-owned) companies, predominantly within health centres.[64] Specialist clinics, so-called *Dispensaires* (the government used the French term, but with reference to the health system in the Soviet Union), were dedicated to screening and prevention campaigns for selected diseases and health problems, including cardiovascular disease.[65] Straube was not the only clinician turned epidemiologist who pioneered the risk factor approach in the GDR. J. Knappe, for example, and his co-workers undertook epidemiological studies of heart disease in the Erfurt area in Thuringia.[66] Most important for the Buch institute, however, was the Berlin Mitte study undertaken by Siegfried Böthig and his colleagues at the Charité in Berlin.[67] All these studies were directly or indirectly modelled on US examples. Kurt Winter's students and successors in the social hygiene tradition remained highly critical of both the clinicians turned epidemiologists and the risk factor approach.[68]

Why then was this Western approach to epidemiology implemented at the Academy's Central Institute for Cardiovascular Research after 1972, bypassing home-grown social hygienists? There are several explanations. First, the risk factor approach matched the changed landscape of domestic politics. The new GDR leadership under Erich Honecker, who succeeded Ulbricht in 1971, put a much stronger emphasis on satisfying the demands of GDR citizens as consumers. This individualist focus in everyday matters also brought with it a stronger emphasis on the responsibility of individuals for maintaining their health and found its expression, for example, in the jogging movement, for which Wollenberger served as a figurehead.

A second reason for the GDR government to support the implementation of Anglo-American informed epidemiological approaches was the desire to create a basis for involvement in international research projects under the umbrella of the World Health Organization (WHO).[69] Getting international recognition for the GDR as an independent state was one of the main priorities of the SED leadership in the 1970s. Both the GDR and the Federal Republic formally joined the WHO in 1973, but already before this date the East Germans frequently sent delegations to WHO conventions. The WHO Committee of the GDR published translations of WHO publications in the journal *Das deutsche Gesundheitswesen* from 1961.

A third factor, concerning specifically the Academy institute, was generational change. The merger of Baumann's and Wollenberger's institutes in 1972 was in fact more of a takeover. Wollenberger's laboratory became the division of molecular cardiology in the new institute, while Baumann was appointed its director. However, the retirement of both Wollenberger and Baumann was imminent, and the institute was changing its character fundamentally. In the 1970s and early 1980s, a group of clinicians moved from the Humboldt University to the Academy institute in Buch, in what critical voices described as a *Kadertanz* (cadre dance).[70] They implemented their own research programmes and made Baumann's post-Pavlovian approaches look more and more like a thing of the past. Horst Heine, who succeeded Baumann as director in 1977, had the reputation of being politically even closer to the GDR government than Baumann. In the 1960s he had worked closely with Dutz at the Charité.

The first clinician who established the risk factor approach and other Anglo-American informed epidemiological approaches at the Academy was Hans Dieter Faulhaber, who moved from the Charité to Buch in 1972. Faulhaber had trained in pharmacology and internal medicine, and specialised in hypertension research. After a pilot study on the incidence of high blood pressure in the Berlin borough of Pankow, Faulhaber and his co-workers designed a hypertension treatment study in the same district. Like Straube's and Knappe's studies, Faulhaber's work profited from the existence of specialist cardiological services for districts and regions in the GDR, with whom he collaborated.[71]

When Heine succeeded Baumann as director, he was joined in Buch by a number of former Charité co-workers, including, for example, Lothar Heinemann, who had worked with Böthig on the Berlin Mitte study and was going to co-ordinate the GDR branch of the World Health Organization's multicentred MONICA study, launched in the early 1980s to MONItor trends in CArdiovascular diseases.[72] In 1985, finally, the institute took over the official co-ordination of cardiovascular research in the GDR, which until then had resided with colleagues at the Charité. Heine changed the emphasis of the institute's work, away from basic research and towards clinical work. Under his directorship, a large diagnostic department and a new intensive care unit were set up, with modern, Western equipment, paid for from the limited Western currency reserves. While this led to resentments in other parts of the institute (for example, the cell biologists and biochemists in what used to be Wollenberger's laboratory still used centrifuges purchased in the 1950s) the institute as a whole came to look more than ever like that envisaged in the original plans of the mid-1950s.

Conclusion

In this chapter I used the stories of two very different institutions within the East German Academy of Science as case studies for the development of cardiovascular research in the GDR at a time when chronic disease gained significantly in visibility. The stories of Albert Wollenberger's *Arbeitsstelle für Kreislaufforschung* and Rudolf Baumann's *Institut für Kortiko-Viszerale Pathologie und Therapie*, and the circumstances of their forced marriage that gave rise to a Central Institute for Cardiovascular Research, point to some of the contingencies and local specificities of this development. Wollenberger and Baumann played different and very distinctive roles in these stories, roles that also shaped the work of their respective institutes: Wollenberger, as a *Westemigrant* who had trained in the USA, was rather cosmopolitan and published the results of his cell biological work predominantly in English and for an international audience. Throughout his career, while he continued to work with the tools of the 1950s and 1960s, and lack of funding prevented him and his co-workers from exploring, for example, molecular biological approaches, Wollenberger's cell biological research programme remained valid in the eyes of colleagues in the West. The questions he addressed were of interest to Western researchers, with whom he maintained regular contact. Baumann and his colleagues, in contrast, pursued local interests and published predominantly in German and for a GDR audience. Wollenberger and Baumann were not a good match. Before the merger there was hardly any collaboration, and this was not helped by the fact that Baumann's institute was located about two kilometres away from the rest of the academy institutes in the grounds of the municipal hospital. But the intellectual distance between the two was still greater, and, even after the merger, the Wollenberger lab never became fully integrated into the new central institute.

Both Wollenberger and Baumann represented and responded to certain policy agendas, foreign and domestic, of the GDR government. The work of

Wollenberger's laboratory was to demonstrate to Western researchers the significance (if not superiority) of East German science when following US-style research programmes, and Baumann's represented the attempt to construct a brand of science modelled on the Soviet Union. Interestingly (but not entirely surprisingly), Wollenberger's memory is cherished until today within the institution that succeeded the Academy institutes in Buch after the Berlin Wall had fallen in 1989, the Max Delbrück Centre for Molecular Medicine, while Baumann, in contrast, is not mentioned.[73] Clearly, the new institution is interested in stressing continuities with what its directors consider good GDR science. Baumann's approach was geared specifically to a 1950s GDR context and quickly looked somewhat anachronistic, long before the end of the GDR. He had supporters in the government, but, as we have seen, fellow medical scientists were critical of his work. His research programme became increasingly marginal in the 1970s when a new generation of researchers, predominantly clinically trained, moved from the Charité to the newly formed Central Institute and brought with them new approaches and plans to install a modern and expensive diagnostic department. Like Wollenberger, these researchers chose to implement Western models (and use Western technologies) in their work. This included their approach to epidemiology, which did not build on the established social hygiene traditions but was modelled on US work.

Henry Sigerist, in his 1937 book, stated that he was 'primarily interested in the principles of Soviet medicine and in those positive achievements which represent a permanent gain. Shortcomings will be remedied sooner or later'.[74] After 1990, the German authorities have chosen to tackle what they saw as shortcomings and inadequacies by largely dismantling all Soviet-style institutions in what used to be the GDR. Similar developments have taken place in other countries of the former Soviet Bloc. So has the legacy of Soviet medicine disappeared, completely and justifiably?

The reality of biomedical research in the Soviet-inspired, socialist system of the GDR, in fact, was a far cry from Sigerist's idealistic projections of purposeful integration. Initially, many researchers remained committed to 'bourgeois science' and showed little enthusiasm for government calls to build and embrace a new, socialist science. Not long after the demise of National Socialism, another totalitarian system that had promoted its own approach to science, this was perhaps not surprising. When finally a new generation took control of biomedicine in the GDR, they were looking for inspiration in the West. This was not only true for Wollenberger's student and later successor, Ernst Georg Krause, who had come to Berlin to study with an 'American'. In the epidemiology of heart disease, many, including the Humboldt University group, followed the Framingham model. Even amongst their critics in the social hygiene tradition, the younger generation were inspired by Western models. In their case the model was social medicine in Britain, which is somewhat ironic considering that this was an approach at least temporarily and partly inspired by Soviet medicine, but developed under the conditions of capitalism. I guess that in systems such as the British National Health Service, built on compromise and with many imperfections, we may find the legacy of Soviet medicine as adapted to the realities of a twentieth-century liberal society. And why not? Sigerist himself, after all, chose to return to the USA to write his book, and Wollenberger, too, would have stayed there, despite his communist convictions, had not McCarthy's activities forced him to leave.

My case studies of the careers of Baumann and Wollenberger suggest that, at least for biomedical technoscience, the Cold War reality did not hold what Soviet medicine had seemed to promise to visitors to the USSR in the very different context of the interwar period. However, this should not lead us towards whiggishly dismissing GDR medicine and biomedical science in its entirety. Scholarship in science studies in the last few decades has taught us to be careful about equating a lost argument with qualitative inferiority and to look at the contexts of a controversy instead. While the ambitions of the GDR government to match and beat the West German competition in the realms of technoscience were unrealistic, especially under increasingly difficult economic conditions, some of the achievements of GDR biomedicine were remarkable. The integrated health system, too, had its strengths, and it leaves a bitter aftertaste that the institutions of GDR medicine were completely disposed of after German reunification, by a medical elite keen to quickly and effectively stamp out all traces of practicable alternatives to individualised medical practice, with devastating consequences for medical care especially in some rural districts. On re-reading Sigerist's book one is tempted to embrace at least some of its assumptions. For the time being, Germans (not only in the East) may have to live with a health system that is, as Sigerist observed for the case of the USA, 'splendidly equipped technically' but somewhat 'backward socially'. What is lacking, however, is a clear and obvious alternative.

Notes

1 Such expectations can only insufficiently be explained by reference to propaganda publications commissioned by the respective governments. See, for example, K. Hecht, *What is Done to Protect People's Health? Information on the Health Service of the GDR*, Berlin: Panorama DDR – Auslandspresseagentur GmbH, 1974.

2 J. Stewart, *'The Battle for Health': a Political History of the Socialist Medical Association, 1930–51*, Aldershot: Ashgate, 1999.

3 For a short, critical review of Western attitudes and literature on Soviet medicine, see M. G. Field, *Soviet Socialized Medicine: An Introduction*, New York: Free Press, 1967, pp. ix-xi.

4 H.E. Sigerist, *Socialised Medicine in the Soviet Union*, London: Victor Gollancz, 1937.

5 Sigerist, *Socialised Medicine*, p. 15. H.E. Sigerist, *American Medicine*, New York: Norton, 1934.

6 Hecht, *What is Done to Protect People's Health?*.

7 T. Schlich, 'Degrees of control: the spread of operative fracture treatment with metal implants: a comparative perspective on Switzerland, East Germany and

the USA, 1950s-1990s', in J. Stanton (ed.), *Innovations in Health and Medicine: Diffusion and Resistance in the Twentieth Century*, London and New York: Routledge, 2002, pp. 106–25.

8 See, for example, A. Beyer and K. Winter (eds), *Lehrbuch der Sozialhygiene*, Berlin: VEB Verlag Volk und Gesundheit, 1959. Cardiovascular disease was the subject of a special issue of the GDR medical journal, *Das Deutsche Gesundheitswesen*, in 1956 (issue 11). Still, as far as public attention and interest by medical scientists and by policy-makers was concerned, cardiovascular disease long remained in the shadow of another so-called 'disease of civilisation', cancer.

9 Cf. E. Fischer, L. Rohland and D. Tutzke (eds), *Für das Wohl des Menschen*, vol. II, *Dokumente zur Gesundheitspolitk der Sozialistischen Einheitspartei Deutschlands*, Berlin: Volk & Gesundheit, 1979, p. 98.

10 For more information on the history of the Academy and the reforms leading to the 1972 restructuring, see H. Bielka, *Die Medizinisch-Biologischen Institute Berlin-Buch: Beiträge zur Geschichte*, Berlin: Springer, 1997; J. Reindl, 'Akademiereform und biomedizinische Forschung in Berlin-Buch,' in G.A. Ritter, M. Szöllösi-Janze and H. Trischler (eds), *Antworten auf die amerikanische Herausforderung: Forschung in der Bundesrepublik und der DDR in den 'langen' siebziger Jahren*, Frankfurt/New York: Campus, 1999, pp. 339–60; P. Nötzold, 'From German academy of sciences to socialist research academy', in K. Macrakis and D. Hoffmann (eds), *Science under Socialism: East Germany in Comparative Perspective*, Cambridge, MA: Harvard University Press, 1999, pp. 140–57.

11 Hecht, *What is Done to Protect People's Health*, p. 48. Hecht was head of the laboratory for experimental physiology and pathophysiology of higher nerve activity in Baumann's institute in the 1950s and early 1960s. Cf. *Jahrbuch der Deutschen Akademie der Wissenschaften*, 1958, p. 594; ibid., 1959, p. 456; ibid., 1960, p. 713; ibid., 1961, p. 717. In subsequent years co-workers are no longer listed.

12 Nötzold, 'From German academy of sciences to socialist research academy'.

13 The Kaiser Wilhelm Society was the precursor of today's Max Planck Society, one of the main umbrella organisations of research institutes in the Federal Republic of Germany. For the history of the Society, see B. vom Brocke and H. Laitko (eds), *Die Kaiser-Wilhelm-/Max-Planck-Gesellschaft und ihre Institute*, Berlin and New York: De Gruyter, 1996.

14 Bielka, *Die Medizinisch-Biologischen Institute Berlin-Buch.*

15 Ibid., pp. 62–8.

16 Nötzold, 'From German academy of sciences to socialist research academy', p. 147.

17 Cf. Fischer, Rohland and Tutzke (eds), *Für das Wohl des Menschen*, vol. II, p. 98.

18 Berlin Brandenburgische Akademie der Wissenschaften, Akademiearchiv (BBAA), Akademieleitung (AKL) 57, Arbeitsstelle für Kreislaufforschung, 1954–65.

19 Until the Berlin Wall was erected and the German–German border closed in 1961, the GDR government had serious problems with the provision of medical care, not least because a constant stream of young doctors, after passing their degrees, left the country for West Germany, where at the same time there was a surplus of doctors. Cf. A.-S. Ernst, *'Die beste Prophylaxe ist der Sozialismus': Ärzte und medizinische Hochschullehrer in der SBZ/DDR 1945–1961*, Münster: Waxmann, 1997; W. Süß, 'Gesundheitspolitik', in H.G. Hockerts (ed.), *Drei Wege deutscher Sozialstaatlichkeit: NS-Diktatur, Bundesrepublik und DDR im Vergleich*, München: Oldenbourg, 1998, pp. 55–100.

20 S. Kutzschmar and U. Hoffmann, 'Erleben, Erfahren, Erkennen: Akademiemitglied Albert Wollenberger erinnert sich', *Spectrum* 14(4), 1983: 14–17.

21 Bundesarchiv Berlin (BAB), DDR, DQ1 (Ministerium für Gesundheit), 2570, Abt. Wissenschaft: Kreislaufforschung 1955 – Protokolle über die Gründung des Arbeitskreises für Kreislaufforschung, März 1955.

22 Clinical (rather than laboratory-based, fundamental) research within the Academy remained a bone of contention. In 1967, the influential professor of clinical biochemistry, Samuel Mitja Rapoport, launched an ultimately unsuccessful initiative in the GDR Research Council to stop clinical research within the Academy and transfer the respective facilities, including Baumann's, into other institutional settings. Cf. BBAA, Forschungsgemeinschaft (FG) 191, Vorsitzender und Ständiger Stellvertreter; Institut für Kortiko-Viszerale Pathologie und Therapie, 1958–68.

23 BBAA, AKL 57, Arbeitsstelle für Kreislaufforschung, Protokoll der Sitzung des Präsidiums vom 1. Dezember 1955.

24 BBAA, AKL 57, Arbeitsstelle für Kreislaufforschung; FG 184, Vorsitzender und Ständiger Stellvertreter, Institut für Kreislaufforschung, 1956–68; FG 79, Vorsitzender und Ständiger Stellvertreter, Institut für Kreislaufforschung, 1956–66.

25 *Jahrbuch der Deutschen Akademie der Wissenschaften*, 1960, p. 751.

26 Cf., for example, I. Rapoport, *Meine ersten drei Leben. Erinnerungen*, Berlin: Edition Ost, 1997; 'Handschlag mit Roosevelt: Junge Welt sprach mit Albert Wollenberger,' *Junge Welt*, 12 January 1998; or S. Heym, *Nachruf*, Munich: Bertelsmann, 1988.

27 Interview with Professor Ernst Georg Krause, Berlin-Buch, 20 June 2001.

28 Ibid.

29 Kutzschmar and Hoffmann, 'Erleben, Erfahren, Erkennen', p. 14.

30 Ibid., p. 15; interview with E.G. Krause.

31 The article that Wollenberger published on the Wollenberger Clamp, jointly with the engineer and chemist Otto Ristau, is one of the most cited publications by a GDR scientist: A. Wollenberger, O. Ristau and G. Schoffa, 'Eine einfache Technik der extrem schnellen Abkühlung größerer Gewebestücke,' *Pflügers Archiv* 270, 1960: 399–412. Cf. E. Garfield, 'Uncitedness III – the importance of not being cited,' *Current Contents* 8, 21 February 1973: 5–6; www.garfield.library.upenn.edu/essays/V1p413y1962–73.pdf, accessed on 7 May 2003.

32 Interview with E.G. Krause.

33 Interview with E.G. Krause.

34 BBAA, AKL 57, Arbeitsstelle für Kreislaufforschung, Mendel an Wittbrodt, 30.1.1956.

35 BBAA, AKL 57, Arbeitsstelle für Kreislaufforschung, Protokoll über die Besprechung des Herrn Sekretärs der Klasse für Medizin, Prof. Lohmann, mit den Herren Kokkalis, Prof. Wollenberger u. Gründel im Beisein des Unterzeichneten [Kneller] am 19.6.1956 im Institut für Medizin und Biologie in Bln.-Buch.

36 BBAA, FG 184, Vorsitzender und Ständiger Stellvertreter, Institut für Kreislaufforschung, 1956–68, Kuratoriumsbeschluß Nr. K/66/13 vom 13. Juni 1962.

37 The publications of the Academy reveal little about Baumann's career before 1945.

38 R. Baumann, ''Klinische Forschungsabteilung für Schlaftherapie' in Berlin-Buch', *Das deutsche Gesundheitswesen* 9, 1954: 1001–3.

39 Cf. Ernst, *'Die beste Prophylaxe ist der Sozialismus'*, pp. 308–32.

40 E. von Skramlik, 'Die Auswirkungen der Lehre Pawlows', *Das deutsche Gesundheitswesen* 6, 1951: 887–907 and 917–40; E.M. Tarejew, 'Die Lehre Pawlows und die Aufgaben der klinischen Medizin', *Das deutsche*

Gesundheitswesen 6, 1951: 953–9; A.G. Iwanow, 'Die Lehre von der höheren Nerven tätigkeit und die pathologische Physiologie', *Das deutsche Gesundheitswesen* 6, 1951: 1337–40 and 1373–9.

41 S. Rapoport, 'Zur Pawlow-Tagung, Leipzig, 15.-16. Januar 1953', *Das deutsche Gesundheitswesen* 8. 1953: 29–31; L. Pickenhain, 'Bericht über die Pawlow-Tagung in Leipzig am 15. und 16. Januar 1953', *Das deutsche Gesundheitswesen* 8, 1953: 218–33; L. Pickenhain, 'Konsequenzen aus der Pawlow-Tagung in Leipzig 1953', *Das deutsche Gesundheitswesen* 8, 1953: 669–72; L. Pickenhain and Matthies, 'Arbeitstagung der Staatlichen Pawlow-Kommission der Deutschen Demokratischen Republik vom 15. bis 17. Januar 1954 in Leipzig', *Das deutsche Gesundheitswesen* 9, 1954: 457–71; 'Erfurt, Pawlow-Tagung am 2. und 3. Juli 1954', *Das deutsche Gesundheitswesen* 10, 1955: 593–5.

42 Quoted after Fischer, Rohland and Tutzke (eds), *Für das Wohl des Menschen*, vol II, p. 98.

43 BBAA, FG 191, Vorsitzender und Ständiger Stellvertreter, Institut für kortiko-viszerale Pathologie und Therapie, 1958–68.

44 *Jahrbuch der Deutschen Akademie der Wissenschaften*, 1960, p. 714.

45 *Jahrbuch der Deutschen Akademie der Wissenschaften*, 1959, p. 460; 1961, p. 727. See BBAA, FG 191 for diagram.

46 R. Baumann and G. Lange, 'Barrieren gegen Stress und Herzinfarkt: Gespräch mit Akademiemitglied Rudolf Baumann', *Spectrum* 9(11) 1978: 24–7.

47 Cf. reports on the work of the institute, BBAA, FG 62, Fachbereich Medizin und Biologie, Institut für Kortiko-Viszerale Pathologie und Therapie, 1961–8, Bericht über das Institut für kortiko-viszerale Pathologie und Therapie, 24.5.65; and Außenstelle Buch (Bu) A75, Rat der Direktoren, Institut für Kortiko-Viszerale Pathologie und Therapie, untitled, 8.8.67.

48 Baumann and Lange, 'Barrieren gegen Stress und Herzinfarkt' and H. Scheel (ed.), *Herz-Kreislauf-Forschung: Rudolf Baumann zum 70. Geburtstag*, Berlin: Akademie-Verlag, 1982.

49 BBAA, AKL 477, Beziehungen zu fremden Institutionen, Persönlichkeiten; BAB, DQ1, 5084, Sekretariat des Ministers, Prof. Friedeberger, Erarbeitung der Generalperspektive der medizinisch-wissenschaftlichen Forschung bis 1980, 1953, 1958–65. See also Hecht, *What is Done to Protect People's Health?*

50 H. Kraatz and W. Scheler, 'Medizinische Wissenschaft', in K. Winter (ed.), *Das Gesundheitswesen in der Deutschen Demokratischen Republik: eine Bilanz zum 25. Jahrestag der Staatsgründung*, Berlin: VEB Verlag Volk und Gesundheit, 1974, pp. 177–91, p. 181.

51 Bielka, *Die Medizinisch-Biologischen Institute*; BBAA, FG 79, Fachbereich Medizin und Biologie, Institut für Kreislaufforschung, 1962–8.

52 Interview with Hans-Dieter Faulhaber, 9 August 2001. See also K.-G. Eickenjäger, 'Zielobjekt: Herz-Kreislauf- und Krebserkrankungen,' *Spectrum* 3(6), 1972: 18–25, for some impressive pictures.

53 BBAA, AKL 477, Beziehungen zu fremden Institutionen, Persönlichkeiten, Thesen zur Entwicklung der medizinischen Wissenschaft in der DDR.

54 BBAA, FG 191, Institut für kortiko-viszerale Pathologie u. Therapie, 1958–68, Klare an Kraatz, 8.10.63.

55 The decentralised approach, interestingly, would have been much more similar to what was going on in West Germany, where plans to build a central cardiovascular research institute were never realised. Cf. Bundesarchiv Koblenz, B142/3634, Zentral-Forschungs-Institut für Herz- und Kreislauferkrankungen – Prof. Wollheim, 1965–7. Instead, the major West German funding body, the *Deutsche Forschungsgemeinschaft* had a *Schwerpunkt* (focus programme) on cardiovascular research and was funding groups at various university medical schools.

56 BBAA, FG 191, Institut für kortiko-viszerale Pathologie u. Therapie, 1958–68, Baumann an Klare, 9.11.1965.

57 Stiftung Archiv der Parteien und Massenorganisationen der DDR im Bundesarchiv (SAPMO), DY 30/vorl. SED/21924, Zur Weiterentwicklung des medizinischen Forschungspotentials.

58 SAPMO, DY 30/vorl. SED/21924, Erfahrungen des Sektors medizinische Wissenschaft und Ausbildung bei der Erarbeitung einer Analyse über die Leistungen und die Entwicklung der medizinischen Forschung als Grundlage für die Forschungskonzeption 1981–90; Diskussion für die Mitgliederversammlung am 20. Juni 1978.

59 For a comparison of the health systems of the GDR, the Federal Republic and Nazi Germany, see Süß, 'Gesundheitspolitik'.

60 A. Wollenberger, 'Kreislaufkrankheiten und Ernährung,' *Das deutsche Gesundheitswesen* 11, 1956: 1410–16; K. Winter, 'Verbreitung der Herz- und Kreislaufkrankheiten in der DDR. Einige Bemerkungen zu dem Artikel von A. Wollenberger, veröffentlicht in Heft 42/1956 dieser Zeitschrift,' *Das deutsche Gesundheitswesen* 12, 1957: 327–31.

61 Cf. H. Enke, 'Zur Entwicklung der medizinischen Statistik in der DDR', *Zeitschrift für die gesamte Hygiene* 23, 1977: 41–3. For Winter, see 'Nachruf', *Charité-Annalen*, 1987: 64–5. On Grotjahn, see D. Tutzke, *Alfred Grotjahn*, Leipzig: Teubner, 1979.

62 Cf. on this issue R.A. Aronowitz, *Making Sense of Illness: Science, Society, and Disease*, Cambridge: Cambridge University Press, 1998.

63 G. Schott, 'Professor Dr. med. habil. Karl Heinz Staube zum 90. Geburtstag', *Ärzteblatt Sachsen* 5, 2001: 191. See also K.-H. Straube, 'Epidemiologie und Dispensairebetreuung der Koronarerkrankungen', *Zeitschrift für die gesamte innere Medizin* 21, 1966: 582–7.

64 Cf. H. Redetzky, *Unsere Polikliniken: Entwicklung, Aufgaben und Ziele*, Berlin: Volk & Gesundheit, 1954.

65 K. Winter, 'Die Bedeutung der Dispensairebetreuung für die Volksgesundheit', *Das deutsche Gesundheitswesen* 12, 1957: 1549–52; H. Harmsen (ed.), *Die Dispensaire-Methode im Ambulatorium, in der Poliklinik und in der Werkgesundheitsfürsorge in der UdSSR und in Mitteldeutschland*, Hamburg: Akademie für Staatsmedizin, 1957; Fritz-Ludwig Schmidt, 'Über die Dispensairebetreuung Kreislauferkrankter,' *Das deutsche Gesundheitswesen* 14, 1959: 352–7.

66 See, for example: J. Knappe, G. Strube, K.-D. Dück and G. Knappe, 'Epidemiologische Untersuchungen zur Prävalenz der Hypertonie in Abhängigkeit von sogenannten Risikofaktoren', *Das deutsche Gesundheitswesen* 26, 1971: 2212–5.

67 S. Böthig, W. Barth and H. Hutzelmann, 'Die Häufigkeit der Koronarkrankheit, der Hypertonie und der peripheren arteriellen Durchblutungsstörungen bei 50- bis 54jährigen Männern einer großstädtischen Population: Ergebnisse der epidemiologischen Studie Berlin-Mitte', *Das deutsche Gesundheitswesen* 25, 1970: 1048–9. Böthig now works for the World Health Organization.

68 Interview with Jens-Uwe Niehoff, 7 August 2001. See also J.-U. Niehoff, 'Risikofaktoren – Risikofaktorentheorie – Risikokonzept: theoretische Voraussetzungen und Schwierigkeiten bei der Interpretation', *Zeitschrift für ärztliche Fortbildung* 72, 1978: 84–9 and 145–9.

69 S. Böthig, J. Knappe, H. Heine and G. Anders, 'Epidemiologie der Herz-Kreislauf-Krankheiten in der Deutschen Demokratischen Republik', *Das deutsche Gesundheitswesen* 27, 1972: 823–9.

70 Rainer Hohlfeld, 'Diskussion Herz-Kreislauf-Forschung', unpublished transcript.

71 Interview with Hans-Dieter Faulhaber, 9 August 2001; H.-D. Faulhaber and E. Manke, 'Gegen den hohen Blutdruck', *Spectrum* 12(5), 1981: 8–9.

72 Lothar Heinemann, 'Gesundheit: auf dem Weg zur Trendwende', *Spectrum* 18(7), 1987: 1–3.

73 'About the MDC: History', www.mdc-berlin.de/englisch/about_the_mdc/e_index.htm, accessed on 7 May 2003.

74 Sigerist, *Socialised Medicine*, p. 325.

Recommended further reading

H. Bielka, *Die Medizinisch-Biologischen Institute Berlin-Buch: Beiträge zur Geschichte*, Berlin: Springer, 1997.

A.-S. Ernst, *'Die beste Prophylaxe ist der Sozialismus': Ärzte und medizinische Hochschullehrer in der SBZ/DDR 1945–1961*, Münster: Waxmann, 1997.

K. Macrakis and D. Hoffmann (eds), *Science under Socialism: East Germany in Comparative Perspective*, Cambridge, MA: Harvard University Press, 1999.

G.A. Ritter, M. Szöllösi-Janze and H. Trischler (eds), *Antworten auf die amerikanische Herausforderung: Forschung in der Bundesrepublik und der DDR in den 'langen' siebziger Jahren,* Frankfurt and New York: Campus, 1999.

T. Schlich, 'Degrees of control: the spread of operative fracture treatment with metal implants: a comparative perspective on Switzerland, East Germany and the USA, 1950s–1990s', in J. Stanton (ed.), *Innovations in Health and Medicine: Diffusion and Resistance in the Twentieth Century*, London and New York: Routledge, 2002, pp. 106–25.

11 Science, markets and public health

Contemporary testing for breast cancer predisposition

Jean-Paul Gaudillière and Ilana Löwy

Introduction

Towards the end of 2000, as the USA was preparing for a new election year, President Clinton's health secretary, Dona Shallaly, received a thick report written by the 'Secretary's Advisory Committee on Genetic Testing'.[1] This committee had been established three years before in order to assess the rapid development of genetic testing in the USA. One of the mandates of the committee was to evaluate risks associated with new forms of medical investigation. In a vein that echoed the postwar discourse in favour of increased government regulation of the drug market, the committee recommended the creation of a special Food and Drug Administration-based review procedure for surveying newly invented genetic tests (FDA). The basic idea was to create marketing authorisations whose delivery would depend on an evaluation of both the technical feasibility, and the medical utility of DNA testing. This proposal did not follow any sort of 'public health' disaster like the Thalidomide scandal, which triggered the 1962 reform on drug evaluation.[2] It originated in the widespread suspicion that testing the genetic constitution of unborn or healthy individuals might be neither beneficial to the individual nor useful when viewed from a public health perspective. One specific medical innovation was at the very centre of the discussion that prepared the committee's task, namely the development of procedures for identifying chromosomal mutations predisposing women to early forms of breast cancer.

The story of the breast cancer (BRCA) genes, as well as the story of their uses, has attracted many comments from health professionals and social scientists. In spite of its exceptional character, the development of breast cancer predisposition testing is highly revealing of the changing relationship between science, medicine and the market. In the 1990s, research conglomerates ranging from pure academic consortia to private biotech start-ups have pursued the identification of these genes. Moreover, as soon as the sequences of the BRCA genes were identified, this new knowledge was patented. This early appropriation resulted in the establishment of a legal monopoly on the uses of the BRCA genes. This in turn deeply affected the development of cancer genetics, facilitating the creation of an autonomous testing market and raising concerns about the consequences of identifying 'high risk' individuals in terms of public health.

From a historical viewpoint, tensions between innovation, markets and public health have resulted in ongoing debates about regulation. Regulatory practices, like marketing permits for drugs, were meant to control and organise market operations. Regulation has however a broader meaning than simply defining the conditions under which medical goods may be sold. As argued in this paper, medical regulation does not focus solely on commercialisation; it also deals with the attribution of intellectual property, the development of professional guidelines, and the public assessment of new technologies. An analysis of BRCA testing thus reveals various forms of regulation and various sets of norms associated with the trajectory of one single innovation.

The BRCA story is also emblematic of another major trend in contemporary biomedicine, namely the mounting importance of health risk management, and more particularly of embodied risks. The main locus of traditional public health has been the 'unhealthy environment' seen as independent of the will of the individual. In the postwar era, the focus of intervention shifted to 'unhealthy behaviours'. With genetic testing, a new category of health risk is coming to the fore, the 'embodied risk', that is the incorporated vulnerability to a disease. The management of such risks is considered to be a matter of 'free' choice rather than a problem deserving state intervention: those who suffer from an increased probability are invited to act in specific ways in order to limit the risk. If they do not follow these recommendations, resulting adverse consequences will somehow be their responsibility. This problematic conjunction of genetic testing and risk management resulted, in the USA at least, in a plea for regulation advanced by a coalition, including doctors, patients/users and officials from public health services. They targeted what they perceived as proof of the inability of market forces to improve public health, and asked for new forms of control.

This chapter focuses on the uses of the BRCA genes as they illustrate the present configuration of medical research, market developments and state-based public health intervention. Compared with the 1960s, when drug evaluation and cancer risks attracted much attention, biomedicine and its conditions of production have changed. New actors have surfaced, and new values and habits have crystallised. We need to analyse afresh evidence and practices in order to discuss and back appropriate forms of regulation. As a contribution to this task, this chapter compares the development of breast cancer genetic testing in France and in the USA. This comparative approach has two advantages. First, it contributes to the identification of alternative systems of action and stimulates a discussion of their origins, since the development of BRCA testing has followed contrasted paths in countries characterised by different medical cultures and different health-care systems. In addition, by revealing alternative regulatory configurations, our comparisons help place in perspective the biotechnological model of innovation – often seen as the up-to-date and normal way of ensuring medical progress.

Models of ownership, models of testing

Until the late 1980s, the hereditary transmission of breast cancer was considered of little importance and was investigated in a limited number of laboratories and medical services.[3] The linkage between genes and cancer was merely a statistical entity. It was used by epidemiologists, who examined large populations of women affected with the disease and computed 'relative risks' for a combination of factors, ranging from age at first pregnancy to number of affected family relatives.[4] However, by the end of the 1990s the situation had changed radically. Thanks to the development of techniques in molecular biology, the cloning of genes responsible for human diseases had become a highly debated topic. In 1990, a group of researchers based in San Francisco and headed by Mary Claire King identified for the first time a gene involved in hereditary forms of breast cancer.[5] Chromosome 17 was the target. This discovery launched a highly competitive race for the identification and sequencing of these genetic factors.

Access to an adequate set of DNA markers, as well as access to families with cancer, are central requisites to the search for 'pathological' genes. Markers are necessary for mapping the genome, and finding a sequence whose transmission is correlated with the appearance of specific diseases within families or populations. Families with cancer are even more critical since they provide the pedigrees and DNA samples that constitute the basis of the quest. One way to access such families was to organise consultations in cancer genetics or 'oncogenetics' as it was often labelled. However, for most researchers the accumulation of interesting and informative cases was a slow process.

One way to accelerate the research process was therefore to participate in the 'International Breast Cancer Linkage Consortium'. This network was initiated in 1989 by researchers at the International Centre for Cancer Research in Lyon (France). It was envisioned as a flexible network for exchanging information and DNA markers. Regular workshops were also planned. Collaboration was nevertheless hampered by severe competition between laboratories and prospects of industrial developments. In the 1970s, human genetic research was free of marketing considerations. But this was no longer the case in the 1990s.[6] A clear sign of the increasing importance of property in biomedical research was the fact that DNA samples and other biological materials were not circulated between laboratories. Each team worked on 'its' families, while circulating (with variable delay) results from linkage analysis. Moreover, it was clear from the beginning that every participating team would pursue its own strategy for cloning and sequencing the genes.[7] As localisation became more and more precise, the intensity of communication scaled down. In other words, localisation was a common problem requiring common goods, while the identification of genetic sequences or their uses triggered strong competition.

A second strategy for gaining quick access to genetic material was developed by the start-up group Myriad Genetics, which actually won the sequencing race in 1994. The company was founded in 1990. The main entrepreneur, Mark Skolnick, a population geneticist and computer scientist, had been hired by the University of Utah to set up and use a familial database gathering information about the ancestors and descendants of the 10,000 Mormons who settled in Utah in the 1880s. In 1990, Skolnick negotiated privileged access to this database for researchers working for his company. Coupling the Utah cancer registry with the Mormon genealogies, Myriad's scientists got access to large and well-documented families with a cancer history. These families gave Myriad a clear edge in the search for BRCA genes.

Taking into account the centrality of property rights within contemporary genetic research, one may oppose two models of research organisation that shaped the history of BRCA gene research. One model may be called the clinical model and is well illustrated by cancer research in France. The second model may be labelled the biotech model. It is exemplified by the collaboration between the University of Utah and the private start-up group, Myriad Genetics.

The first breast cancer gene (BRCA1) was cloned and sequenced by this company, which also invented a new system of development and use of genetic knowledge. The success of Myriad was based not only on its privileged access to genetic resources. It was also based on the use of a novel strategy, which isolated the practice of molecular genetics from risk analysis and clinical work. Like most start-ups, Myriad was not financially viable. The creation and management of an important research infrastructure was only made possible by the collection of venture capital, both through specialised firms (after the early success of the mid-1990s) and through direct access to the Nasdaq. Development also depended on research contracts with large pharmaceutical companies. Initially the firm was selling preliminary results and promises of patents. For instance, Myriad started to work on BRCA after a large contract with Eli Lilly was signed. The division of labour and of proprietary rights between the pharmaceutical company and the start-up group was such that Eli Lilly would receive exclusive rights on all therapeutic developments, while Myriad kept all the rights on more short-term diagnostic developments. This agreement was based on the assumption that Myriad would be the first one to sequence the breast cancer genes, and that the company could secure large 'umbrella' patents on the use of such data.

Winning the race for the sequencing of BRCA1 was a major achievement, but this was not sufficient to control its medical applications. BRCA1 mutations were viewed as responsible for only 30–40 per cent of family-linked cases of breast cancer. A second gene, BRCA2, was eagerly sought. The results of the new race were controversial. Both Myriad and a group of British workers associated with the international consortium, and supported by the British charity Cancer Research Campaign (CRC), claimed priority. The US patent office attributed BRCA2 rights to the British group. Looking for partners, CRC sold an exclusive licence for all uses outside the UK to Oncormed, a US biotechnology company. Myriad contested Oncormed's rights in court, but, as is often the case, the dispute was settled by a financial agreement before the trial took place. Myriad acquired Oncormed's intellectual property rights. The Utah firm thus became the owner of 'umbrella' patents protecting the uses of BRCA sequences, putatively worldwide with the exception of the UK.

These financial intricacies are not only of interest for local investors since Myriad's patents are not ordinary patents. They may be called 'sequence' or 'gene' patents as they include a very broad definition of the invention. This may be illustrated by a rapid description of the main patent application regarding the BRCA1 gene.[8] The basic information documenting the invention – and its novelty – is the description of the molecular sequence of the gene. Half of the text actually consists of sequence data. The first claim is accordingly an umbrella demand covering all uses of both the nucleotide sequence of BRCA1 and the derived protein sequence. Specific claims then focus on all possible applications of the sequence: the design of mutation tests for cancer predisposition, the production of genetically modified animals, or the development of gene therapies. Such gene patents would not have been granted fifteen years ago. Their mere existence is vivid testimony to the very broad redefinition of patentability which has taken place since 1985.[9] The understanding of two criteria – novelty and industrial usefulness – has accordingly been revised.

First, gene patents tend to blur – if not eliminate – the distinction between invention and discovery. They provide a proprietary status for entities, which for a long time had been perceived as natural objects. Genes, like hormones or bacteria, could be discovered but not invented. The argument, which nowadays justifies the appropriation of DNA sequences, is that the work involved in identifying DNA and finding its chemical structure produces laboratory artefacts that are different from the gene in the organism. The same argument can however be applied to almost any experimental system. Historically it was at the very centre of the debates about the appropriation of chemicals derived from natural products.

A second point of contention is the necessity of an 'industrial usefulness' of the invention. Myriad patents provided limited insight into the technological uses of the sequence. Whereas diagnostic prospects could be described in some detail (although there was nothing new in the testing techniques proposed) nothing specific could be written about 'gene therapy', or 'transgenic animals'. As the function of the BRCA gene was not – and is still not – known, the nature of most industrial and medical applications could barely be specified. As argued by many legal specialists, this situation can easily lead to complex legal battles due to overlapping rights.

In 1998 when Oncormed's legal situation was settled, Myriad was free to exploit its monopoly on BRCA testing. Myriad considered developing the diagnostic market as a way of getting quick revenues from knowledge regarding predisposing genes. Because it was not possible to rapidly find out the function of BRCA genes diagnostic activities were not only more straightforward but also the only available applications. Usually holders of patents for diagnostic procedures either commercialise diagnostic kits or sell licences. Myriad decided, in contrast, to centralise BRCA testing, to create a sister firm, and to construct a local 'test factory'. This decision was partly based on technical reasons. The BRCA gene is very large, about ten times the size of an average gene, and its mutations are nearly exclusively 'private', that is mutations found in a single family. This situation made the manufacture of kits complex. Moreover, having successfully established a large sequencing platform for research purposes, Myriad could readily expand on this experience and the available facility, to offer diagnostic procedures based on an automated and complete analysis of the BRCA genes. This option materialised in a new sequencing platform, which was soon coupled with a mutation database bringing together all the mutations in BRCA1 or 2. Selling a service rather than a kit was, in addition, a cheap way to avoid regulation. Contrary to kits that are evaluated by the FDA, medical services in the USA are neither reviewed nor subjected to marketing authorisations.[10]

The development of Myriad's testing service reflects another important dimension of the start-up model of genetic innovation, namely the consumer-based organisation of access. In 1997, Myriad Genetics started an aggressive promotion of tests for BRCA mutations in the USA. The campaign included direct marketing to potential users. Under the slogan 'understanding your risk can save your life', the company put great emphasis on the fact that women have the right to access their genetic information, i.e. they have a right to know whether they are mutation carriers or not. Myriad's diagnostic service is advertised on the web.[11] Women can therefore assess their family status in order to determine whether they are part of the group that 'should' consider testing. If this is the case, the person can find the address of cancer centres or physicians who might write a prescription. Such broad access to tests is not only justified by women's 'right to know', but also by the possible benefits of early detection of malignancies in high-risk women, and better targeting of preventive measures for mutation carriers. However, 'high risk' is a problematic and unstable category. Boundaries depend on mathematical models used to calculate risk of breast cancer, and on the cut-off point used for defining 'high' risk.[12] Myriad's marketing practices have accordingly being criticised for pushing the notion of risk far beyond what may be considered reasonable.[13]

The service model is based on current practice in the field of medical biology: laboratory procedures are conducted in specialised units, which have no direct connection with clinical services. Testing for blood glucose or cholesterol level is done in financially autonomous units that operate within a particular segment of the medical market. The extension of this configuration to BRCA testing in the USA is illustrated by the following three features. First, Myriad's officials do not consider that they should limit writing of prescriptions to specialists in genetics or cancer. They argue that genetic testing is just like any other biological examination, the one single requirement of competency being that it be carried out by a doctor in medicine. Second, and more importantly, it is not the role of a service centre such as Myriad to organise follow-up and care. The service laboratory provides controlled, accurate results on the mutations. The rest of the procedure is up to the person tested and her physician. Genetic counselling is therefore not required to obtain a BRCA test. It is only strongly recommended by oncologists, geneticists and patient advocacy groups. These organisations are concerned that the lack of professional help in interpreting and accepting the results of genetic tests may be harmful. It is difficult to know how many tested women actually follow these recommendations. Early studies tended to indicate that one-third of the test prescriptions are filled out without organising any access to genetic counselling.[14] Finally, in order to stabilise the market, Myriad has looked for global testing contracts with insurance companies and large care providers, HMO being the most important one. Organisations like Kaiser in California, or Aetna nationwide, have included BRCA testing in their health packages.[15] In 2000, 38 per cent of insurers covered BRCA testing in women.[16] For them, offering the test is a way to attract healthy middle-class women who are still young. It is also an interesting management tool, even in the absence of premium modulation.

Knowing how many insured persons are at risk is interesting when planning future costs and prevention services. It is also valuable for rationalising clinical trajectories as BRCA-caused breast cancer may in the future prove to require different therapeutic approaches from those used in sporadic breast cancers.

The start-up model of genetic testing that prevails in the USA is centred on the activities and commercial strategies of the new biotechnological companies.[17] These firms act on a knowledge market, which expanded in the 1990s with the development of a new legal framework for defining the appropriation of genes and other biological entities. These firms manage research and development laboratories, while trading their knowledge base. This fragile status has pushed some medical start-up firms towards the independent development of genetic testing. They defend views from recent predictive medicine models, which favour individual autonomy, consumer choice as well as the postulated link between market competition and efficient technology.

In France, testing practices expanded on a different basis. Most cancer research in the country is conducted either in public hospitals or in the Centre de Lutte contre le Cancer (CLCC). These centres are hybrid organisations operating at the interface between the public and private sectors, i.e. they are charity-based centres although most of the money comes from the state.[18] They were created on a regional basis, and allocate laboratory research facilities and hospital beds for patients who participate in clinical trials or receive more routine treatments. In the 1990s, as the search for BRCA genes became more visible, some centres (Paris, Lyon and Marseille) established specialised oncogenetic clinics. The initial purpose was to enhance research. Persons with significant family histories would come to these services. They would give samples, help track other members of the family, and in return receive information on their risk status. As these clinics opened in treatment centres, the majority of the women followed for inherited forms of breast cancer already had the disease.

French laboratories thus combine routine tests for mutations in BRCA genes, the search for new predisposing genes, genetic counselling for individuals perceived to be at risk, the establishment of pedigrees, the collection of DNA samples, and the centralisation of data.[19] Since cancer genetics services are part of cancer centres, they exclusively perform tests for mutations, which increase susceptibility to malignancies. They are not concerned with predisposition to other diseases. Moreover, French physicians who follow women with a family history of breast cancer are not interested in non-genetic risks of cancer such as reproductive history or abnormalities of the breast tissue. Because of this type of division of labour between these centres and public hospitals, the supervision of women with hyperplasia, Ductal Carcinoma in Situ or Lobular Carcinoma in Situ, clustered calcifications or dense breast tissue may be delegated to radiologists, oncologists or breast surgeons within the same facility.

In France, the search for mutations is made through partial sequencing of the gene. In contrast to Myriad's total sequencing approach, partial sequencing is considerably cheaper. It is efficient when applied to the DNA of a family with high prevalence of breast cancer, but much less so when the probability of finding a mutation is low. This 'French' technical choice originated in the 'low-tech' nature of local genetics laboratories, which did not possess large sequencing facilities. The clinical context of the centres also explains this choice since the search for mutations starts as a rule with a person diagnosed with cancer. If the person who initiates the search is a woman who is free of cancer, but worried about the high incidence of breast or ovarian cancer among her relatives, she then needs to convince a family member who is already affected to undergo testing.

Another specific feature related to the unique clinical context of the French centres is the autonomy of the settings. Technical collaboration between cancer centres is minimal. Each regional unit is – as is the case in most clinical services – operating according to its own logic, something physicians view as a sign of competence and medical responsibility. Autonomy pervades the handling of patients, as well as the taking on of cases. As is the case for clinical records, family material does not circulate between centres. Moreover each oncogenetic unit tends to develop its own set of procedures for genetic analysis, without much interest for standardisation.[20]

Finally, one critical aspect of this model of oncogenetics is the near invisibility of a profit motive in research.[21] French physicians working in cancer genetic units did not, in our interviews, express a particular distrust of commercial operations; they simply did not say much about commercialisation of tests and the development of their practices. Tests are paid with research funds, which are allocated on the basis of grants and umbrella appropriations for cancer centres. Like most clinicians working in elite research hospitals in France, cancer specialists do not need to take into account strong cost/benefit constraints, or to handle the administrative and commercial development of their inventions. The prevailing feeling is that everything that is medically justified should somehow be made available. Consequently, neither technological nor proprietary issues have attracted much attention. For instance, in contrast to molecular biologists working in local state research agencies (INSERM and CNRS), who have been more influenced by new trends in biotechnology, gene patents remained outside the scope of action of those French physicians working in the field of cancer genetics. No patent applications for the 'invention' of BRCA sequences, or the development of testing techniques, were made in France. Moreover, as a powerful indication of this reluctance to participate in the new research market, several thousand clinicians signed a petition in 1999 asking for a revision of the European patent law that would forbid the ownership of DNA sequences from human genes. This move was finally echoed in the decision made by the Institut Curie (a leading cancer centre in Paris) to challenge Myriad patents in court.[22]

The contrast between US and French modes of testing calls for two additional comments. The first is that this clinical model is not specific to France. It may be found in the USA as well. Close integration of research on breast cancer families, assessment of cancer risk, and treatment of existing tumours have surfaced in medical schools of various universities such as Harvard University, University of Pennsylvania or the University of California San Francisco (UCSF). The case of UCSF is worth mentioning as M.C. King's group was the first group to localize BRCA1 in the 1990s.

The UCSF breast cancer genetics unit practised counselling, but did not combine genetic analysis with clinical care. As practised by French physicians, this group balanced cancer genetics with cautious involvement in the research market. They did not engage in any sort of industrial collaboration beyond the classical academic practice of trading some results for instrumentation. The Berkeley team developed a perspective on BRCA genes that excluded short-term applications. They believed that the main use of BRCA sequences would be the implementation of new treatments, something that would only become possible once the biological functions of predisposing genes were clarified. Accordingly, they focused research on the biology of the gene, while considering that therapeutic developments would take place within or in collaboration with large pharmaceutical firms.

A second comment is that the start-up model would not have prevailed, if it had been exclusively rooted in market forces. The culture of medical risk is an equally powerful incentive for its development. This culture has a long history in the USA where it is more visible in public debates.[23] The strong emphasis placed on medical risk provided a ready-made 'demand' for what Myriad could offer. In the case of breast cancer, the notion of risk was at first promoted by the women's health movement. 'Breast cancer risk clinics', which were opened by several major hospitals in the 1980s, may be seen as specialised offshoots of the women's health centres established during the previous decade. These risk clinics deal with all aspects of breast cancer risks (heredity, suspicious mammographic images, pre-cancerous conditions). They can provide psychological support, advise women about preventive as well as financial options, and help them negotiate with their insurance companies and HMOs. Risk clinics are directed to middle-class, educated and health-conscious women, who manage their health risks through a judicious consumption of medical resources. Such 'enlightened consumerism', which includes, when appropriate, genetic tests, is encouraged rather than opposed by medical experts. The part played by the contemporary culture of risk in the BRCA story brings up another question, which is the issue of how these contrasted forms of research organisation are related to the medical meaning of genetic testing.

Managing genetic predisposition: what to do once the 'at risk' status has been determined

The principle of autonomy is often presented as crucial to the legitimacy of genetic testing. Women have a 'right to know'. They also have a 'right not to know'. This principle does not extend, however, to risk management. Physicians exercise strong pressure on the persons 'at risk' to follow medical recommendations to undergo regular clinical tests, mammographic and ovarian echographic procedures. A woman who tests positive for BRCA mutation, and then decides to opt out and refuses intensive medical supervision, is seen as displaying deviant behaviour that warrants psychological consultation. The supervision issue is however complicated by the absence of consensus on the efficacy of preventive measures in diminishing mortality from breast cancer in BRCA mutation carriers. Three options are usually mentioned, i.e. intensive mammographic monitoring, hormonal chemoprevention, and preventive mastectomy, but specific recommendations vary greatly from one country to the other, and among centres in the same country.

Cancer experts uniformly consider intensive mammographic, echographic and clinical monitoring of women at risk to be a basic requirement. In France, cancer centres have opened special services for BRCA mutation carriers, especially for young women who are not usually followed for breast cancer risk.[24] These services are presented as an extension of oncology clinics. Their existence is justified by the need to follow this specific population and accumulate epidemiological data on risk management. In the USA the resources open to women at risk reflect a generally heterogeneous medical situation. The management of BRCA mutation carriers is not distinct from the supervision of women 'at risk' in general. The level of supervision may vary from simple mammograms to the use of sophisticated imagery such as Nuclear Magnetic Resonance techniques. It varies according to the techniques available in the institution where follow-up takes place. It depends on the views of the physicians in charge, and to a great extent on the financial resources and health insurance plan of the diagnosed person.

There is widespread agreement among professionals regarding the preventive value of oophorectomy to prevent ovarian cancer.[25] By contrast, attitudes toward preventive mastectomy vary greatly.[26] In France, this proce-dure is exceptional and was not, until recently, actively encouraged by experts. It is provided if a woman requests it. BRCA-positive women who have developed a small cancer or pre-cancerous cells are however frequently advised to undergo a preventative mastectomy of the unaffected breast. This choice is justified in terms of a higher risk for developing a tumour in the other breast. In the USA, more BRCA-positive women undergo prophylactic mastectomy, considered to be the most effective means of prevention.[27] Differences may be related to cultural factors, and body image issues. They are also the product of local professional cultures. For instance, in the USA, the improvement of cosmetic results from breast reconstruction may have contributed to a better acceptance of prophylactic mastectomies, and to stronger working relationships between oncologists and surgeons.

One of the main criticisms concerning the introduction of genetic tests for BRCA mutations has been the absence of efficient (and acceptable) preventive measures for individuals identified as being 'at risk'. As a result, there was a strong interest in the 1990s in the preventive potential of selec-tive oestrogen receptor modulators (SERM) such as Tamoxifen, thought to be a promising avenue for chemoprevention of breast cancer. Tamoxifen (an anti-oestrogen) was initially administered to prevent local recurrence of breast cancer. At first, only post-menopausal women with tumours positive for oestrogen receptors were viewed as good candidates for Tamoxifen therapy. The recent tendency to intensify drug therapy of breast cancer led to an increased use of a combination of chemotherapy with Tamoxifen (previously women were treated by either chemotherapy or Tamoxifen), as well as the administration of Tamoxifen to pre-menopausal women and women with oestrogen receptor-negative tumours. It finally led to attempts to use this drug to prevent breast cancer in 'high risk' women.

In the USA, women were classified 'at risk', following a model (the Gail model) that takes into account hereditary and non-hereditary risk elements. In Europe women were recruited on the basis of their family history alone. Both European trials and the US trial reported identical findings. Tamoxifen did prevent breast tumours in high-risk women, but the treatment was asso-ciated with iatrogenic complications, such as endometrial cancer, thrombosis and lung embolism, and possibly stroke.[28] The conclusions drawn from the European and the US trials were, however, very different. The FDA approved the use of Tamoxifen in 1998 for reducing breast cancer risk. The Europeans concluded that this type of use of Tamoxifen was not justified and recommended the continuation of clinical trials.

The FDA's approval of the preventive use of Tamoxifen (Novaldex®) was followed in the USA by an aggressive publicity campaign conducted by the manufacturer of this drug. Advertisements in magazines and on billboards urged women 'to know their breast cancer assessment number', and, if this number is higher than 1.7 (that is, more than 1.7 per cent chance to develop breast cancer in the next five years), to consider prophylactic use of Novaldex. The publicity was written in an 'empowering' style: women were invited to collect information by talking with competent professionals, then to take their own, informed decisions.[29] Cancer activists who criticised the Novaldex campaign argued that it exploited women's fears of breast cancer and preyed on their often highly exaggerated representation of their risk level. Breast Cancer Action sponsored counter-publicity aimed at sensitising women to the danger of being manipulated by drug manufacturers. Paradoxically, however, women (white, middle class) considered it was this counter-campaign rather than the Novaldex publicity that was dishonest and manipulative, a telling illustration of the success of an individualised 'risk management' approach among some strata of the US population.[30]

In spite of this push towards chemoprevention, the uncertainties of breast cancer risk management have been the subject of numerous public debates and, in the USA at least, led to proposals for increased surveillance of the field of medical genetics.

Regulation practices: the state, the medical profession and patient advocacy groups

The notion that molecular genetics should be regulated can be traced back to debates about the risks associated with early transfer of DNA between species, i.e. the genetic engineering controversy in the 1970s.[31] In the 1970s, critics considered laboratory work as a possible source of danger. They distrusted the ability of professional scientists to recognise and control the risks they created, especially when pursuing technological aims and/or when collaborating with industry. In the 1990s, critics of biomedicine are more concerned about failure, bureaucratic entrenchment, identities and domination than about capitalism and the quest for profit. This displacement has led to new alliances and practices, best illustrated by the mobilisation of AIDS advocacy groups, especially in their attempt to control the aims and methods of clinical research.[32] As a result, the whole issue of how one should regulate innovations in molecular medicine has been redefined, leaving space for new modes of intervention, which overlap with, and sometimes oppose, the classical arenas, i.e. professional committees and governmental agencies. These displacements are aptly reflected in contemporary discussions over the regulation of genetic testing.

Questions regarding the legitimate uses of genetic knowledge have been rampant since the launch of the Human Genome Project.[33] They have generally focused on two sets of issues: 1) the possible discrimination related to the use of test results by insurers and employers; 2) the consequences and expected limitations of prenatal diagnosis. Interestingly, breast cancer predisposition testing has introduced a different type of problem since the practice gains its legitimacy by investigating healthy individuals in order to reduce individual risks. Among women and medical practitioners, concerns about the consequences of expanding the practice of diagnosing BRCA mutations have consequently been reinforced by the above-mentioned uncertainty concerning medical follow-up. Debates about regulation have been much more visible in the USA than in France. Factors contributing to this difference may include contrasting political systems, the US tradition of public lobbying, or the traditional French alliance between the state and professional corporations. New developments associated with the politics of identity, its medical translation, and the search for more democratic forms of expertise have however played an increasing role, as genetic testing has become a public health issue.

The discussion on predisposition testing has, in the USA, developed in two stages. The first step was a professional phase that focused on issues of quality control. It was followed by a second debate initiated by public health authorities, which targeted problems of marketing, clinical utility and efficacy. The first phase started in the mid-1990s (before Myriad achieved its large-scale testing platform) with an accumulation of guidelines produced by various medical groups. These guidelines were written for those practitioners who prescribe and interpret BRCA mutation data. One typical and widely discussed example concerns the guidelines published by the American Society of Clinical Oncology (ASCO).[34] An appropriate level of access was envisioned wherein all women for whom the probability of finding a mutation was 10 per cent should be targeted. ASCO barely discussed the issue of medical follow-up or risk reduction strategies and insisted upon the importance of providing genetic counselling. Patients' freedom of choice rather than regulation or administrative evaluation was perceived as the most important principle for handling the potentially adverse consequences of the innovation. In parallel, ASCO quite unambiguously endorsed the model of a free medical market and the idea of privately organised testing services. The only issue considered to be a target for regulation was quality control. The basic proposal defended by ASCO leaders was to extend and modify the CLIA system of approval already in operation for all laboratories doing medical tests. These CLIA norms define conditions for running a biological facility. They specify basic requirements such as proper sterilisation or refrigerating equipment, as well as minimal personnel training. ASCO's objective was to add specific requirements in order to ensure the quality of genetic tests.

During the second phase, regulations developed along very different lines. One major difference with the French situation was the mobilisation of patient advocacy groups. For instance, ASCO's rules were first published and discussed in a special issue of the *Journal of Clinical Oncology*. Mark Skolnick from Myriad Genetics, who was invited to comment, stressed that the proposal was quite reasonable. In his view, regulation should remain a matter of self-accepted professional recommendations that respect women's freedom of choice. This plea for informed *laissez-faire* came under attack in the same issue by Frances Visco, from the National Breast Cancer Coalition (NBCC), a powerful organisation of women activists. She argued in favour of less rather than more testing, as the fate of those women labelled at risk was totally uncertain. The women's health organisation thus opposed the professional suggestion of wide access to BRCA testing in all cancer clinics, explaining that genetic screening should only be organised in clinical research centres, and made available only to individuals who agree to join peer-reviewed and approved research protocols.

This critical perspective from NBCC must be understood within the framework of a more general move towards the practice of getting second opinions, which has affected the cancer scene in the USA, with no comparable trend in continental Europe. This move has complex roots including the rise of environmental activism and its associated interest in carcinogenic chemicals, as well as the feminist movement. The women's health movement developed autonomous evaluations of medical claims, and a form of woman-centred medical culture. This in turn put pressure on medical practitioners. In the area of cancer, one major change was the gradual disappearance of radical mastectomy after a diagnosis of breast cancer.[35]

In the 1990s, a new wave of mobilisation in favour of women's health issues emerged in the form of local breast cancer organisations, created in large cities like Boston, Los Angeles, San Francisco and New York City. Many of these organisations originated in self-help or support groups sometimes linked with specialised cancer clinics. As mentioned above, these groups were led by a new generation of patients: middle-aged women. Following the example of AIDS activists, they were critical of existing cancer policies and cancer treatment practices.[36] Activists participating in Save Ourselves, Breast Cancer Action, or Bay Area Breast Cancer Network thus articulated new themes that diverged from the classical approach followed by organizations like the American Cancer Society, which played a critical role in the rise of biomedical research after 1945.[37] First, they argued that breast cancer had become an epidemic with a (rapidly) increasing incidence. Second, they explained that – in spite of all claims to the contrary – treatments have not been much improved over the past thirty years. Chemotherapy in particular has become a dubious field, characterised by massive research investment, great benefit for the pharmaceutical industry, temporary positive effects in many forms of breast cancer, and multiple adverse side-effects for the patients. Finally, breast cancer support groups claimed that this situation should be compared with other medical areas, where important advances have been made since the 1960s (for instance cardiovascular disorders). According to these women's groups, this contrast is explained by the fact that the existing biomedical complex does not consider women's health as a priority.

In 1990, these local groups decided to establish an umbrella organisation, which would help co-ordinate their action at the federal level. This umbrella structure became the National Breast Cancer Coalition. One of the targets of their co-operative action was to lobby the Congress and the Federal Administration for 'more money' to fight breast cancer. This proved highly successful as the coalition managed, in 1993 (in the early days of the Clinton era), to reroute 300 million dollars from the defence budget into cancer research. Following this achievement, the NBCC initiated a discussion about the type of research that should be supported. As the coalition became an obligatory partner for the health administration, it developed its own criteria for evaluating projects, innovations and their uses. This led the NBCC to collaborate with specific groups of researchers and clinicians, to increase the giving of advice, organise controversial debates, acculturate members to the biomedical discourse, and develop their ability to participate in various evaluation committees, both at local and federal level. A discussion about genetic testing emerged out of these practices of scientific empowerment.

The culture of advocacy and lay expertise shared by many NBCC members was echoed in an alternative set of guidelines constructed by a panel from the Program in Genomics, Ethics and Society at the University of Stanford.[38] Although it was a pluralistic academic gathering, the Stanford panel was strongly influenced by participants from the West Coast women's health movement. The Stanford recommendations were first presented in the *Journal of Women's Health*, as a tacit alternative to the above mentioned ASCO guidelines. The Stanford committee questioned the benefits of the innovation, the new economy of knowledge, and the misuses of genetic information. For instance, it made a specific connection between appropriation and the practice of testing.[39] Echoing NBCC views, the Stanford group looked cautiously if not suspiciously at the usefulness of BRCA testing outside the research context.[40] Moreover they considered that marketing might well aggravate the problem.[41] Members of the Stanford panel were suspicious of the logic of consumerism and special-interest parties, and preferred to follow the powerful example of drug regulation. Thus they suggested that the FDA or another federal agency monitor the testing market and establish a system of marketing authorisations.[42]

The quest for some sort of government regulation was not specific to the Stanford panel, since the NIH Task Force on Genetic Testing was also thinking along similar lines. This group was established in 1994 as part of the Ethical, Legal and Sociological Investigations (ELSI) section of the NIH-based human genome program (National Institute of Health).[43] This semi-official structure brought together a large body of interested parties:

governmental agencies, medical societies, patient associations as well as representatives from health insurance companies and the biotech industry. The aim was to investigate the status of genetic testing in the USA and suggest recommendations for improving the safety and efficiency of testing. Between 1995 and 1998, debates focused on delineating the nature of the relationship between the federal government and professionals. Regulation was understood in terms of governmental initiative, focusing on the issue of whether the FDA should or should not oversee the testing market. Advocates of regulation, public health officials and academic experts argued that such surveillance, including a system of marketing permits and collective standards, was indispensable in order to limit the adverse effects of commercialisation, achieve high quality, and medical usefulness. Most actors operating on the medical market opposed this perspective. They considered that the most important risk for society was that a small group of bureaucrats decide in the place of interested parties, slow down innovation, and deprive patients of the benefits of testing in order to complete endless studies of efficiency. Not too surprisingly, no consensus on the possible role of the FDA could be reached. The Task Force merely decided that another advisory body should be mandated in order to conduct more specific recommendations.

The Task Force on Genetic Testing nonetheless framed the US regulatory debate in one essential way: it specified why genetic tests should require a particular form of surveillance. The argument was that these tests provide a special form of information with wide-ranging effects in terms of personal identity, as well as medical and social status. This view implied that some tests (predisposition testing in particular) would require 'stringent scrutiny', one of the aims being the evaluation of the clinical usefulness of the test under consideration.

In 1998 the Health Secretary announced the establishment of a Secretary's Advisory Committee on Genetic Testing (SACGT).[44] The administration took one year to decide about its composition. In contrast to the Task Force, most of its members were users and producers of tests rather than governmental and public health officials. SACGT's activities were not limited to the congressional model of lobbying. Following a preliminary report, steps were taken in the direction of setting up a public forum and included an official call for comments published in the Federal Register as well as the organisation of a one-day assembly during which the work of the committee was discussed by patients and their organisations.[45]

These events and discussions generated three types of comments. First, start-ups and test manufacturers unambiguously resented the proposed draft of recommendations. All involved companies criticised the idea that the FDA should somehow regulate the supply of tests. They all stressed that performing genetic testing is equivalent to the measurement of any other biological parameter, such as the blood concentration of glucose. Second, medical associations were very cautious about state intervention. One group grudgingly accepted the need for some federal regulation of the testing market while arguing that research activities as well as routine testing for rare pathologies should not be submitted to legal restrictions. Another group of professionals – including medical geneticists – opposed a general regulatory framework. Only one professional body, the National Society of Genetic Counselors, echoed the committee's commitment to pre- and post-marketing clinical evaluation. In its comments, the society strongly recommends the creation of a permanent genetic advisory panel to help the FDA develop criteria 'to assess benefit and risk of genetic tests', 'to differentiate categories of tests' and 'establish criteria for regular review'. Finally, few patient organisations discussed the question of usefulness and efficacy. The NBCC was in this respect quite isolated. Most patient activists concentrated on problems of access and confidentiality. Fears of having results from genetic tests used to deny or to raise insurance premiums (something the very structure of the US healthcare system makes quite plausible) were the main topics of inquiry and the source of numerous pleas for governmental intervention.

Following these debates, the SACGT adopted a first set of proposals, which were sent to the Health Secretary.[46] This white paper clearly stated that 'the FDA should be involved in the review of all genetic tests', but 'the review should be appropriate to the level of complexity of the information generated by the test'. BRCA-like tests were perceived as being the most problematic.[47] Possible adverse consequences of testing included feelings of anxiety for the persons labelled at high risk, the multiplication of useless operations, the existence of irreversible and controversial means of prevention, and the social stigma associated with the status of a person at risk. The final report from the committee was made public in the fall of 2000: it again stressed that genetic tests raise specific issues and require particular scrutiny in view of their potential harmfulness.[48] Two mechanisms for evaluation were detailed. The first one summarised debates about data collection. The inventors were considered responsible for the first phase of data collection. During test development, when problems involve the quantification of mutation frequencies and technological performances, the biotechnological and pharmaceutical developers should organise their own studies in order to collect enough information to support the application for a marketing permit. Clinical usefulness should be evaluated during a second phase on a more long-term basis by means of a new structure, a genetic testing data bank that would be run by public health services and by the industry. Moreover:

> FDA should be the federal agency responsible for the review, approval and labeling of all new genetic tests that have moved beyond the basic research phase. The level of review applied by FDA should correlate with the level of scrutiny warranted by the test. Using criteria informed by standards already in place in professional organizations and based on and integrated with existing regulations, such as CLIA, FDA must

delineate review processes for pre-market evaluation of genetic tests. These processes should focus on evaluation of the data regarding the analytical and clinical validity, as well as on claims made by the developer of the tests about its clinical utility.

Genetic test surveillance would accordingly be aligned with drug regulation, thus remaining a domain of professional expertise. In order not to completely eliminate the participation of 'final users of tests', another level of regulation was proposed:

> Because the FDA's review will focus on assuring the analytical and clinical validity of a test, the agency's capacity to assess the ethical and social implication of a test may not be sufficient. The Secretary should consider the development of a mechanism to ensure the identification and appropriate review of tests that raise major social and ethical concerns.[49]

These recommendations were endorsed by the administration shortly before the 2001 presidential elections. Following the return of a Republican administration that is hostile to the development of state 'control', SACGT's proposals were not implemented. Testing for BRCA mutations remains as now in the domain of market and professional regulation.

Compared to the US situation, the French regulatory debates offer an interesting combination of similarities and differences. Equivalent professional rules of good practice were produced by a group of geneticists and oncologists assembled by INSERM and the national federation of cancer centres.[50] In contrast to the US framework, French specialists insisted that BRCA testing be completed by specialised multidisciplinary services. The basic plan was a *consultation d'oncogénétique* combining molecular analysis, risk assessment, psychological support and medical follow-up. In contrast to ASCO's recommendations, the French recommendations took the form of guidelines for hospital clinicians. For instance, when discussing medical options for different groups of women at risk, i.e. patients already diagnosed with ovarian cancer or breast cancer, or persons with no symptoms, French researchers reluctantly raised surgical options. Echoing the view that hospital work has to do neither with commercial activities nor with industrial standardisation, French experts avoided issues of marketing and organised quality control.

The latter issue nonetheless surfaced. The possibility of creating a legal framework for genetic tests was actually raised by another professional group: the French association of medical geneticists. Pointing to the vast heterogeneity of competencies among laboratories, geneticists from this group felt that the health administration should participate in the regulation of practices.[51] They pleaded for the organisation of a national system of quality control based on two processes. The first one involved a general certification procedure for deciding whether a given laboratory may or may not perform genetic tests (one may compare this with the CLIA system in the USA). The second process involved a nationwide system of quality checks organised for the tests that were most frequently requested. A special committee connected with the Ministry of Health implemented both recommendations. This committee brought together a majority of medical geneticists, a few officials from the public health administration, but did not include representatives from either the industry or from voluntary organisations. The regulatory alliance has therefore taken the classical form of a convergence of elite clinicians and state administrators. This alliance pushed forwards the internal organisation of the profession, imposing on clinicians minimal rules of quality control. Two fears justify the idea of a state-based surveillance system. First, molecular geneticists feared that anyone could begin testing without having the necessary (analytical) knowledge. This typical issue of expert knowledge was linked to another organisational issue, namely the fear that after the first wave of creation of medical genetics laboratories within research hospitals, the increase in the number of small centres would result in technical inefficiency and inaccurate results. Both concerns were articulated as public health concerns, i.e. problems of accuracy leading to poor management of the patients, but they remained framed in terms of collective intra-professional organisation. Ironically, in order to establish this type of technical control by professional organisations, the intervention of the state proved indispensable.

Conclusion

In a recent article on the technoscientific transformations of US medicine, the historian Adele Clarke and her collaborators discuss a second wave of medicalisation of health and illness, which they describe as a process of *biomedicalisation*.[52] Many aspects of the 'second transformation of American medicine' resonate with those issues investigated in this paper. According to Clarke and her co-authors, biomedicalisation consists of several interactive processes including the increasing privatisation of research, the development of managed care-dominated systems, the focus on risk and surveillance, increasingly molecular and technological forms of intervention, and the customisation of bodies and means of intervention. This work analyses how processes that are typical of this biomedicalisation, i.e. new forms of intellectual property and research organisation, the development of patient advocacy groups, or the redefinition of risk at the genetic and molecular level, have coalesced in new regimes of testing. Although this new trend towards biomedicalisation may be a global phenomenon, our comparison also shows that the practice of BRCA testing, as well as its economic and legal status, are shaped by technical and administrative arrangements that are different in France and in the USA. These differences between national contexts thus illustrate the notion that different, and sometimes conflicting, regimes of production and use of biomedical knowledge may co-exist.

Our paper focused on the changing relationship between science, medicine and the market. From a historical perspective, the relationships between innovation, markets and public health are defined in terms of regulation. Regulatory practices, like the establishment of marketing permits for drugs, are aimed at controlling and organising market operations for the good of the public. These practices are deemed necessary since market operators pursue their own economic interests. As argued above, medical regulation – when approached through the analysis of practices – not only focuses on commercialisation, but also deals with the attribution of intellectual property, the creation of professional guidelines, or the public assessment of technologies. Issues related to intellectual property are intertwined with professional and institutional arrangements that shape the use made of medical innovations.

Debates about BRCA testing suggest that the contemporary reorganisation of the research system has created a configuration in which new ways of defining 'public health' compete with the old professional regime. The latter is well illustrated by the French configuration. It is characterised by the professional nature of medical regulation, with expert clinicians acting on behalf of the state and mistrusting market developments as well as the industrialisation of medical services. The first mode has its roots in the new market economy of the gene characterised by gene patents, and the start-up system of research. It is a technological and consumer-oriented approach to regulation. Within this framework, genetic procedures are like any other bioassay or technical service. Testing for hereditary predisposition is an option, which should be offered to individuals, who collect information from various sources and make their best personal choices. Freedom of access is therefore essential to the public good and the advancement of health. Collective regulation should take the form of guidelines whose application may be controlled by professional bodies. This approach may be shared by advocacy groups, which are operating as collectively organised consumers of biomedical goods. These groups consider that their responsibility is to facilitate access to up-to-date technologies. The same type of organisation may, as shown by the activities of the NBCC, favour another framework, a third mode of definition of public health, which stresses patients' autonomy and self-help, and favours practices of lobbying and getting second opinions. The latter practices, at least as long as there is political space for such activity, make controversies visible, and open spaces for discussion. Regulation consequently focuses on the creation of committees and management bodies that reflect the plurality of interests in the biomedical arenas and their unequal power, and help construct compromises in the form of contextualised recommendations. Mistrust in market forces as well as mistrust in the capacity of biomolecular innovations to solve health problems accordingly gave birth to a vision of risk technologies as being technologies at risk.

Notes

1 Secretary's Advisory Committee on Genetic Testing, *Enhancing the Oversight of Genetic Tests: Recommendations of the SACGT*, Washington: NIH, 2000.
2 H.M. Marks, 'Confiance et méfiance dans le marché: les statistiques et la recherche clinique', *Sciences sociales et santé* 18(4), 2000: 9–28.
3 H.T. Lynch, *Dynamic Genetic Counseling for Clinicians,* Springfield: Charles C. Thomas, 1969.
4 E. Anderson, H.O. Goodman and S.C. Reed, *Variables Related to Human Breast Cancer*, Minneapolis: The University of Minnesota Press, 1958; B. Lerner, *The Breast Cancer Wars*, New York: Oxford University Press, 2001.
5 K. Davis and M. White, *Breakthrough: the Quest to Isolate the Gene for Hereditary Breast Cancer*, London: Macmillan, 1995.
6 P. Dasgupta and P. David, 'Towards a new economics of science', *Research Policy* 23, 1994: 487–521; R. Eisenberg, 'The move towards the privatization of biomedical research', in C.E. Barfield and L.R. Smith (eds), *The Future of Biomedical Research*, New York: AEI Press, 1997, pp. 123–46.
7 This statement, as well as many others in this paper, is based on a series of interviews we conducted with various actors involved in the BRCA gene story. Interviews were completed both in France and in the USA. The series included eighteen molecular geneticists and breast cancer specialists, ten patent lawyers or intellectual property managers, seven health administrators or public health specialists, six officials in breast cancer patient advocacy groups (in the USA only).
8 US PTO, Patent application by Myriad Genetics, '17q-Linked Breast and Ovarian Cancer Susceptibility Gene'.
9 A. Thackray (ed.), *Private Science: Biotechnology and the Rise of the Molecular Sciences*, Philadelphia: University of Pennsylvania Press, 1998; D. Kevles, *A History of Patenting Life in the United States; with Comparative Attention to Europe and Canada*, Report to the European group on Ethics, Bruxelles: European Community, 2002; B. Coriat (ed.), *Les Droits de propriété intellectuelle: nouveaux domaines, nouveaux enjeux*, special issue, *La Revue d'economie industrielle* 99, 2002.
10 N. Holtzman, 'Are genetic tests adequately regulated', *Science* 286, 1999: 409.
11 www.myriad.com.
12 M.H. Gail, L.A. Brinton, D.P. Byar, *et al.*, 'Projecting individual probabilities of developing breast cancer for white females who are being examined annually', *Journal of the National Cancer Institute* 81, 1989: 1879–86.
13 Following these critical comments, particularly those expressed by the National Breast Cancer Coalition (see below), Myriad's site has been modified, leading to a very significant reduction of the population of women who might consider taking a test.
14 M.K. Cho, P. Sankar, P.R. Wolpe and L. Godmilow, 'Commercialization of BRCA testing: practitioner awareness and use of a new genetic test', *American Journal of Medical Genetics* 83, 1999: 157–63.
15 S. Kutner, 'Breast cancer genetics and managed care: the Kaiser Permanente experience', *Cancer* 86, 1999: 1750–4. S. Parthasarathy 'Regulating Risks: Defining Genetic Privacy in the US and Britain' *Science, Technology and Human Values* 9, 2004: 332–352.
16 H.M. Kuerer, E.S. Hwang, J.P. Antony, *et al.*, 'Current national health insurance coverage policies for breast and ovarian cancer prophylactic surgery', *Annals of Surgical Oncology* 7, 2000: 325–32.
17 S. Hilgartner and N. Holtzman, 'State of the art of genetic testing in the United States: survey of biotechnology companies and nonprofit clinical laboratories and interviews of selected organization', Washington: ELSI, NIH, 1997.
18 P. Pinell, *Naissance d'un fléau: la lutte contre le cancer en France,* Paris: Métallié, 1994.

19 M. Cassier and J.-P. Gaudillière, 'Recherche, médecine et marché: la génétique du cancer du sein', *Sciences sociales et santé* 18, 2000: 29–49.

20 J.-P. Gaudillière and M. Cassier, *Production, valorisation et usages des savoirs: la génétique du cancer du sein*, Paris: MIRE, 2001.

21 Cassier and Gaudillière, 'Recherche'.

22 In 2004 the procedure led to the cancellation of Myriad's European patents on BRCA genes. Information on the judicial process may be found on the site of Institut Curie (www.curie.net/actualities/myriad).

23 M. Hayes, 'On the epidemiology of risk: language, logic, and social science', *Social Science and Medicine* 35, 1992: 401–7; R. Aronowitz, *Making Sense of Illness: Science, Society, and Disease*, Cambridge: Cambridge University Press, 1998; R. Aronowitz, 'Do not delay: breast cancer and time', *The Millbank Quarterly* 79, 2001: 355–86.

24 D. Stoppa-Lyonnet, C. Blandy and F. Eisinger, 'Cancer du sein: évaluer le risque. Les tests génétiques donnent naissance à une médecine de l'incertain', *La Recherche* 294, 1997: 72–6; D. Stoppa-Lyonnet, 'Pour quelles raisons pourrait-on conseiller une mastectomie prophylactique à une femme à risque?' *Bulletin du Cancer* 86, 1999: 754–9.

25 T. Rebbecj, H.T. Lynch and S.L. Neuhasen, 'Prophylactic oophorectomy in carriers of BRCA1 and BRCA2 mutations', *New England Journal of Medicine* 346, 2002: 1616–22.

26 N. Janin, 'Pour quelles raisons devrait-on s'abstenir de conseiller une mastectomie prophylactique chez les femmes à risque?' *Bulletin du Cancer* 86, 1999: 760–6.

27 L.C. Hartmann, T.A. Sellers, D.J. Schaid, *et al.*, 'Efficacy of bilateral prophylactic mastectomy in BRCA1 and BRCA2 gene mutation carriers', *Journal of the National Cancer Institute* 93, 1998: 1586–7.

28 B. Fisher, J.P. Constantino, D.L. Wickerham, *et al.*, 'Tamoxifen for prevention of breast cancer: report of the National Surgical Adjuvant Breast and Bowel Project P-1 study', *Journal of the National Cancer Institute* 90(18), 1998: 1371–88; T. Powles, R. Eccles, S. Ashley, *et al.*, 'Interim analysis of the incidence of breast cancer in the Royal Mardsen Hospital Tamoxifen randomised chemo-prevention trial', *Lancet* 352, 1998: 98–101.

29 Direct publicity of drugs to consumers is now legal in the USA, but is not (yet?) allowed in Europe; it was found to be an efficient means of increasing drug sales. M.S. Wilkes, R.A. Bell and R.L. Kravitz, 'Direct to consumer prescription drug advertising: trends, impact and implications', *Health Affairs* 19, 2000: 110–28.

30 L.F. Hogle, 'Chemoprevention for healthy women: harbinger of things to come?' *Health* 5(3), 2001: 311–33.

31 S. Wright, *Molecular Politics: Developing American and British Regulatory Policy for Genetic Engineering*, Chicago: University of Chicago Press, 1994.

32 N. Dodier, *Le désenclavement de la science et de la médecine,* Paris: Editions de l'EHESS, 2003; S. Epstein, *Impure Science: Aids, Activism and the Politics of Knowledge*, Berkeley: University of California Press, 1996.

33 D. Kevles and L. Hood (eds), *The Code of Codes: Scientific and Social Issues in the Human Genome Project*, Cambridge, MA: Harvard University Press, 1992; R. Cook-Degan, *The Gene Wars: Science, Politics, and the Human Genome Project*, New York: Norton & Co., 1994.

34 American Society of Clinical Oncology, 'Genetic testing for cancer suscepti-bility', *Journal of Clinical Oncology* 14, 1996: 1730–6.

35 Lerner, *Breast Cancer Wars*.

36 M.H. Casamayou, *The Politics of Breast Cancer*, Washington: Georgetown University Press, 2001. S. Parthasarathy 'Knowledge is Power: Genetic Testing for Breast Cancer and Patient Activism in the US and Britain' in T. Pinch and N. Oudshoorn (eds), *How Users Matter*, Cambridge, MA: MIT Press, 2003.

37 J.T. Paterson, *The Dread Disease*, Cambridge, MA: Harvard University Press, 1987; J.P. Gaudillière, *Inventer la biomédecine: la France, l'Amérique et la production des savoirs du vivant, 1945–1965*, Paris: La Découverte, 2002.
38 Stanford Program in Genomics, Ethics, and Society, 'Genetic testing for BRCA1 and BRCA2', *Journal of Women's Health* 7, 1998: 531–45.
39 'BRCA1 and BRCA2 are the subjects of several patents and patent applications. To the extent that they are granted, these patents would give the institutions that employed the inventors substantial power to control how genetic testing is conducted and by whom.' Ibid., p. 543.
40 'The effects of genetic testing for BRCA1 and BRCA2 mutations are complicated. The tests may have both positive and negative consequences for individuals and families. At our present level of knowledge, the tests should be offered, and taken only with great care.' Ibid., p. 535.
41 'It is easy to imagine an advertisement for BRCA1 and BRCA2 mutation testing that preys on women's fear of breast cancer and then offers testing as a solution to this heightened concern.' Ibid., p. 541.
42 Stanford Program in Genomics, Ethics and Society, 'Genetic testing'.
43 N. Holtzman and S. Watson, *Promoting Safe and Effective Genetic Testing in the United States, Final Report of the Task Force on Genetic Testing*, Baltimore: The Johns Hopkins University Press, 1998.
44 www4.od.nih.gov./oba/sacgt.html.
45 Secretary's Advisory Committee on Genetic Testing, *A Public Consultation on Oversight of Genetic Tests*, Washington: NIH, 2000.
46 Secretary's Advisory Committee on Genetic Testing, *A Public Consultation*.
47 'The FDA should give particular attention to the review of genetic tests for predictive purposes in diseases and conditions for which a safe and effective intervention has not been established.'
48 Secretary's Advisory Committee on Genetic Testing, *Enhancing the Oversight of Genetic Tests: Recommendations of the SACGT*, Washington: NIH, 2000.
49 Secretary's Advisory Committee on Genetic Testing, *Enhancing the Oversight of Genetic Tests*, pp. 27,31.
50 INSERM, Expertise collective, *Risques héréditaires des cancers du sein et de l'ovaire. Quelle prise en charge?* Paris: INSERM Editions, 1998; F. Eisinger, N. Alby, A. Bremond, *et al.*, 'Recommendations for medical management of hereditary breast and ovarian cancer: the French National Ad Hoc Committee', *Annals of Oncology* 9, 1998: 939–50.
51 Association des praticiens de génétique moléculaire, *Livre blanc*, Paris: Association des praticiens de génétique moléculaire, 1998.
52 A. Clarke, J. Shim, L. Mamo, J. Fosket and F. Fishman, 'Biomedicalization: technoscientific transformations of health, illness, and US biomedicine', *American Sociological Review* 68, 2003: 161–94.

Recommended further reading

S. de Chadarevian and H. Kamminga (eds), *The Molecularization of Biology and Medicine,* Amsterdam: Harwood Academic Publishers, 1998.
A. Clarke *et al.*, 'Biomedicalization: technoscientific transformations of health, illness and US biomedicine', *American Sociological Review* 68, 2003: 161–94.
R. Cooter and J. Pickstone (eds), *Medicine in the Twentieth Century*, London and Melbourne: Harwood Publishers, 2000.
B. Lerner, *The Breast Cancer Wars*, New York: Oxford University Press, 2001.
M. Lock, A. Young and A. Cambrosio (eds), *Living and Working with New Medical Technologies: Intersections of Inquiry*, Cambridge: Cambridge University Press, 2000.

Index